Pathways and Barriers to Parenthood

Orit Taubman – Ben-Ari
Editor

Pathways and Barriers to Parenthood

Existential Concerns Regarding Fertility, Pregnancy, and Early Parenthood

Springer

Editor
Orit Taubman – Ben-Ari
Bar-Ilan University
Ramat Gan, Israel

ISBN 978-3-030-24863-5   ISBN 978-3-030-24864-2 (eBook)
https://doi.org/10.1007/978-3-030-24864-2

This Springer imprint is published by the registered company Springer Nature Switzerland AG
The registered company address is: Gewerbestrasse 11, 6330 Cham, Switzerland

*To my mother, **Lea**, who has always been my ultimate model of the perfect mother, and who paved the way to the mother I became; and to my children, **Liron**, **Adi**, and **Nir**, who teach me every day how precious this life transforming transition has been to me.*

Preface: The Complex Multidimensional Pathways and Barriers to Parenthood

Much has been written over the years concerning the transition to parenthood. Some authors relate only to the joy it brings, while others concentrate on psychopathology in the pre- and postnatal periods. Some look only at women, whereas others consider couples. Many address infertility as a medical obstacle on the path to becoming a parent, while others explore its psychological consequences for women, men, and their offspring's development. Little attention, however, has been devoted to an attempt to consider the medical, psychological, ethical, epidemiological, cultural, and clinical aspects of the journey to parenthood in parallel, and to view this challenging journey from the beginning, the desire to become parents, through pregnancy and the expectations and experience of childbirth, to actual parenthood. This book attempts to do just that, offering a multidimensional look at these highly complex and sensitive issues.

The first section is dedicated to the quest for parenthood, along the barriers it may carry. It includes chapters relating to the meaning of parenthood and its effect on meaning in life, as well as fertility, infertility, and reproductive technology from different angles and theoretical perspectives, including psychological, medical, and cultural implications, the couple and the individual, the impact of the media, the short- and long-term consequences of treatment, and alternative methods of pursuing parenthood.

In Chap. 1, Jessica L. Morse and Michael F. Steger present the most recent conceptualizations of meaning in life, which they consider the feature that most distinguishes us as human beings. Second to this, they claim, is humans' need to understand their role as parents. Interestingly, though meaning in life and parenthood have each been studied extensively, only few authors address their interconnections. Morse and Steger argue that regarding parenthood as an existential issue may yield new insights into the profound impact that parenting—or trying to become a parent—has on people's lives.

In Chap. 2, Brennan Peterson and Jean Marie S. Place delve into one of the most painful and frustrating barriers to becoming parents: infertility. Focusing on the couple level, they claim that infertility represents an interruption in a couple's normative life course. As they attempt to resolve this medical problem, they experience substantial emotional, physical, psychological, and financial stress. The authors review coping strategies as well as counseling strategies that may provide tools to help navigate the infertility experience, strengthen the couple relationship, assist in decision-making, and moderate feelings of grief and loss. In addition, they discuss the evolving issue of fertility awareness, stressing that infertility can also be addressed by enhancing primary, secondary, and tertiary prevention strategies.

In Chap. 3, Vera Skvirsky and Orit Taubman – Ben-Ari deal with the damage to the individual's identity and well-being resulting from infertility. We show how coping with this problem can generate distress, anxiety, and sense of loss, failure, and pain throughout the process, from the initial consultation with a fertility specialist to achieved pregnancy and parenthood. The chapter examines the infertility experience at different stages in the journey to becoming a parent, with special emphasis on the beginning of fertility consultation, and relates to a number of contributors to both positive and negative outcomes for the individual.

In Chap. 4, Henny M. W. Bos and her colleagues discuss infertility from a cultural perspective, stressing that fertility care for involuntarily childless couples is not a high priority for governments in developing countries, where population growth and life-threatening diseases are of greater concern. Nevertheless, fertility problems may have an enormous negative effect on the life and well-being of couples in these countries. The authors examine the case of Kenya, presenting the findings of a mixed method study among individuals dealing with infertility.

In Chap. 5, Shirley Ben Shlomo and Oneg Kabizon-Pery analyze the issue of infertility within the sociological framework of modern media, showing how the media influences the shaping of social perceptions of fertility and fertility treatment. The authors present a study based on the theory of social construction of values and perceptions in which they performed a semiotic analysis of items relating to childbirth and fertility in the Israeli media. They demonstrate how the linguistic and visual aspects of these items reflect a specific cultural point of view and shared values.

In Chap. 6, the outcomes of fertility treatment from a medical standpoint are considered by Adel Farhi, Saralee Glasser, and Liat Lerner-Geva. They present statistical evidence of the frequency of assisted reproductive technology (ART) treatments worldwide, as well as in Israel, and raise concerns regarding their safety and their effect on the infant's physical health and emotional well-being. Reviewing the literature on long-term outcomes for children born following ART, the authors conclude that despite variations in assessment scales, the growth, development, and cognitive functioning of these children are similar to those of spontaneously conceived children.

The first section ends with Chap. 7, by Olga van den Akker, who considers the growing phenomenon of transitioning to parenthood using third-party-assisted conception and surrogate motherhood. Although a solution to various barriers to parenthood, this approach evokes problematic issues, including commercialization and commodification, inequality in access to assisted conception services and choice of third-party input, and questionable human rights and psychosocial welfare practices. In addition, the anonymity and marginalization of the donors and surrogates raise psychological, social, health, and ethical questions for donors and recipients, and potentially for others in the extended family. The author describes the implications of these concerns and calls on future research, policy, and practice to address them.

The second section of the book is dedicated to prenatal issues and the path to parenthood. It includes chapters relating to resilient ecologies for the prevention of parenting stress, decisions about a new family model, and concerns regarding selecting the sex of the newborn. The final chapter in this section discusses the desire for parenthood and relevant parental decisions through the lens of Terror Management Theory, an existential view of individuals' discourse with the threat of death.

In Chap. 8, Michael Ungar, Kristin Hadfield, Nicole Bush, Amélie Quesnel-Vallée, and Igor Pekelny discuss the social ecology of resilience as a framework for understanding how prenatal stress impacts child development. The authors consider several protective and promotive factors and processes associated with resilience, particularly those involved in mitigating the impact of prenatal programming of maternal stress. They claim that the problem of stress on mothers should be viewed multi-systemically, on the genetic, neurological, psychological, social, and economic levels, and that solutions need to be equally complex.

In Chap. 9, Dorit Segal-Engelchin, Sarah Jen, and Pauline I. Erera deal with one of the new family configurations, the "hetero-gay family," comprised of a gay man and a heterosexual woman who choose to conceive and raise a child together outside of marriage. Though not sharing a residence, both birth parents are actively involved in their child's daily life and in child-related decisions. The authors discuss the motivations for choosing the hetero-gay family and show that they are largely similar for men and women, with both sides tending to hold a traditional view of the ideal parental model.

In Chap. 10, Gil Siegal provides an extensive review of the medical possibility of choosing the sex of an unborn child and discusses the legal and ethical issues involved, as well as additional issues, including gender stereotypes, discrimination of women, personal and parental reproductive autonomy, and abortion. These concerns have led different societies to come up with diverse solutions, reflecting their particular circumstances, social norms, culture, history, and religion. Siegal considers the Israeli solution in depth, describing how it demonstrates Israel's unique autonomous status among Western liberal democratic nations.

In Chap. 11, Sheldon Solomon presents Terror Management Theory, which holds that humans are unique in their awareness of the inevitability of death. As death awareness gives rise to potentially debilitating existential terror, it is managed by embracing three devices: cultural worldviews, self-esteem, and close relationships with significant others. Viewed from this perspective, becoming a parent may have social and psychological benefits on the one hand, and frightening aspects on the other. Solomon provides not only a theoretical overview, but also an empirical account of how parenthood arouses and lessens existential anxieties.

The last section of the book revolves around perceptions of childbirth and their effect on women's later distress and well-being, as well as early parenthood and the concerns it brings with it. The chapters in this section relate to challenges in promoting health among new parents, personal growth in the transition to parenthood, an existential psychotherapeutical view of new parenthood, and new insights into attachment theory and its relation to parenthood.

In Chap. 12, Susan Ayers and Alexandra Sawyer consider the changes inherent in the transition to parenthood in terms of mental health problems, whether pre-existing or new. They show how for some women, pregnancy and childbirth can be traumatic, perhaps even leading to posttraumatic stress disorder (PTSD). The authors stress the importance of identifying factors that determine a woman's experience of birth and its impact on her and her infant's mental health. They argue that viewing childbirth and its consequences from both a risk and a resilience and personal growth perspective will enable the design of interventions which ensure that women adapt and thrive, and note the practical and political advantages of adopting this approach in healthcare systems.

In Chap. 13, Miri Scharf, Pnina Isenberg-Borenstein, and Rachel Marcow Rosenberg focus on difficult experiences associated with childbirth, and their imagined and actual implications on future parenting. They contend that struggling with difficulties might result in a higher level of functioning than previously exhibited. The authors present two studies, one on the experience of stillbirth and the other on traumatic labor, which reveal factors that may promote positive change and increased strength in the face of adversity on the road to motherhood.

In Chap. 14, Noga Levin-Keini and Shirley Ben Shlomo present an existential approach to the transition to parenthood. Relying on Irvin Yalom's theoretical existential model, they show how first-time mothers and fathers are confronted with basic concerns of death, freedom, isolation, and meaninglessness. The authors provide two clinical examples, using them to demonstrate the way in which the challenges associated with the transition to parenthood arouse such concerns. They conclude by proposing a therapeutic intervention model based on existential concepts.

In Chap. 15, Martin S. Hagger and Kyra Hamilton relate to the transition to parenthood as a period of considerable challenge and stress (e.g., loss of sleep, limited "leisure" time, restrictions on social life, and difficulties in managing a work–life balance and maintaining health habits). These challenges can have deleterious effects on parents' health and well-being. The authors review social cognitive theories and call for the identification of strategies that parents can adopt in order to initiate and maintain both their own and their offspring's health behaviors at this time, thereby increasing their physical and psychological health.

In Chap. 16, Orit Taubman – Ben-Ari presents the latest findings regarding the personal growth (also known as posttraumatic growth or stress-related growth) of men and women during the transition to parenthood. The chapter reviews associations between level of stress, personal and external resources, and demographic characteristics on the one hand, and personal growth on the other, and considers the development of personal growth over time. It relates to normative parenthood to a single baby, as well as special circumstances, such as delivering twins or preterm babies or being a single mother by choice.

The last two chapters in this section call on attachment theory to explain the transition to parenthood and early parenting. In Chap. 17, W. Steven Rholes and Ramona L. Paetzold discuss the transition to parenthood from the perspective of adult attachment theory, revealing the way attachment styles relate to new parents' experiences. The authors consider not only problems that dysfunctional or insecure attachment styles can arouse, but also the possibility of a shift from an insecure to a secure attachment style, and show that growth in attachment security can result from support for one's relationship partner. They conclude by proposing new directions for the study of attachment theory in the transition to parenthood.

In Chap. 18, the final chapter in the book, Mario Mikulincer and Phillip R. Shaver, claims that parenting is managed by two behavioral systems: attachment and caregiving. The authors review theoretical and empirical evidence concerning the link between these systems and the ways in which individual differences in each shape functioning in the other. They show that heightening attachment security yields sensitive and responsive caregiving, which may be translated into positive and growth-oriented parenting. They therefore suggest that enhancing children's sense of security not only has numerous benefits for the children, but also serves as a positive modeling of parenthood, which in turn can make them good parents in the future.

Paulo Coelho wrote that "life is not about good answers, it is about interesting questions." The forty-five contributors to the 18 chapters in this book not only give voice to established knowledge and well-known theories, but also raise awareness of highly important questions and new paths waiting to be explored. I am grateful and indebted to all these remarkable experts, who generously agreed to take part in the journey toward an understanding of the challenges and obstacles in the pursuit of parenthood, the life-changing decisions, basic perceptions, and coping strategies involved in one of the most demanding and impactful roles in the world: being a parent. Having gotten to know these people personally, I can confidently say that they are not only concerned with the advancement of science, but are equally imbued with the mission of making our reality better, more meaningful, and more empathic.

With the help of the contributing authors, I have sought to paint a broad and insightful picture of the experience of becoming a parent, from the desire to have a child, through pregnancy and childbirth, and to early parenthood. My aim was to enable as many voices as possible to be heard. Parenthood is frequently portrayed as a blessing, as pure joy, ignoring the fact that it may also be experienced as overwhelming, frustrating, debilitating, and/or distressing. This book seeks to give expression to the array of feelings aroused in women and men by this major life transition, as well as to their courage, strengths, and resilience, their positive outlook on life, and their potential to develop and thrive from this experience. Hopefully, the book will also pave the way for greater attention being paid to the complexity of the transition to parenthood on the theoretical, empirical, and clinical levels.

I am grateful to Esther Otten and Hendrike Tuerlings from Springer Publishing for seeing the value and importance of this book and for their professional and generous assistance throughout its birth. Finally, I would like to express my gratitude and appreciation to Sara Kitai and Vera Skvirsky for their help and attention to detail. Having both of you in my life is a blessing.

On a personal note, I would like to thank my family (my mother, Lea, my husband, Rami, and my children, Adi, Liron, and Nir) for their support, for accompanying me on my own journey, and for being the source of an infinite experience of love.

Acknowledgements Supported by the Schnitzer Foundation for Research on Israeli Economy and Society.

Ramat Gan, Israel Orit Taubman – Ben-Ari

Contents

Contributors

Susan Ayers Centre for Maternal and Child Health Research, City, University of London, London, UK

Shirley Ben Shlomo The Louis and Gabi Weisfeld School of Social Work, Bar Ilan University, Ramat Gan, Israel

Aida Bilajbegovic Amsterdam Institute for Social Science Research, University of Amsterdam, Amsterdam, The Netherlands

Henny M. W. Bos Research Institute of Child Development and Education, University of Amsterdam, Amsterdam, The Netherlands

Nicole Bush Center for Health and Community, University of California, San Francisco, California, USA

Pauline I. Erera School of Social Work, University of Washington, Seattle, WA, USA

Tammary Esho Department of Community and Public Health, Technical University of Kenya, Nairobi, Kenya

Adel Farhi Women and Children's Health Research Unit, Gertner Institute for Epidemiology and Health Policy Research (Ltd.), Sheba Medical Center, Tel Hashomer, Israel

Trudie Gerrits Amsterdam Institute for Social Science Research, University of Amsterdam, Amsterdam, The Netherlands

Saralee Glasser Women and Children's Health Research Unit, Gertner Institute for Epidemiology and Health Policy Research (Ltd.), Sheba Medical Center, Tel Hashomer, Israel

Kristin Hadfield Positive Psychology, Queen Mary University of London, London, UK

Martin S. Hagger Health Psychology and Behavioral Medicine Research Group, Faculty of Health Sciences, School of Psychology and Speech Pathology, Curtin University, Perth, WA, Australia;
School of Applied Psychology, Griffith University, Mt. Gravatt, QLD, Australia;
Faculty of Sport and Health Sciences, University of Jyväskylä, Jyväskylä, Finland

Kyra Hamilton Health Psychology and Behavioral Medicine Research Group, Faculty of Health Sciences, School of Psychology and Speech Pathology, Curtin University, Perth, WA, Australia;
Health and Psychology Innovations (HAPI) Lab, School of Applied Psychology, Griffith University, Mt. Gravatt, QLD, Australia

Pnina Isenberg-Borenstein Department of Counseling and Human Development, University of Haifa, Haifa, Israel

Sarah Jen School of Social Work, University of Washington, Seattle, WA, USA

Oneg Kabizon-Pery The Louis and Gabi Weisfeld School of Social Work, Bar Ilan University, Ramat Gan, Israel

S. Kemunto Migiro Department of Community and Public Health, Technical University of Kenya, Nairobi, Kenya

Benjamin Kioko Department of Community and Public Health, Technical University of Kenya, Nairobi, Kenya

Luca Koppen Amsterdam Institute for Social Science Research, University of Amsterdam, Amsterdam, The Netherlands

Liat Lerner-Geva Women and Children's Health Research Unit, Gertner Institute for Epidemiology and Health Policy Research (Ltd.), Sheba Medical Center, Tel Hashomer, Israel;
Sackler Faculty of Medicine, School of Public Health, Tel Aviv University, Tel Aviv, Israel

Noga Levin-Keini The School of Social Work, Ashkelon Academic College, Ashkelon, Israel

Rachel Marcow Rosenberg Department of Counseling and Human Development, University of Haifa, Haifa, Israel

Mario Mikulincer School of Psychology, Interdisciplinary Center (IDC) Herzliya, Herzliya, Israel

Jessica L. Morse Center for Meaning and Purpose, Department of Psychology, Colorado State University, Fort Collins, CO, USA

Solomon Mwendah Department of Community and Public Health, Technical University of Kenya, Nairobi, Kenya

Wanjiru Ndegwa Footsteps for Fertility Foundation, Nairobi, Kenya

Ramona L. Paetzold Department of Management, Texas A & M University, College Station, TX, USA

Igor Pekelny Resilience Research Centre, Dalhousie University, Halifax, Canada

Brennan Peterson Crean College of Health and Behavioral Sciences, Department of Marriage and Family Therapy, Chapman University, Orange, CA, USA

Jean Marie S. Place Department of Nutrition & Health Science, Women's and Gender Studies Affiliate, Ball State University, Muncie, IN, USA

Amélie Quesnel-Vallée Canada Research Chair in Policies and Health Inequalities, McGill University, Montreal, Canada

W. Steven Rholes Department of Psychology, Texas A & M University, College Station, TX, USA

Alexandra Sawyer School of Health Sciences, University of Brighton, Brighton, UK

Miri Scharf Department of Counseling and Human Development, University of Haifa, Haifa, Israel

Dorit Segal-Engelchin The Spitzer Department of Social Work, Ben-Gurion University of the Negev, Beer-Sheva, Israel

Phillip R. Shaver Department of Psychology, University of California, Davis, CA, USA

Gil Siegal University of Virginia School of Law, Charlottesville, VA, USA;
The Israeli National Committee for Non-Medical Sex Selection, Jerusalem, Israel;
Center for Health Law, Bioethics and Health Policy, Ono Academic College, Kiryat Ono, Israel

Vera Skvirsky The Louis and Gabi Weisfeld School of Social Work, Bar Ilan University, Ramat Gan, Israel

Sheldon Solomon Skidmore College, Saratoga Springs, NY, USA

Michael F. Steger Center for Meaning and Purpose, Department of Psychology, Colorado State University, Fort Collins, CO, USA;
Optentia Research Programme, North-West University, Vanderbijklpark, South Africa

Orit Taubman – Ben-Ari The Louis and Gabi Weisfeld School of Social Work, Bar Ilan University, Ramat Gan, Israel

Michael Ungar Canada Research Chair in Child, Family and Community Resilience, Resilience Research Centre, Dalhousie University, Halifax, Canada

Olga van den Akker Middlesex University, Hendon, London, UK

Floor B. van Rooij Research Institute of Child Development and Education, University of Amsterdam, Amsterdam, The Netherlands

Chapter 1
Giving Birth to Meaning: Understanding Parenthood Through the Psychology of Meaning in Life

Jessica L. Morse and Michael F. Steger

Ah, babies! They're more than just adorable little creatures on whom you can blame your farts. Like most people who have had one baby, I am an expert on everything and will tell you, unsolicited, how to raise your kid!

—Tina Fey

Marge, don't discourage the boy! Weaseling out of things is important to learn. It's what separates us from the animals! Except the weasel.

—Homer Simpson

1.1 Introduction

Parenthood. Biological imperative? Spiritual calling? Naturally facile role? Impossible labyrinth of madness? Legacy of joy or despair? Fodder for comedy? Creating and raising a child is probably all of the above and more.

It seems as if humans often struggle most with the natural behaviors that animals seem to breeze through: sex, sleep, eating, eliminating our waste, reproducing. There is not an easy answer about why we struggle with these tasks, but it does seem that attaching abstract values, significance, and expectations to such functions is part of it. We do not simply have sex when provoked by seasonal and hormonal changes, we seduce, we make love, we hook up, and if research is to believed, we regret quite a lot of it (Roese et al., 2006). Similarly, we need machines, medicines, behavioral hygiene programs, motorized beds, and careful self-talk in order to obtain sleep at

J. L. Morse · M. F. Steger (✉)
Center for Meaning and Purpose, Department of Psychology, Colorado State University, Fort Collins, CO 80523, USA
e-mail: michael.f.steger@colostate.edu

J. L. Morse
e-mail: Jessica.Morse@colostate.edu

M. F. Steger
Optentia Research Programme, North-West University, Vanderbijklpark, South Africa

O. Taubman – Ben-Ari (ed.), *Pathways and Barriers to Parenthood*,
https://doi.org/10.1007/978-3-030-24864-2_1

some times, and to resist it at others. Parenting seems to be one of these puzzles, too. Some parents fall far short of even reptiles in terms of nurturing young, whereas many fret over whether their children will truly achieve their dreams on the world's stage. Some of us anguish over whether we are ready to become parents; others of us give years and wealth to try to address fertility challenges. Most of us appear concerned that we are doing some part of it wrong and feel guilty over having kids, not having kids, saying yes, saying no, or simply not knowing what to say next. Lemmings, with their pea-brains, glide through the very elements of life that give our massive, gelatinous super-computer-brains so much trouble. We suggest that it is the ascription of meaning, on an individual and collective level, that turns up the intensity of these functions.

1.2 Meaning in Life

In its most fundamental form, meaning can be viewed simply as the unfolding web of informational associations and links people attach to stimuli. Thus, the meaning of a word is the information its visual, tactile, or spoken form elicits in our thought. The meaning of an aroma, a facial expression, or a sound may function similarly, activating a network of stored associations. There are, of course more complex stimuli; an aroma of decomposing meat emanating from a birthday cake, an expression of rage on the face of a lover, or the sound of a friend's surprise seeing you in a café halfway around the world. As the complexity of the stimuli increases, more information is called forth from storage and we have the (perhaps irresistible) ability to reconstruct and recombine a much greater array of possibilities. At this level, we might refer to episodic meaning, or the set of interpretations, lessons, or associations we carry forth from discrete events, days, or thematically linked stretches of time. Episodes might be as short as the announcement of a pop quiz in class, or as long as the frightening weeks parents spend by the bedside of their hospitalized child. Somehow, we have the ability to aggregate all the stimuli, the episodes, even the phases of life and the frenetic churn of the world around us into some even larger kind of meaning: meaning in life.

If we agree with the argument that the more complex the stimuli the greater the complexity, range, variety, depth, and facets of the meaning that people may make of it, then parenthood is a prime candidate for analysis from a meaning perspective. Parenthood not only delivers myriad momentary stimuli, it delivers them in often ambiguous and complex servings. Many parents have wondered out loud, "Is she smiling or farting?" or "Is she asleep or standing silently in her crib with an evil, expectant smile on her face waiting for us to check to see if she is sleeping?" Or "He needs me so much!" (smiling) and "He needs me SO MUCH!" (crying). Further, parenthood seems perfectly designed to create episodes, which express a seemingly natural human inclination to combine discrete events into thematic time capsules. Some episodes are age-dependent: newborns, toddlers, terrible twos, teenagers. Some are maturation-dependent: learning how to eat, learning how to eat solid food, learning how to eat with utensils, learning how to eat quinoa. Some are ability-oriented: elementary school, driving lessons, earning and losing responsibility, earning money. Some combine all of that: dating and break-ups, attitudes toward law and law enforcement, drugs.

In the meaning literature, the process of meaning-making is presumed to lead to what is loosely referred to as meaning (e.g., Steger, 2012; Steger & Park, 2012). Meaning is the entire network of associations, beliefs, goals, conclusions, and perceptions regarding a particular domain. Meaning-making, then, is the way in which experiences and information are integrated into pre-existing and ever-evolving networks. To the degree that parenthood is meaningful, it conveys to that particular parent a particular network of associations, beliefs, etc. that are relatively stable. Meaning, or meaningfulness, generally conveys a positive and valued network, whereas meaninglessness generally conveys negative meaning rather than an absence of meaning. A final distinction is worth making, between the subjective experience meaning, sometimes referred to as the *presence of meaning*, and the *search for meaning* (Steger, Frazier, Oishi, & Kaler, 2006). Presence of meaning captures this idea that people have a generally positive set network of associations and beliefs, whereas search for meaning captures people's strivings and efforts to obtain greater, or qualitatively deeper, meaning than they already experience.

By far, the greatest amount of meaning research has focused on presence of meaning in life as a whole. Thousands of studies have been published on meaning in life, and the overwhelming message is that viewing one's life to be meaningful is fundamental to well-being and positive mental health (for reviews, see Steger, 2009, 2012). One might extrapolate that viewing parenthood to be meaningful would be similarly positive (cf. research on meaningful work; Steger, Dik, & Duffy, 2012). Perhaps more importantly, meaning in life has been the subject of substantial theoretical scrutiny, which might be applied to understanding the psychological impact of parenthood. Meaning in life is thought to be comprised of three distinct dimensions—*coherence, purpose*, and *significance*—which correspond with cognitive, motivational, and evaluative psychological processes (George & Park, 2017; Martela & Steger, 2016; Steger, in press).

Our suggestion here is that these three dimensions also might be useful in understanding parenthood. Parenthood might be analyzed in terms of the degree that one's role as a parent is understandable, and its demands can be made sense of, which we might call *coherence*. Similarly, parents may have specific, valued goals for what they hope to achieve, or see achieved, throughout their children's lives, on their own behalf or on behalf of their children, which we might call *purpose*. Finally, people might view the role of being a parent as being important, valuable, and worthwhile, which we might call *significance*. To the extent that people are able to buttress their parental coherence, purpose, and significance with direct experience, or through psychological adaptation, then parenting overall would be meaningful to them. In contrast, threats to the well-being of parents might lie in how these three dimensions are thwarted, whether such threats occur in efforts to parent children, in efforts to conceive children in the first place, or in the loss of a child, as just a few examples. Further, the meaning of parenthood has roots that precede childbirth, and that people who face difficulties in having children also struggle in ways that are related to meaning. We would suggest that the dimensions of coherence, purpose, and significance may provide new insights into these processes as well. Additionally, we suggest that examining the processes by which parenting does (or does not) contribute to these three dimensions may provide valuable insight into variations in people's experiences of parenthood as meaningful. For some people, becoming a parent may initiate a process of searching for meaning, understanding, and fulfillment in one's new role of parent. For others, difficulty conceiving or not being able to become a parent, may initiate a process of searching for meaning in other valued roles to compensate. And, on a daily basis, living with a child might unexpectedly confront parents with a search for meaning, sometimes quite literally, as when children ask existential questions like, "What happens when we die?" or "Who made the world?" or just, "Why (fill in the blank)?".

1.3 Meaning and Parenthood

Our argument is that because parenthood is a complex life event, people confront an open field of possibilities for the meaning they may derive from the experience. Research and anecdotal evidence indicates that parenthood can both positively and negatively influence people's overall well-being, life satisfaction, and happiness (e.g., Buckles et al. 2015; Nelson, Kushlev, English, Dunn, & Lyubomirsky, 2013; Nelson, Kushlev, Dunn, & Lyubmirsky, 2014a; Kahneman, Krueger, Schkade, Schwarz, & Stone, 2004; Twenge, Campbell, & Foster, 2003). Experiences of parenting, similar to any major life task, are impacted by many factors (i.e., situational/contextual supports and barriers, personality traits, beliefs and expectations about parenting, etc.), all of which influence the parent's affect and well-being. Researchers and laypeople frequently comment on the complexity of parenthood and the seemingly inconceivable phenomenon that people continue to bear children despite widespread lamentations about parenthood as challenging, stressful, and constraining (Hansen, 2012). This phenomenon, referred to as the "parenting paradox" (Baumeister, 1991), captures the unique picture of parenthood: a fruitful experience which contributes to one's sense of purpose and mattering in a way that cannot be achieved in any other domain AND an experience that comes with many costs that detract from one's personal well-being. This paradox also encapsulates individuals' expectations that parenthood will be fulfilling and blissful, when in fact it is also often experienced as stressful, exhausting, and thankless (Rizzo, Schiffrin, & Liss, 2013).

If parenting is so resource-draining, one might wonder what the appeal is of having children. We approach this point from the perspective of meaning in life. Several studies have investigated correlations between parenting, well-being, overall meaning in life, and meaning associated with parenting. Generally, findings indicate that perceiving a sense of meaning in parenting is associated with higher levels of well-being (e.g., Nelson et al., 2013; Nomaguchi & Milkie, 2003; Palkovitz 2002; To, 2015). In their examination of the relation between parenting and well-being,

Nelson, Kushlev, and Lyubomirsky (2014) found that when parents, in comparison to nonparents, experience high levels of meaning in life, they are more likely to experience well-being (e.g., joy and happiness). They suggest that parenting serves as a source of meaning, contributing to parents' overall sense of meaning in life when parenting aligns with individuals' understanding of their purpose and valued goals.

Research supports this contention, as experiencing one's role as a parent as meaningful seems to contribute to higher levels of overall meaning in life (e.g., Baumeister, Vohs, Aaker, & Garbinsky, 2013; Nelson et al., 2013). Baumeister et al. (2013) found that the more time parents spent taking care of children, the more meaningful they reported their lives to be. Additionally, results suggest that parents think about meaning in life more frequently than nonparents (Nelson et al., 2013, Study 1), that parents report more meaningful moments in their daily lives than nonparents (Nelson et al., 2013, Study 2), and parents experience more meaningful and personally rewarding moments while spending time with their children (Nelson et al., 2013, Study 3; White & Dolan, 2009). Thinking about meaning could indicate engagement in a process of searching for meaning. One potential explanation of this result is that parents might seek to understand their parenting experiences—the disruptions and impacts both negative and positive that they and their children create in each other's' lives—which may contribute to them attributing and/or deriving a greater sense of meaning in the moments they spend with their children. As an example, a parent at work may juxtapose the time they spend on apparently pointless menial tasks with their child being cared for by others at the moment, enabling them to derive more meaning from the everyday moments they spend as a parent, such as cooking dinner with the child, reading him a story, or putting her to bed. Overall, research indicates that parenting seems to promote a sense of meaning that is attached to the parenting role, which further contributes to parents' overall sense that life is meaningful.

There are, of course, many factors that influence people's experiences of parenthood, and thus it is mistaken to conclude that this association between parenting and meaning in life holds true for all parents, or for all times in a parent's experience. As with any role or major life domain, many factors influence the experience of parenthood, and changes occur over time as the child matures and parents age. Research indicates a number of factors that may increase the likelihood of parents finding meaning in parenting and experiencing an overall enhancement in their sense of meaning in life as parents. Examples of factors that promote meaning in parenting include: intrinsic motivation to parent (e.g., To, 2015), perceiving parenting as a valued goal (e.g., Grolnick & Apostoleris, 2002), high level of involvement in childcare (Palkovitz, 2002), engaging in child-centric parenting (Ashton-James, Kushlev, & Dunn, 2013), low levels of "intensive mothering beliefs" (Rizzo et al., 2013), high sense of competence and efficacy in parenting (e.g., Ngai, Chan, & Holroyd, 2007 in To, 2015), and high levels of community and social support (e.g., Taubman – Ben-Ari, Ben Shlomo, & Findler, 2012).

Much of the existing research in the field of meaning and parenthood suggests that parenthood is a complex task that generally conveys enhanced meaning; however, very little elaboration appears as to how and why parenting may promote a stronger sense of meaning in life. Like any major life transition, adding a child to one's life (or planning to do so) initiates changes across domains. Based on the theory of meaning in life detailed above, we explore how having children may impact parents' understanding of themselves and their world (comprehension), their sense of purpose (purpose), and their feelings of mattering (significance). Throughout the following discussion, we focus on how people experience the presence of meaning in these three dimensions; however, parents may also search for meaning in any of these dimensions.

The *comprehension* facet of meaning in life refers to individuals' understanding of themselves—their identity, strengths, and values—and their sense that their life makes sense (Martela & Steger, 2016). For most people, becoming a parent involves a significant shift in how they view themselves and the world around them. New responsibilities, expectations, and information must be accommodated into one's existing understanding of the self, one's role as a parent, and the world of parenting. At a basic level, parenthood appears to interact with other forms of identity. For example, the roles and experiences of mothers and fathers differ, and accordingly, research suggests fathers and mothers differ in their experiences of parental meaning (To, 2015). However, research results are mixed, suggesting that individual perspectives may supersede more general social identities. Some research indicates that fathers show fewer changes than mothers in various aspects of mental health and well-being (e.g., Nomaguchi & Milkie, 2003), whereas some results indicate that fathers exhibit more positive changes in well-being than mothers (e.g., Nelson et al., 2013).

Becoming a parent involves a role shift in which salient identities as a worker, spouse, etc. are modified to make room for developing an identity as a parent (e.g., Nomaguchi & Milkie, 2003). Time and resources are necessarily taken away from these other roles and dedicated to parenting. Individuals' interpretations of the meaning of this nascent identity, and the importance they attach to it, differ. It is likely that the meaning attached to the role of "parent" is different for a teenage mother with limited resources who unexpectedly becomes pregnant and a thirty-five year old woman who has been trying to conceive for years. For some people, identifying with, or incorporating, "parent" into one's understanding of oneself may be more challenging. For example, individuals who do not perceive of themselves as adequate parents, never expected to become a parent, or experience the parenting role as threatening other valued roles, may be less likely to make sense of this role and integrate "parent" into their understanding of themselves. If taking on parental responsibilities does not fit with one's perception of oneself or one's reasons for existing, then becoming a parent would likely detract from one's sense of coherence or might initiate a search for meaning conducted through identity development to accommodate such a role. On the other hand, for some individuals, the role of parenthood is long sought after and positively adds to or complements one's view of oneself, contributing to coherence.

From a developmental perspective, parenting aligns with the developmental period of adulthood wherein the primary task is "generativity" (Erikson, 1950). Generativity is conceptualized as growth, self-esteem, and self-efficacy often derived from effective caring for and nurturing of one's children (Erikson, 1950; Nomaguchi & Milkie, 2003). Effective engagement in the parenting role fosters feelings of personal growth and self-efficacy and the development of an identity as an effective, reliable, supportive caregiver. Research suggests that feeling efficacious in fulfilling valued tasks and roles contributes to a sense of competence and likely promotes a sense of comprehension of oneself in a prescribed role (e.g., Hirschi, 2012; Steger, Bundick, & Yeager, 2012). To's (2015) research reveals that people derive meaning in parenting through feelings of self-enhancement, wherein parents report raising children promotes their own growth, and thus parenting feels meaningful. Additionally, having children fulfills what many societies expect of adults, thus when individuals become parents, they may experience an enhancement in their view of themselves due to this alignment with or fulfillment of cultural values (Dunlop, Walker, Hanley, & Harake, 2017). Kenrick, Griskevicius, Neuberg, and Schaller's (2010) revision of Maslow's hierarchy of needs replaces the *need for self-actualization* with the *need for parenting* as the ultimate purpose to which humans aspire, highlighting the value placed on parenting as a fundamental undertaking of adulthood. Dunlop et al.'s (2017) results lend support to parenting as a fundamental human motive, as the majority of their sample referenced parenting at the top of their list of personal future goals. Furthermore, they found individuals who reported a higher proportion of parenting goals in relation to all future personal goals expressed greater well-being (Dunlop et al., 2017). It seems that parenting can enhance meaning through encouraging a shift in one's self, the roles one is able to play, and by integrating those changes into a recognizable aspiration to forge down a path that brings to life one's role as a parent.

It is the fusion of identity and coherence into a durable set of highly valued goals that links parenthood to the meaning dimension of *purpose*. Purpose, which refers to an individual's core aims and life direction (Martela & Steger, 2016), can thus be shaped by the task of parenting, if not largely directed by parenting goals. People find purpose from work, community involvement, and other activities, like parenting, that provide valued goals to pursue. There are numerous factors that contribute to and detract from people finding purpose in parenthood. One's reasons or motivations for parenting influence the sense of purpose experienced. People who become parents to seek external rewards like higher social status, wherein parenting serves as an instrument to achieving some other desired reward, find parenting less personally meaningful and are more likely to experience perceived strain and lower levels of well-being from parenting (To, 2015). On the other hand, people who perceive of parenting as a valued goal in and of itself that aligns with and contributes to their personal growth tend to view parenting as more satisfying and meaningful (e.g., Grolnick & Apostoleris, 2002). For example, in Chinese culture, rearing children to continue one's lineage is perceived as a primary task of the marital relationship, and is perhaps even the ultimate purpose of marriage (To, 2015). Furthermore, Chinese parents who reported being motivated to parent in order to foster the growth of their children, to cultivate deep relationships with their children, and to guide their children to become quality citizens, reported experiencing parenting as particularly meaningful (To, 2015). Thus, the motivation behind and values associated with parenthood impact the experience of purposefulness related to parenting.

Given the potential scope and importance of parenthood as a lever of purpose, it should not be surprising that there are a variety of factors that detract from people's sense of purpose in parenting. According to Cheung (2000), when parents experience problems related to parenting (i.e., a child's behavioral challenges, perceived inability to provide children with access to desired opportunities), their sense of purpose in executing parenting tasks is diminished. Parental attitudes also impact sense of purpose derived from parenting. A line of research investigating the association between socioeconomic status and parents' experiences of meaning in life suggests highly educated and/or high SES parents report finding less value and fulfillment in parenting (Nelson & Lyubomirsky, 2015) and experience less meaning in life when spending time with their children (Kushlev, Dunn, & Ashton-James, 2012). Kushlev (2011) conceptualizes these findings from the perspective of "opportunity cost" wherein time spent parenting is seen as taking time away from other important tasks, such as work. Thus, when parenting is perceived of as conflicting with and taking time away from other valued goals, parents may experience less meaning from parenting (Nelson & Lyubomirsky, 2015).

Parenting may also influence an individual's overall sense of meaning in life through the facet of *significance*, or the sense that one's life matters, is worthwhile, or makes a difference. Generally, research on meaning in life indicates that people feel the desire to leave a legacy or to have an impact on the world that lasts beyond their limited years on earth (e.g., King & Napa, 1998; Reker, 2000). Parenthood provides an opportunity for living beyond one's earthly years, in a sense attaining the satisfaction of symbolic immortality (e.g., St. Aubin, 2013; see also Solomon, Chap. 11 in this volume). By investing oneself and one's resources into promoting the well-being of future generations, parents may experience a sense that their actions matter.

Parenthood provides many opportunities to make a difference through serving others—one's own children and spouse as well as others within one's community (i.e., coaching children in a sport, volunteering at a child's school). In fact, some individuals may view parenthood as a calling, or "a strongly held belief that one is destined to fulfill; a specific life role, regardless of sacrifice, that will make a meaningful contribution to the greater good" (Coulson, Oades, & Stoyles. 2012, p. 84). Coulson et al. (2012) developed a scale to measure subjective sense of calling in parenting and found three factors that contribute to parental calling: life purpose, awareness, and passion. When individuals identify parenting as aligning with their life purpose, demonstrate an awareness of their children's needs and the sacrifice necessary to meet those needs, and feel passionate in their belief that they are meant to or called to raise children, then they have a high sense of calling to parent (Coulson et al., 2012). A high sense of calling is related to implementing an authoritative parenting style, reporting that parenting is important, pleasurable, and satisfying, and endorsing high levels of presence of meaning in life, and satisfaction with life (Coulson et al., 2012). Thus, people who feel called to parent are likely to find parenting as highly meaningful and satisfying.

1.4 When Complications Arise

As Nelson, Kushlev, and Lyubomirsky (2014) indicate in their examination of the relation between parenting and well-being, the relationship between parenting and meaning in life is highly complex. Many contextual, personality, and motivational factors of parents and children must be accounted for in examining the relation between people's experience of parenting as contributing to meaning in life. Much of the above discussion assumes a somewhat "normative" parenting experience; however, there are many factors that can make parenthood much more challenging and complex. Common challenges to parenthood include infertility or difficulty conceiving (See also Peterson & Place, Chap. 2; Skvirsky & Taubman – Ben-Ari, Chap. 3, in this volume), single parenting, unplanned pregnancy, illness of mother or child, birth defects or preterm delivery, birth of twins or multiples (See also Taubman – Ben-Ari, Chap. 16, in this volume), infant mortality, genetic or medical disease (See also Farhi et al., Chap. 6, in this volume), and psychological illness, as well as feelings of being a failure as a parent, experiencing conflicts between parenthood and other life domains, and simply being overwhelmed by the experience. We suggest that such factors may be viewed as exerting their effects by challenging people's comprehension, purpose, or significance. For example, struggles to conceive might challenges one's sense of comprehension insofar as one anticipated stepping into the parent role, or it might conflict with a sense of significance insofar as parenthood represents a way to make an impact and leave a positive legacy. Work-family conflicts may be viewed as competition for scarce resources among incompatible purposes. One of the advantages of taking a meaning framework to parenthood—in contrast to a positivity, happiness, well-being, or satisfaction framework—is that meaning is inherently complex, and its roots as a topic of study lie in the human response to tragedy (Frankl, 1963). Thus, meaning can provide a flexible framework that integrates both desirable and undesirable manifestations of parenthood in a person's life.

Adjusting to new roles and responsibilities is highly challenging when parenting a typically developing baby, and research suggests that parenting becomes even more demanding when a baby has special needs (e.g., Vaughan, Feinn, Bernard, Brereton, & Kaufman, 2013). Several studies have focused on such challenges in the context of parenting a child with specific emotional and behavioral concerns. Parents of children with high levels of internalizing and externalizing symptoms (i.e., emotional and behavioral disturbance) experience the highest levels of caregiver strain and stress (Vaughan et al., 2013). Studies indicate that making sense of or finding meaning in parenting and identifying benefits in parenting predict better parental adjustment (e.g., Pakenham, Sofronoff, & Samios, 2004), use of adaptive coping skills (e.g., Pakenham et al., 2004), and greater application of a compassionate parenting style (e.g., Conti, 2015). At the same time, some research indicates that parenting can be perceived of as more meaningful and promoting greater personal growth amongst parents of children who face developmental or medical challenges (Taubman – Ben-Ari, 2014). Personal growth occurs when one encounters a stressor and meets the demands of the stressor despite perhaps not feeling capable to do so at first (Tedeschi

& Calhoun, 1996). Research suggests that parenthood leads to personal growth in a number of domains (e.g., Sawyer & Ayers, 2009; Taubman – Ben-Ari, 2014), including positive changes in self-perception (i.e., sense of competence, awareness of one's positive attributes) and interpersonal relationships (i.e., awareness and use of social resources). When additive stressors such as illness accompany parenthood, the potential for personal growth may be even greater and may occur in additional domains such as spiritual development (Taubman – Ben-Ari, 2014), self-actualization (McMahon, Gibson, Leslie, Cohen, & Tennant, 2003), and enhanced gratitude and appreciation for life (Taubman – Ben-Ari, 2014).

However, just as with any stressful event or undertaking, not everyone experiences personal growth, enhanced meaning in life, or other benefits in the wake of difficulty. People's capacity for resilience may be limited by their ability to find meaning in challenging circumstances and make sense of the situation. For example, difficulty conceiving and miscarriage are two common distressing experiences that can perpetuate a variety of negative emotional responses in expectant mothers and fathers (e.g., Nelson, Robbins, Andrews, & Sweeny, 2017; Sweeny, Andrews, Nelson, & Robbins, 2015). In a sample of women trying to conceive, Sweeny et al. (2015) found that presence of meaning predicted engaging in more adaptive coping in the face of uncertainty around conception (i.e. more positive expectation management and information seeking), whereas search for meaning predicted rumination, suppression of thoughts, bracing one's self against expectations, in addition to more benefit finding and information seeking. Thus, presence of meaning related to skills that helped women trying to conceive buffer from the uncertainty and distress of the experience. Search for meaning, as often indicated in the literature, seems to convey some protective benefits as well as some risk for anxiety and distress. To the extent that parenthood triggered a search for meaning, it seems possible that the uncertainty of trying to have a child was difficult to integrate into the aspects of life that predated beginning on the path toward hopeful conception. It also is possible that these expectant mothers were prone to searching for meaning in life all along. In this case, it seems possible that having a child represented a desired path toward greater meaning, with potentially higher perceived psychological stakes in the outcome. Either interpretations highlights the value that might be derived in fertility treatment professionals and those seeking to become parents of assessing both presence of meaning and search for meaning throughout the process.

Similarly, research on the psychological impact of undergoing in vitro fertilization treatment (IVF) indicates that women experience anxiety, distress, and depressive symptoms throughout the IVF process (Verhaak et al., 2006). Although in their systematic review of the literature, Verhaak et al. (2006) found women generally demonstrate good short-term psychological adjustment after unsuccessful IVF, the long-term emotional impact is less clear (See also Peterson & Place, Chap. 2; Skvirsky & Taubman – Ben-Ari, Chap. 3, in this volume). Studies investigating women's emotional adjustment after two years of unsuccessful IVF treatments reveals they experience grief related to childlessness, grief about the loss of a desired future, and that they begin engaging in efforts directed toward identifying other valued purposes in their lives (Johansson & Berg, 2005). Thus, in the case of unsuccessful

IVF, women may experience distress and grief while also engaging in the process of searching for meaning in other domains. These results suggest that helping expectant mothers and their partners enhance their overall sense of meaning and develop a perspective that enables them to find meaning in the challenging events surrounding conception may protect them from the anxiety and distress that such uncertainty and challenge stimulates.

Women struggling to conceive (with or without IVF) may experience miscarriage(s). Nelson et al. (2017) reported that experiencing a miscarriage is associated with anxious, depressive, and grief symptoms with the experience of more than one miscarriage correlating with greater distress. Further, women in the study reported that future attempts to conceive were tainted by the experience of their miscarriage(s). Nelson et al. (2017) suggest that women who have had a miscarriage experience greater uncertainty than those who have not experienced a miscarriage. Thus, experiencing a miscarriage or unsuccessful round of IVF treatment could represent additional hurdles that women and their partners must cope with, and perhaps make sense of, as they strive to become parents.

Overall, when parents find themselves in especially difficult circumstances, such as struggling to conceive or miscarrying, those who are able to make sense of and find meaning in their experience tend to report better adjustment to the stressor, greater personal growth, and more overall meaning in life (Park, 2010). In fact, we would suggest that those who choose to pursue parenthood may have expectations regarding the meaning they will derive, as well as how parenthood fits with their sense of coherence, purpose, and significance in life. Difficulties conceiving, and the protracted nature of IVF—where success is not guaranteed but where sacrifices and time commitment are—are likely to rupture the vessel that holds people's meanings, initiating a search for meaning along a more difficult path to parenthood than imagined, or to a future life without genetic children.

As with prolonged efforts to conceive, single parenthood also has the potential to bring unique challenges to parenthood, most or all responsibilities fall upon one individual. Meier, Musick, Flood, and Dunifon (2016) found that single mothers tend to report less happiness, more sadness, stress, and fatigue than mothers with partners. However, within their sample of single mothers, they found this to be largely true only for unemployed single mothers. Overall, they suggest that motherhood may provide single mothers with a source of love, intimacy, and a source of competence, and, those mothers who choose single motherhood because of their strong childbearing desires may experience motherhood as more meaningful and purposeful than partnered mothers. This indicates that although there may be differences in many aspects of well-being for single and partnered mothers, meaning derived from time spent with children is one dimension in which single parents report equal or higher levels as compared to partnered parents. Thus, parenthood may be experienced as a meaningful activity regardless of partnership or employment status for both single and partnered parents (Meier et al., 2016).

1.5 Conclusions

Parenthood would seem to be an ideal part of life for seeing signs of how people confront the matter of meaning. We have introduced the concept of meaning, and its three dimensions of coherence, purpose, and significance. We also have reviewed the research that has been conducted on how people experience meaning in their roles as parents, how they may search for meaning when complications arise in their pursuit of parenthood, and how finding meaning itself may serve as a resource in facing disappointments and challenges in parenthood. Although we can report that there are important data-points in this literature, there seems to be a need for some initial conceptualizing about what the psychology of meaning can reveal about parenthood. We suggest that the three dimensions of meaning provide this starting point.

Table 1.1 presents a set of examples for how a variety of parenthood domains may nest within the three dimensions of meaning (dimensions from Martela & Steger, 2016). Each parenthood domain is broken down into a small number of tasks within that domain, and each task is briefly portrayed in terms of the way in which it might be viewed from a meaning perspective. For example, coming to terms with one's role as a parent includes the anticipation of becoming a parent at some future point, which, from a meaning perspective, would likely be seen as involving the integration of the parent role into the self-concept that forms the foundation of the coherence dimension of meaning. Similarly, raising a child to independence might be thought of as a long-term set of aims and aspirations that will unfold across many years, requiring parents to apply effort and motivation in working flexibly with their child across many years. Consistent application of effort and motivation over long periods of time, while flexibly adapting approaches to changing circumstances is a hallmark of the purpose dimension of meaning.

We do not intend to suggest that parenthood domains may only link to one dimension of meaning, or vice versa. It is beyond the scope of this chapter to comprehensively lay out each of the possible connections or various feedback loops that might exist. As we have noted already, parenthood is extremely complex, and with higher complexity comes a deeper richness of potential meaning. Instead, our limited intent in presenting this table is simply to suggest one way of conceptually organizing future research on meaning and parenthood. If we take seriously the idea—and the research evidence—that parenthood is a major contributor to and beneficiary of meaning in people's lives, then more systematic investigations of the pathways between meaning and parenthood are needed. These much-needed investigations would help us understand how the joys and sorrows, ups and downs, and moments both mundane and miraculous help give birth to meaning.

Table 1.1 Linking the three dimensions of meaning to domains and tasks of parenthood

Dimension of meaning	Possible domains of parenthood	Tasks related to parenthood domains	Examples of meaning-based interpretations of task
Coherence—a sense of comprehensibility and one's life making sense	Role as parent	Anticipation of being a parent	Integration of parent role into self-concept
		Conflicts with other roles	Clarifying values and priorities; effectively anticipating conflicts; gauging deviations from comfortable balance
		Difficulty becoming parent	Understanding, and potentially revising, centrality of parent role to self-concept
	Understanding child	Learning how to manage behavior	Identifying behavioral preferences of child, desired targets, parent's interaction strengths and child's incentives
		Forming relationship with child	Viewing child as individual, managing distance and boundaries between self and child, conceptualizing differences in child-as-child, child-as-peer, and child in other roles, understanding child's view of self
Purpose—a sense of core goals, aims, and direction in life	Raising child	Setting and pursuing parenting goals	Articulating and discussing aims for child in terms of education, occupation, socialization

(continued)

Table 1.1 (continued)

Dimension of meaning	Possible domains of parenthood	Tasks related to parenthood domains	Examples of meaning-based interpretations of task
		Raising child to independence	Applying effort and motivation over time to achieve aims for child, incorporating developmental and life changes, setting markers for successful progress
		Confronting challenges/obstacles	Maintaining and adjusting aims for child in midst of obstacles, developing subsidiary shorter-term goals to work through obstacles while preserving aims for child
Significance—a sense of life's inherent value and having a life worth living	Building a good life for child	Passing on values, traditions, character	Teaching a moral world view, demonstrating that world view through behavior, helping child to develop own moral character
	Leaving a legacy	Knowing child will remember parents, and will contribute	Seeing parenting efforts make a difference to child, maintaining relationships over time, symbolic life extension through the impact child will have on world

References

Ashton-James, C. E., Kushlev, K., & Dunn, E. W. (2013). Parents reap what they sow: Child-centrism and parental well-being. *Social Psychological and Personality Science, 4*(6), 635–642.

Aubin, E. D. S. (2013). Generativity and the meaning of life. In J. A Hicks & C. Routledge (Eds.), *The experience of meaning in life* (pp. 241–255). New York: Springer.

Baumeister, R. F. (1991). *Meanings of life*. New York: Guilford Press.

Baumeister, R. F., Vohs, K. D., Aaker, J. L., & Garbinsky, E. N. (2013). Some key differences between a happy life and a meaningful life. *The Journal of Positive Psychology, 8*(6), 505–516.

Buckles, E. E., Beall, A. T., Hofer, M. K., Lin, E. Y., Zhou, Z., & Schaller, M. (2015). Individual differences in activation of the parental care motivation system: Assessment, prediction, and implications. *Journal of Personality and Social Psychology, 108,* 497–514.

Cheung, S. K. (2000). Psychometric properties of the Chinese version of the parental stress scale. *Psychologia, 43,* 253–261.

Conti, R. (2015). Compassionate parenting as a key to satisfaction, efficacy and meaning among mothers of children with autism. *Journal of Autism and Developmental Disorders, 45*(7), 2008–2018.

Coulson, J. C., Oades, L. G., & Stoyles, G. J. (2012). Parents' subjective sense of calling in childrearing: Measurement, development and initial findings. *The Journal of Positive Psychology, 7*(2), 83–94.

Dunlop, W. L., Walker, L. J., Hanley, G. E., & Harake, N. (2017). The psychosocial construction of parenting: An examination of parenting goals and narratives in relation to well-being. *Journal of Happiness Studies, 18*(6), 1729–1745.

Erikson, E. (1950). *Childhood and society*. New York: Norton.

Frankl, V. E. (1963). *Man's search for meaning: An introduction to Logotherapy*. New York, NY: Washington Square Press.

George, L. S., & Park, C. L. (2017). The multidimensional existential meaning scale: A tripartite approach to measuring meaning in life. *The Journal of Positive Psychology, 12*(6), 613–627.

Grolnick, W. S., & Apostoleris, N. H. (2002). What makes parents controlling? In E. L. Deci & R. M. Ryan (Eds.), *Handbook of self-determination research* (pp. 161–181). Rochester, NY: University of Rochester.

Hansen, T. (2012). Parenthood and happiness: A review of folk theories versus empirical evidence. *Social Indicators Research, 108,* 29–64.

Hirschi, A. (2012). Callings and work engagement: Moderated mediation model of work meaningfulness, occupational identity, and occupational self-efficacy. *Journal of Counseling Psychology, 59*(3), 479–485.

Johansson, M., & Berg, M. (2005). Women's experiences of childlessness 2 years after the end of in vitro fertilization treatment. *Scandinavian Journal of Caring Sciences, 19*(1), 58–63.

Kahneman, D., Krueger, A. B., Schkade, D. A., Schwarz, N., & Stone, A. A. (2004). A survey method for characterizing daily life experience: The day reconstruction method. *Science, 306,* 1776–1780.

Kenrick, D. T., Griskevicius, V., Neuberg, S. L., & Schaller, M. (2010). Renovating the pyramid of needs: Contemporary extensions built upon ancient foundations. *Perspectives on Psychological Science, 5*(3), 292–314.

King, L. A., & Napa, C. K. (1998). What makes a life good? *Journal of Personality and Social Psychology, 75*(1), 156–165.

Kushlev, K. (2011). *Exploring parental well-being: Is childcare associated with parental well-being and what factors can enhance it*. Doctoral dissertation, University of British Columbia.

Kushlev, K., Dunn, E. W., & Ashton-James, C. E. (2012). Does affluence impoverish the experience of parenting? *Journal of Experimental Social Psychology, 48*(6), 1381–1384.

Martela, F., & Steger, M. F. (2016). The three meanings of meaning in life: Distinguishing coherence, purpose, and significance. *The Journal of Positive Psychology, 11*(5), 531–545.

McMahon, C. A., Gibson, F., Leslie, G., Cohen, J., & Tennant, C. (2003). Parents of 5-year-old in vitro fertilization children: Psychological adjustment, parenting stress and the influence of subsequent in vitro fertilization treatment. *Journal of Family Psychology, 17,* 361–369.

Meier, A., Musick, K., Flood, S., & Dunifon, R. (2016). Mothering experiences: How single parenthood and employment structure the emotional valence of parenting. *Demography, 53*(3), 649–674.

Nelson, S. K., Kushlev, K., Dunn, E. W., & Lyubomirsky, S. (2014a). Parents are slightly happier than nonparents, but causality still cannot be inferred. *Psychological Science, 25,* 303–304.

Nelson, S. K., Kushlev, K., English, T., Dunn, E. W., & Lyubomirsky, S. (2013). In defense of parenthood: Children are associated with more joy than misery. *Psychological Science, 24,* 3–10.

Nelson, S. K., Kushlev, K., & Lyubomirsky, S. (2014b). The pains and pleasures of parenting: When, why, and how is parenthood associated with more or less well-being? *Psychological Bulletin, 140,* 846–895.

Nelson, S. K., & Lyubomirsky, S. (2015). Juggling family and career: Parents' pathways to a balanced and happy life. In K. Page, R. Burke, & C. Cooper (Eds.), *Flourishing in life, work, and careers: Individual wellbeing and career experiences* (pp. 100–118). Cheltenham, UK: Edward Elgar Publishing.

Nelson, S. K., Robbins, M. L., Andrews, S. E., & Sweeny, K. (2017). Disrupted transition to parenthood: Gender moderates the association between miscarriage and uncertainty about conception. *Sex Roles, 76*(5–6), 380–392.

Ngai, F. W., Chan, S. W. C., & Holroyd, E. (2007). Translation and validation of a Chinese version of the parenting sense of competence scale in Chinese mothers. *Nursing Research, 56,* 348–354.

Nomaguchi, K. M., & Milkie, M. A. (2003). Costs and rewards of children: The effects of becoming a parent on adults' lives. *Journal of Marriage and Family, 65*(2), 356–374.

Pakenham, K. I., Sofronoff, K., & Samios, C. (2004). Finding meaning in parenting a child with Asperger syndrome: Correlates of sense making and benefit finding. *Research in Developmental Disabilities, 25*(3), 245–264.

Palkovitz, R. (2002). Involved fathering and child development: Advancing our understanding of good fathering. In C. S. Tamis-LeMonda & N. Cabrera (Eds.), *Handbook of father involvement: Multidisciplinary perspectives* (pp. 119–140). Mahwah, NJ: Lawrence Erlbaum.

Park, C. L. (2010). Making sense of the meaning literature: An integrative review of meaning making and its effects on adjustment to stressful life events. *Psychological Bulletin, 136*(2), 257–301.

Reker, G. T. (2000). Theoretical perspective, dimensions, and measurement of existential meaning. In G. T. Reker & K. Chamberlain (Eds.), *Exploring existential meaning: Optimizing human development across the life span* (pp. 39–55). Thousand Oaks, CA: Sage.

Rizzo, K. M., Schiffrin, H. H., & Liss, M. (2013). Insight into the parenthood paradox: Mental health outcomes of intensive mothering. *Journal of Child and Family Studies, 22*(5), 614–620.

Roese, N. J., Pennington, G. L., Coleman, J., Janicki, M., Li, N. P., & Kenrick, D. T. (2006). Sex differences in regret: All for love or some for lust? *Personality and Social Psychology Bulletin, 32*(6), 770–780.

Sawyer, A., & Ayers, S. (2009). Post-traumatic growth in women after childbirth. *Psychology and Health, 24*(4), 457–471.

Steger, M. F. (2009). Meaning in life. In S. J. Lopez (Ed.), *Oxford handbook of positive psychology* (2nd ed., pp. 679–687). Oxford, UK: Oxford University Press.

Steger, M. F. (2012). Experiencing meaning in life: Optimal functioning at the nexus of spirituality, psychopathology, and well-being. In P. T. P. Wong (Ed.), *The human quest for meaning* (2nd ed., pp. 165–184). New York: Routledge.

Steger, M. F. (in press). Meaning in life: A unified model. In S. J. Lopez, L. M. Edwards, & S. C. Marques (Eds.), *Oxford handbook of positive psychology* (3rd ed.). Oxford, UK: Oxford University Press.

Steger, M. F., Bundick, M., & Yeager, D. (2012). Understanding and promoting meaning in life during adolescence. In R. J. R. Levesque (Ed.), *Encyclopedia of adolescence* (pp. 1666–1677). New York: Springer.

Steger, M. F., Dik, B. J., & Duffy, R. D. (2012b). Measuring meaningful work: The work and meaning inventory (WAMI). *Journal of Career Assessment, 20*(3), 322–337.

Steger, M. F., Frazier, P., Oishi, S., & Kaler, M. (2006). The meaning in life questionnaire: Assessing the presence of and search for meaning in life. *Journal of Counseling Psychology, 53*(1), 80–93.

Steger, M. F., & Park, C. L. (2012). The creation of meaning following trauma: Meaning making and trajectories of distress and recovery. In T. Keane, E. Newman, & K. Fogler (Eds.), *Toward an integrated approach to trauma focused therapy: Placing evidence-based interventions in an expanded psychological context* (pp. 171–191). Washington, DC: APA.

Sweeny, K., Andrews, S. E., Nelson, S. K., & Robbins, M. L. (2015). Waiting for a baby: Navigating uncertainty in recollections of trying to conceive. *Social Science and Medicine, 141,* 123–132.

Taubman – Ben-Ari, O. (2014). Well-being and personal growth in emerging motherhood: And what about meaning? In A. Batthyany & P. Russo-Netzer (Eds.), *Meaning in positive and existential psychology* (pp. 415–434). New York: Springer.

Taubman – Ben-Ari, O., Ben Shlomo, S., & Findler, L. (2012). Personal growth and meaning in life among first-time mothers and grandmothers. *Journal of Happiness Studies, 13*(5), 801–820.

Tedeschi, R. G., & Calhoun, L. G. (1996). The posttraumatic growth inventory: Measuring the positive legacy of trauma. *Journal of Traumatic Stress, 9*(3), 455–471.

To, S. M. (2015). Development and validation of a quantitative measure for Chinese sources of parental meaning. *Journal of Child and Family Studies, 24*(12), 3580–3594.

Twenge, J. M., Campbell, W. K., & Foster, C. A. (2003). Parenthood and marital satisfaction: A meta-analytic review. *Journal of Marriage and Family, 65,* 574–583.

Vaughan, E. L., Feinn, R., Bernard, S., Brereton, M., & Kaufman, J. S. (2013). Relationships between child emotional and behavioral symptoms and caregiver strain and parenting stress. *Journal of Family Issues, 34*(4), 534–556.

Verhaak, C. M., Smeenk, J. M. J., Evers, A. W. M., Kremer, J. A., Kraaimaat, F. W., & Braat, D. D. M. (2006). Women's emotional adjustment to IVF: A systematic review of 25 years of research. *Human Reproduction Update, 13*(1), 27–36.

White, M. P., & Dolan, P. (2009). Accounting for the richness of daily activities. *Psychological Science, 20*(8), 1000–1008.

Chapter 2
The Experience of Infertility: An Unexpected Barrier in the Transition to Parenthood

Brennan Peterson and Jean Marie S. Place

2.1 Introduction

Becoming a parent is one of the most universal goals of men and women throughout the world. However, worldwide estimates indicate approximately 72.4 million women are diagnosed with infertility (Boivin, Bunting, Collins, & Nygren, 2007), meaning 9% of couples who desire to become biological parents will face an inability to establish a clinical pregnancy after 12 months of regular unprotected sexual intercourse (Zegers-Hochschild et al., 2017). A medical diagnosis of infertility is frequently accompanied with unexpected stresses and difficulties (see also Skvirsky & Taubman – Ben-Ari, Chap. 3 in this volume), most of which couples feel unprepared to face. This chapter will highlight the stresses of the infertility experience, the impact of coping with infertility, and the types of fertility counseling offered to help women and men reduce distress. The chapter will also examine the growing effect of delayed childbearing and the importance of fertility awareness, as well as discuss public health strategies for the prevention of infertility and infertility-related distress. As these topics are discussed, the chapter will evolve from a focus on individual- and interpersonal-level concerns to broader recommendations for the organizational, community, and public arenas.

B. Peterson (✉)
Crean College of Health and Behavioral Sciences, Department of Marriage and Family Therapy, Chapman University, Orange, CA 92866, USA
e-mail: bpeterson@chapman.edu

J. M. S. Place
Department of Nutrition & Health Science, Women's and Gender Studies Affiliate, Ball State University, Muncie, IN 47306, USA
e-mail: jsplace@bsu.edu

O. Taubman – Ben-Ari (ed.), *Pathways and Barriers to Parenthood*,
https://doi.org/10.1007/978-3-030-24864-2_2

2.2 Causes and Impact of Infertility

It is commonly believed that women are primarily responsible for an infertility diagnosis, however, only half of infertility cases worldwide are caused by female factors, while 20–30% are caused by male factors, and the remaining 20–30% are caused by a combination of male and female factors (Agarwal, Mulgund, Hamada, & Chyatte, 2015). For women, the most common causes of infertility are polycystic ovary syndrome (PCOS) causing irregular ovulation, damage to the fallopian tubes, difficulties with implantation in the uterine wall, damage to the reproductive organs resulting from sexually transmitted infections (STIs), diminished ovarian reserve due to age, and endometriosis (a condition in which the tissue lining the inside of the uterus also grows outside the uterus). For men, low sperm count, poor sperm motility, and abnormal sperm morphology are common causes. Disruption of testicular function, treatments for testicular cancer, and lifestyle factors such as alcohol use, smoking, or steroids can also play a role (Centers for Disease Control and Prevention [CDC], 2017).

It is estimated that 56% of couples worldwide with an infertility diagnosis seek medical treatment (Boivin et al., 2007). Initial, first-line medical treatments for infertility include medications or corrective surgery, much of which is successful. However, if these treatments do not result in pregnancy or a live birth, couples are referred to a reproductive endocrinologist—a physician who specializes in the treatment of infertility. Reproductive endocrinologists use a variety of Assisted Reproductive Technologies (ARTs) to facilitate pregnancy including intrauterine insemination (IUI) and in vitro fertilization (IVF) with intracytoplasmic sperm injection (ICSI). These procedures are physically and emotionally taxing, and are associated with individual and relational distress, sexual dissatisfaction, depression, and lowered life-satisfaction (Schmidt, 2006). In addition, depending on where one resides, insurance may or may not cover these treatments which can add a significant financial burden to the couple. Finally, the success rates of treatment are not as high as many believe as the live-birth rate from a single non-donor ART cycle for women of all ages is between 20–29% worldwide (Center for Disease Control and Prevention, 2014a; Ferraretti et al., 2013).

The emotional impact of infertility is significant. Couples diagnosed with infertility experience a host of unwanted stressors including psychological distress, changes to their social and family networks, and potential threats to their relationship—all of which are influenced by their social and cultural contexts (Greil, Slauson-Blevins, & McQuillan, 2010). In pronatalist societies, couples often feel marginalized as they sit invisibly on the periphery of the normative cultural experience of childbirth and parenting. Couples often suffer in silence as they encounter well-intentioned, but unhelpful friends and family who ask insensitive questions and offer unsolicited advice. When friends and family move forward in their parenting journey, couples commonly experience a feeling of loss and a profound sense of being left behind. Feelings of depression, anger, anxiety, social isolation, shame, guilt, helplessness, and brokenness are common for women and men.

2.3 Lifecycle Developmental Framework

According to the life course perspective, the world is experienced through a series of developmental transitions across the lifespan that are embedded within a constellation of financial, social, cultural, historical, and physical influences (Hutchinson, 2015; McGoldrick, Garcia Preto, & Carter, 2016). For most people throughout the world, biological parenthood is a central life-goal and represents one of the normative and expected life-cycle transitions they plan to experience. Infertility, however, blocks the attainment of this life transition, and as such, represents a significant developmental interruption in their expected life course. In this regard, infertility can be perceived as a failed life course transition, or a 'transition to nonparenthood' (Matthews & Matthews, 1986).

The developmental interruption of infertility can disrupt identity formation, destabilize social relationships, and cause a questioning of one's self concept. As such, infertility is associated with long-term distress among women who never become a biological or adoptive parent (McQuillan, Greil, White, & Jacob, 2003), lending strong evidence to the idea that parenthood, and particularly motherhood, is central to many women's life identity. Women experiencing infertility commonly report being unable to contribute to group conversations on childbirth and parenting which contribute to cohesion among women. An inability to share in this experience or relate personal stories about biological children may lead to isolation and feelings of inauthenticity or inadequacy (Loftus & Andriot, 2012). Furthermore, many women experiencing infertility feel misunderstood by others as they try to cope with immense grief and fear.

Men also report challenges to identity formation as part of the infertility experience. Men commonly report significant emotional distress, threats to their perceptions of masculinity, and feelings of failure in their role of protector of their spouse—often struggling with feelings of helplessness when they are unable to solve the problem (Martins et al., 2016; Petok, 2015). They also experience grief associated with confronting unfulfilled expectations related to not having their own biological child to mentor, teach, and nurture.

Taken together, the interruption of the expected developmental life course for women and men represents a time of disconnection from others who continue onward, with accompanying feelings of brokenness and grief. When couples experience infertility in societies where the normative life-course to parenthood is emphasized through ubiquitous triggers and reminders, finding respite from emotional distress can seem all but impossible (Remennick, 2000).

2.4 Stress & Coping with Infertility

According to Lazarus and Folkman's stress and coping theory (1984), stress occurs when events in a person's life are perceived to exceed one's resources and threaten their well-being. Coping is defined as cognitive or behavioral strategies that are used to manage that stress. Gender differences can play a large role in how women and men manage this unexpected life stressor, and while some coping strategies are effective in reducing stress, others can also be related to increased distress (Peterson, Newton, Rosen, & Skaggs, 2006). For example, women seek social support from others going through infertility, as well as from medical professionals, which buffers the negative impact of infertility on psychological health. However, women also use more avoidance coping strategies, such as avoiding women with young children and other reminders of infertility, which is related to increased stress. Men, on the other hand, use more problem-solving strategies which fit commonly socialized norms of masculinity of working to solve problems in relationships. However, men are also more likely to cope using emotional distancing, which may create a barrier to relational health.

While the majority of studies have examined the individual coping strategies of men and women experiencing infertility, there has also been a growing body of research examining the relational impact of coping using the couple as the unit of analysis (Peterson, Pirritano, Christensen, & Schmidt, 2008; Volmer, Rösner, Toth, Strowitzki, & Wischmann, 2017). In these studies, the impact of a partner's coping pattern is studied in light of its impact on the other partner's infertility-stress. Because of the shared nature of the infertility experience and because one partner's ways of coping may have a direct impact on the well-being and stress levels of the other partner, examining the relational coping processes of couples experiencing infertility is vital. By conceptualizing infertility as a 'couples level stressor' we can better understand the relational impact of coping with infertility. Such a view is the first stage of broadening the lens from an individual to a relational perspective. By focusing on a relational context, clinicians, researchers, and policy makers can gain a more complete picture of the relationship between coping and infertility stress.

One way to examine the impact of partner coping is to examine the agreement or congruence both partners have about the levels of stress they are experiencing. Prior studies have found that agreement in the level of stress the other is experiencing can be an antidote for infertility stress as couples who show agreement related to infertility stress reported higher levels of marital satisfaction and decreased levels of depression compared to couples who did not show agreement in the levels of stress each experience (Peterson, Newton, & Rosen, 2003). However, not all couples agree on the stresses of the infertility experience and often cope with infertility in different ways.

Results of relational studies of coping with infertility suggest that individual coping strategies, which might be beneficial to an individual, could also be stressful to one's partner. For example, a male partner might use emotional distancing to limit the psychological discomfort of infertility, but this coping strategy may be related to his partner's feelings of isolation, which can lead to increased depressive symptoms for the female partner (Peterson, Newton, Rosen, & Schulman, 2006). Men who use emotional distancing to cope with infertility reported making light of the situation, refused to get too serious about infertility, and lived their lives as if nothing had happened. Men may view distancing as an attempt to change the meaning of infertility and gain some perspective about their situation. However, women in these couples may view their partners' actions as an inadvertent form of denial or minimization which limits their willingness to communicate about the problem and work toward its resolution.

For couples, coping strategies that are characterized by a lack of emotional intimacy and acceptance can negatively impact the relationship (Peterson, Newton, Rosen, & Schulman, 2006). Relational coping strategies which cause one partner to experience increased psychological distress can also be related to feelings of emotional isolation and partner resentment, and it has been found that if a spouse is unavailable to offer support and understanding regarding the difficulty of coping with a stressor, support received from other sources is not an adequate replacement. For example, in couples where women used high amounts of emotional self-controlling coping (keeping their feelings to themselves, keeping others from knowing how bad things were), and male partners used low amounts of emotional self-controlling coping, men reported higher levels of infertility stress and decreased levels of marital satisfaction. It is possible that the decreased levels of men's marital adjustment in these couples is related to a perceived lack of social and partner support. Because women in these couples are emotionally isolating themselves from others, male partners may endure an undesired level of emotional burden that could further martial disagreements and create barriers to emotional closeness.

Studies examining the impact of partner coping have also found that active avoidance coping strategies are related to higher depression and anxiety for individuals and partners, while meaning-based coping strategies can be beneficial to both individuals and partners (Peterson et al., 2009; Volmer et al., 2017). Couples who coped using active-avoidance strategies avoided being with pregnant women, kept their feelings regarding infertility stress to themselves, and turned to outside activities such as work to take their mind off of their infertility. Studies have consistently found that active-avoidance coping is significantly associated with personal, social, and marital distress for men and women at the individual and partner level (Peterson et al., 2009). Although avoidance is linked with increased distress in individuals and their partners, when one partner engages in less avoidance-related behavior, this can result in decreased feelings of distress for both partners. Perhaps one reason for this is that a partner's low use of active-avoidance coping acts as a buffer to increased distress for his or her partner. If both partners actively avoided coping with the stressor, it may lead to isolation and a lack of support. Having a partner who does not practice avoidance, although incongruent with his or her partner's coping, may add a protective component to his or her partner's individual distress levels.

A final coping strategy that has individual and relational influences is meaning-based coping. This type of coping is demonstrated when individuals or couples think about infertility in a positive light, discover other goals in life, or begin to view the experience of infertility as something that helped them grow as a person. The impact of gender is especially salient with meaning-based coping. Studies have found that when men use more meaning-based coping, their female partner's distress can increase. However, when a woman uses more meaning-based coping, men's distress decreases. Thus, it appears that a redefinition of the infertility experience by one's partner may be more beneficial for men than for women (Peterson et al., 2009).

Researchers have noted that these gender differences may be related to the pacing and timing of treatment decisions related to the infertility experience, as well as the gender-specific view on the importance of parenthood (Peterson et al., 2009). For example, women have greater difficulty deciding whether to stop treatments and accept infertility as a life-long condition. It is possible that men who try to find new meaning through infertility are doing so before their partner is prepared to do so, thus increasing her distress. Meaning-based coping is one of the few strategies that is related to individual benefit for women as well as benefits for their male partners. When an individual is ready to make new meaning of the experience, they may be more open to accepting the losses associated with the infertility experience. Furthermore, it may also signify the couple's joint readiness to create new meaning and move forward together to find new avenues of purpose for their time, energies, and dreams.

2.5 Fertility Counseling

The field of fertility counseling has evolved over the past several decades from offering general patient education and support to providing an integrated, evidence-based approach to patient care (Boivin & Gameiro, 2015; Domar, 2015). Since the publication of the first comprehensive handbook on infertility counseling in the late 1990s, significant strides have been made in the clinical application of therapeutic interventions and empirically-supported treatments for a wide range of fertility-related issues (Covington, 2015). Interventions for large, multi-disciplinary systems of care have also been developed by organizations such as the European Society of Human Reproduction and Embryology (ESHRE) that provide comprehensive, empirically-supported guidelines for psychosocial care for fertility treatment staff and providers (ESHRE, 2015).

Women and men experiencing infertility have been shown to benefit from psychosocial interventions aimed at reducing depression, anxiety, and infertility stress (Frederiksen, Farver-Vestergaard, Skovgård, Ingerslev, & Zachariae, 2015). Mental health professionals such as psychologists and family therapists are routinely called upon to provide couple counseling (Peterson, 2015), tools for coping with the two-week IVF waiting period (Ockhuijsen, van den Hoogen, Eijkemans, Macklon, & Boivin, 2014a), and psychosocial interventions that are aimed at decreasing emotional distress and improving patient decision-making, particularly as they relate to discontinuation of treatment (Gameiro, Boivin, Peronace, & Verhaak, 2012).

Cognitive-behavioral interventions for individuals and groups as well as mindfulness-based individual, couple, and group therapies have been found effective in reducing distress (Domar et al., 2000; Galhardo, Cunha, & Pinto-Gouveia, 2013; Peterson & Eifert, 2011; Shargh et al., 2016). Other effective forms of counseling include pre-IVF counseling, stress management, integrative body-mind-spirit interventions, psychoeducational support, supportive therapy, emotion-focused therapy, expressive writing interventions, and web-based coping programs (Frederiksen et al.,

2015). Connecting patients to providers who can implement psychosocial supports, as well as continuing to develop evidence-based psychosocial treatments remain important goals for providers and researchers in the field.

An important element of fertility counseling is helping individuals and couples cope with grief and loss. The number of losses couples experience is high and include losses of privacy, feelings of normalcy, cherished expectations of parenthood, relationships with family and friends, financial savings intended for other life goals, and meaningful connections to cultural and religious groups. Counselors can help couples grieve losses through the sharing of stories and emotions that allow couples to make contact with sadness, disappointment, and anger, thus facilitating grief and acceptance (Pascual-Leone & Greenberg, 2007). Experiential interventions, such as expressive writing, can provide a cost-effective, easy-to-administer way to facilitate emotional expression in individuals and couples (Frederiksen et al., 2017). The use of therapeutic rituals can provide an effective way for couples to grieve and mark non-normative life-cycle transitions like miscarriages or failed IVF attempts (Peterson, 2015). Such non-normative transitions often lack a clearly defined ritual, such as a funeral, that normative life transitions have. Marking these transitions with carefully constructed symbolic rituals can facilitate the expressions of emotions that are essential to healing and letting go.

End-of-treatment counseling is also important for couples who consider stopping treatment without achieving their reproductive goal (Klock, 2015). At this stage of the infertility journey, couples are confronted more fully with the possibility that they may never have a biological child. For some couples, the decision to stop treatment comes after years of unsuccessful treatment. In a qualitative study with 65 couples who underwent unsuccessful treatments, most couples believed in hindsight that there were tremendous costs associated with infertility which not only included emotional distress, but included the costs of putting their lives, as well as other important relationships, on hold (Daniluk, 2001). Counselors can help those ending treatment develop self-compassionate responses to their decisions to stop treatment and confront hindsight bias (i.e. I should have stopped treatments sooner) as they examine other life goals and family building options such as third-party reproduction, adoption, foster parenting, or child-free living (Klock, 2015).

Counselors can also incorporate meditation and mindfulness training into their work with couples. Mindfulness is a state of non-judgmental awareness that is open to experience and attuned to the present moment (Atkinson, 2013). It can also include compassionate acceptance of oneself and others through the exercise of loving kindness (Germer, 2009). Couples experiencing infertility commonly find themselves dealing with psychological distress, anger, and excessive self-criticism. Mindfulness has been found to be effective in reducing these emotional states (Davis & Hayes, 2011), and has also been shown to be effective in reducing distress in patients experiencing infertility (Galhardo et al., 2013). While mindfulness can be commonly confused with cognitive-behavioral relaxation strategies, the goal of mindfulness is not to promote relaxation, but to increased awareness of experience through focusing on one's breath or body sensations. Paradoxically, the ability to increase awareness and be present with distress in an accepting way can result in a person's increased capacity to be present with distressing thoughts and emotions related to infertility.

Mindfulness may also be associated with stronger couple relationships. Prior studies have found more mindful individuals demonstrate improved awareness of a partner's emotional states, increased empathy for a partner's experiences, and less emotional reactivity towards their partner (Atkinson, 2013). While couples experiencing infertility typically report strong relationship satisfaction, chronic infertility-related stress can take a toll on the couple's satisfaction levels over time. Mindfulness-based cognitive group therapy for couples has been shown to contribute to improvements in marital satisfaction and mental health (Shargh et al., 2016), and increased interpersonal presence and acceptance towards a partner's experience can improve relationship attunement and satisfaction. In a very real way, increased contact with the present moment in a mindful, non-judgmental way has the potential to increase each partner's ability to meet the needs of the other, which becomes a central resource to couples facing infertility-related stress. Additional resources and tools for use by fertility counselors, researchers, and patients are found in the appendix of the book.

2.6 Infertility at the Societal Level: Fertility Awareness

Individual and interpersonal infertility-related concerns expand to organizational and societal level concerns when we look at delayed childbearing as a potential cause of infertility. Women throughout the world are delaying the age when they have children. This is primarily due to societal changes including the increased availability of effective contraception, gender equality, the deferral of parenthood to pursue educational and career opportunities, and the postponement of marriage (Mills, Rindfuss, McDonald, & Te Velde, 2011). While these changes provide women with increased options to balance work and family responsibilities, delaying childbearing also carries risks including increased chance of miscarriage and trisomy, decreased probability a couple will achieve their desired family size, and an increased possibility of infertility due to age-related fertility decline (Schmidt, Sobotka, Bentzen, & Nyboe Andersen, 2012). In some developed countries, infertility intersects with societal concerns over low fertility and below replacement fertility, making it a population-level issue rather than solely an individual or interpersonal one (Morgan, 2003; Smallwood & Chamberlain, 2005).

Studies have consistently found that women and men throughout the world, in both the general population and in university students, possess an inadequate knowledge of fertility-related issues (Bunting, Tsibulsky, & Boivin, 2013; Chan, Chan, Peterson, Lampic, & Tam, 2015; Hashiloni-Dolev, Kaplan, & Shkedi-Rafid, 2011; Lampic, Svanberg, Karlström, & Tydén, 2006; Peterson, Pirritano, Tucker, & Lampic, 2012). Studies have also found a lack of fertility knowledge in health care professionals, medical students, obstetrics and gynecology residents, and even practicing gynecologists (Garcia, Vassena, Prat, & Vernaeve, 2017; Revelli, Razzano, Delle Piane, Casano, & Benedetto, 2016; Yu, Peterson, Inhorn, Boehm, & Patrizio, 2016). A misunderstanding of basic reproductive facts by both the public and health care providers can lead to uninformed reproductive decision-making which can put women at risk for possible infertility and its accompanying psychological stresses and age-related risk factors.

Fertility awareness was defined in the 2017 *International Glossary on Infertility and Fertility Care* as "the understanding of reproduction, fecundity, fecundability, and related individual risk factors (e.g. advanced age, sexual health factors such as sexually transmitted infections, and life style factors such as smoking and obesity) and non-individual risk factors (e.g. environmental and work place factors); including the awareness of societal and cultural factors affecting options to meet reproductive family planning, as well as family building needs" (Zegers-Hochschild et al., 2017, p. 8). The addition of fertility awareness in the glossary solidifies its importance as a global issue that should be given consideration by clinicians, health care providers, researchers, and policy makers. The Danish Council of Health and Disease Prevention argued that fertility awareness is a form of infertility prevention and recommended increasing the population's knowledge at both the societal and individual levels about the impact of age on fertility (Nielsen et al., 2016). At the societal level, this can be done by including fertility awareness in sexual education curriculums and existing public health campaigns that target related risk factors such as STIs, body weight, alcohol use, and smoking. It can also be accomplished by the inclusion of family friendly policies in the labor force including remote work opportunities, generous and flexible parental leave, affordable housing, and on-site, low-cost day care centers to make it possible for those who wish to have children to do so before the impact of age decreases the chances of fertility (Nielsen et al., 2016).

Fertility awareness can be effectively promoted on an organizational level as health care providers such as obstetricians and gynecologists engage in patient discussions related to fertility (Peterson, 2017; Yu et al., 2016). Studies have found that a woman's health care provider is her preferred source of information about reproductive health, but engagement in reproductive conversations is severely limited as most patients rarely talk about fertility issues with providers (Hodes-Wertz, Druckenmiller, Smith, & Noyes, 2013; Lundsberg et al., 2014). In addition, many physicians are reluctant to engage in these discussions as they fear they might be perceived as pushing childbearing on patients and increase their emotional distress (Yu et al., 2016).

Physicians must weigh these concerns against the benefits that can result from physician-initiated preconception discussions at ages when patients' fertility is at its peak (Wyndham, Figueira, & Patrizio, 2012). By engaging in value-free discussions aimed at patient education, physicians can educate patients about their reproductive options so that they can make intentional reproductive choices. Physicians can also emphasize that whether or not a patient decides to have a child, and at what age they plan to do so, it is a decision made by the patient; but it is the responsibility as a physician to provide patients with the comprehensive reproductive information and encourage autonomy in their decision-making.

Preconception counseling and patient/physician discussions of fertility awareness are essential for all patients, especially highly educated, older couples who may have unrealistic expectations about fertility (Van Voorhis, 2007). For example, a couple in their mid-30s who wants to have biological children, but who believes that healthy living and advances in science have lengthened a woman's biological clock, might continue to delay childbearing until their late 30s or even early 40s. The failure to try to have a biological child before the age of 40 may result in involuntary childlessness, as well as increase the risks associated with pregnancy if conception occurs. Couples often possess inaccurate perceptions of the impact of age on fertility given the influence of media reports that highlight high profile pregnancies at advanced ages. Such reports, however, are often incomplete and do not include correct data about the steep decline in fertility to women in their late 30s and the declining success rates of ARTs to women after age 40. In addition, for privacy reasons, media reports likely fail to discuss that children born to women after age 45 have likely been conceived using donor oocytes (which precludes the mother from having a genetic link to the child).

In addition to discussions on age-related fertility decline, an important aspect of fertility awareness is fertility preservation, particularly oocyte cryopreservation (egg freezing). This procedure has the potential to expand reproductive decision-making as women balance the competing interests of education, career, and the desire to have biological children. While oocyte cryopreservation historically has been accepted for use in patients diagnosed with cancer (Noyes et al., 2011), it has only recently begun to be more widely available and accepted for patients seeking elective fertility preservation (Mertes & Pennings, 2011; Stoop, Cobo, & Silber, 2014).

Because improvements in a rapid freezing technology called 'vitrification' have led to improved success rates similar to those achieved with fresh oocytes, in 2012 the American Society for Reproduction (ASRM) removed the experimental label from this procedure, but also noted that data on the safety, efficacy, and emotional risks were insufficient to fully recommend and support elective cryopreservation to delay childbearing (ASRM Practice Committee, 2013).

Many ethical considerations concerning oocyte cryopreservation continue to be debated, including concerns about commercial exploitation and pressure on women to use the technology (Harwood, 2015). Such ethical considerations have taken on increased importance with the inclusion of egg freezing in employee-sponsored benefit packages. Ethical analysis of such benefits propose that they may not best serve women's reproductive autonomy unless women are fully informed about the procedure, women do not feel pressure to use the benefit, and that the benefit does not negatively affect other family-friendly policies (Mertes, 2015). Still others have cautioned that even though survival and fertilization rates using oocyte cryopreservation are comparable to those with fresh oocytes, women should be aware of the safety, efficacy, and lack of long-term outcome data of the procedure (Potdar, Gelbaya, & Nardo, 2014).

Despite these concerns, there is growing acceptance and use of egg freezing for elective purposes. A 2017 study of 663 women aged 18–44 found that 90% of participants were aware of oocyte cryopreservation, and 72% agreed they would consider freezing their eggs to preserve their fertility (O'Brien, Martyn, Glover, & Wingfield, 2017). In addition, there were no significant differences in attitudes towards using the procedure between women who were single or in a relationship, nor were there significant differences between younger and older women. In a study among 973 women in Denmark and the United Kingdom (UK), 89% of women considered it acceptable to freeze oocytes for elective reasons; however, participants were only likely to accept the procedure if the success rate was 50% or greater and it would not adversely impact future fertility (Lallemant, Vassard, Nyboe Andersen, Schmidt, & Macklon, 2016).

Although this technology is available for women of all ages, women who freeze their eggs for elective purposes commonly do so at an age when their peak reproductive potential has passed. A recent study of 183 women who used oocyte cryopreservation found the mean patient age at the time of freezing was 38, and 79% wished they had frozen their eggs at an earlier age (Hodes-Wertz et al., 2013). To maximize one's reproductive potential, a woman would need to freeze her oocytes in her late 20s or early 30s before the onset of age-related fertility decline. Decision-analysis models propose that the highest probability of achieving a live birth may be when women undertake elective oocyte cryopreservation at <34 years of age (Mesen, Mersereau, Kane, & Steiner, 2015), and cost-effectiveness studies show that freezing oocytes by age 35 in women who plan to delay childbearing until age 40 effectively reduces the cost per live birth (Devine et al., 2015).

2.7 Infertility and Public Health

From a public-health perspective, the treatment of infertility requires the collective efforts of governments and societies. For example, in the United States, the Centers for Disease Control published the *National Public Health Action Plan for the Detection, Prevention, and Management of Infertility* which highlighted the need to understand and address issues at a population level that contribute to and are caused by infertility (CDC, 2014b). In this sense, it has been proposed that a call to public health practitioners be initiated in order to rally collective action and promote primary, secondary, and tertiary prevention by, respectively, (1) encouraging healthy behaviors that can help maintain and preserve fertility and reducing environmental exposures that can threaten it; (2) endorsing early detection; and (3) improving access to and quality of infertility services and treatments. These efforts are not limited to any one country and can be applied to societies based on their unique needs and resources. The following sections will outline the relevant issues at the primary, secondary, tertiary levels of prevention.

2.7.1 Primary Prevention

From a public health perspective, primary prevention aims to reduce the incidence of a disease by removing associated risk factors. In a nationally probabilistic sample of married or cohabitating women from the United States, findings suggested that modifiable risk factors, such as a history of undiagnosed and untreated STIs, smoking, and obesity were directly related to infertility status (Kelly-Weeder & Cox, 2006). A primary prevention approach would promote provider-initiated discussions with at-risk individuals on lifestyle and behavioral risk factors that are tailored, motivational, and supportive. This approach can also apply to health care professionals and OBGYNs who have been found to have low or incomplete fertility awareness (Kudesia, Chernyak, & McAvey, 2017; Yu et al., 2016). Improvements or additions to medical education, residency training, and continuing medical education programs on fertility awareness, including education on the modifiable risk factors for infertility, has the likelihood of enhancing physicians' knowledge base and practice (Will, Maslow, Kaye, & Nulsen, 2017).

Other primary prevention strategies that could reduce underlying risk factors in the socio-cultural environment include understanding that adolescents are disproportionately affected by untreated STIs such as chlamydia and gonorrhea. Thus, advocating for comprehensive sex education and reframing awareness campaigns for condom-use as 'triple protection,' (which communicates condoms as protection from unplanned pregnancy, HIV, and infertility) can be effective primary prevention strategies (Brady, 2003).

2.7.2 Secondary Prevention

Secondary prevention aims to detect a disease in its earliest stages in order to slow, stop, or reverse its progression. The central task of secondary prevention is screening. While there is a lack of conformity in the standard case definitions for infertility, impaired fecundity and related issues—complicating clinical detection and public health surveillance across systems and countries—there is a general rule that women under age 35 trying to achieve pregnancy should consult a specialist after one year of unprotected, vaginal intercourse with the same partner. Women are encouraged to see a specialist after 6 months if they are 35 or older. Early diagnosis and treatment of underlying medical conditions may restore fertility or enhance the probability of treatment success.

Studies suggest younger women who have high fertility knowledge and who suspect a fertility problem have a higher likelihood of working towards fertility-optimizing behavior change such as losing weight or seeking medical help (Fulford, Bunting, Tsibulsky, & Boivin, 2013). Evidence-based messages could be leveraged by the media to inform the public on reproductive health, the ovulatory cycle, and procreative success, as well as the frequency, causes, signs, and repercussions of infertility. These efforts could increase knowledge, reduce stigma, and facilitate early access to diagnosis and treatment.

2.7.3 *Tertiary Prevention*

Tertiary prevention strategies are used to help people appropriately manage or improve their health problem over the long-term. In the case of infertility, ART can help couples to resolve biological childlessness. There is a slightly higher demand for infertility services in developed countries compared to less developed countries, however availability of care is markedly unequal due to allocation of health care resources, regulations, and lack of services in lower-income countries (Boivin et al., 2007). Nevertheless, from 2000 to 2010, IVF services grew from being available in only one-quarter of the world's nations to being available in more than half of the nations, although sub-Saharan Africa is still largely underserved (Inhorn & Patrizio, 2015).

An important public health issue is the racial and ethnic disparities in access to such services. For example, in the United States, a nationally representative survey from 2006–2010 found that only 38% of nulliparous women aged 25–44 who reported fertility problems had ever used infertility services; among those, the users were disproportionally non-Hispanic White women with higher levels of education and household income, despite non-Hispanic Black or Hispanic women without a college degree being the group most affected by infertility (Quinn & Fujimoto, 2016). Studies have also found that Black and Asian women who pursue ART present with infertility for a longer duration than non-Hispanic White women (Lamb et al, 2009; Seifer, Frazier, & Grainger, 2008). If minority couples successfully overcome the challenges to accessing care and receive ART services, Asian, Black, and Hispanic women still report lower rates of live birth compared to White women (Quinn & Fujimoto, 2016). Although there is a myriad of confounding factors to consider, significant research is needed to better understand the potential mechanisms of this disparity. Working to ensure insurance coverage, lower costs, expand ART services in low resource settings, and address social and cultural concerns is paramount.

2.8 Conclusion

Because biological parenthood is a central life-goal for the majority of women and men throughout the world, infertility represents a developmental interruption in a couple's expected life course and is related to substantial stress and emotional challenges. At the intrapersonal and interpersonal levels, individuals and couples use a variety of coping strategies to manage this unexpected stressor. Coping strategies must be viewed in the context of one's relationship to understand the effectiveness for individuals and partners. Furthermore, counseling services offered by mental health and medical professionals can provide much needed relief for women and men undergoing treatment. At the societal level, while there are growing number of women and men having children at older ages throughout the world, fertility awareness is lacking in both the general population and among medical professionals. As such, increasing awareness of age-related fertility decline, as well as fertility preservation options, is needed to ensure patients have the opportunity to make informed reproductive choices. Finally, from a public health perspective, primary, secondary, and tertiary prevention strategies can be used to prevent infertility and reduce the significant burden it places on women and men, communities, and societies.

Appendix 2.1: Additional Fertility Resources

Screen IVF

Screen IVF is a 34-item instrument designed to screen infertility patients prior to treatment in order to identify those at risk for emotional distress and pre-treatment dropout (Verhaak, Lintsen, Evers, & Braat, 2010). It was originally developed for Dutch fertility patients, has been translated into English, and has been found to have both construct and criteria validity. The measure includes 10 items for anxiety (state and trait), 7 items for depression, 12 items for cognitions regarding fertility problems, and 5 items for social support. Recommended cut-off scores are provided to assist in the identification of at-risk patients. It has also been recommended for use by fertility clinics at the beginning of treatment (Ockhuijsen, van Smeden, van den Hoogen, & Boivin, 2017).

FertiCalm

FertiCalm is a smart phone app developed by Alice Domar and Elizabeth Grill, two of the world's leading experts in reproductive psychology. The app is a repository of over 500 coping options that can be accessed by women whenever and wherever they feel distressed by infertility-specific life situations. There are more than 50 specific life situations women are likely to encounter, each with custom-made solutions to increase well-being in that moment. The solutions include cognitive techniques to restructure thoughts, behavioral suggestions, social solutions, relaxation techniques that include 10–20 different guided relaxations, and links to ideas for humor and self-nurturing. For more information, please see http://www.ferticalmapp.com/.

FertiSTAT

FertiSTAT is a 22-question, online fertility status awareness tool developed and validated by Cardiff University researchers Jacky Boivin and Laura Bunting (Bunting & Boivin, 2010). Based on a woman's responses to her age, lifestyle, and health, it provides personalized guidance about reducing risk, optimizing behaviors, and seeking timely medical advice. The tool is aimed at women but includes an opportunity to assess male partner risk. For more information, please see http://www.fertistat.com/.

FertiQoL

FertiQoL is the first validated instrument to reliably measure the impact of fertility problems and its treatment on quality of life for men and women (Boivin, Takefman, & Braverman, 2011). The tool has 36 items, covering emotional, mind-body, relational and social domains, as well as the impact of treatment quality and tolerability on quality of life. The instrument is available in over 20 languages. For more information, please see www.fertiqol.org.

PCRI (Positive Reappraisal Coping Intervention)

Research suggests that the two-week waiting period between embryo transfer and the pregnancy test is a particularly stress-inducing time (Boivin & Takefman, 1995). The PCRI is a self-help, at-home intervention, consisting of a single pocket-sized card or flyer with statements designed to help patients cognitively redefine difficult situations to find more positive meaning. Studies have found that use of the PCRI can increase positive affect (Lancastle & Boivin, 2008; Ockhuijsen, van den Hoogen, Eijkemans, Macklon and Bovin, 2014b), as well as significantly reduce anxiety levels during the waiting period and up to 6 weeks after the start of the waiting period (Ockhuijsen et al., 2014a).

References

Agarwal, A., Mulgund, A., Hamada, A., & Chyatte, M. R. (2015). A unique view on male infertility around the globe. *Reproductive Biology and Endocrinology, 13,* 1–9.

American Society for Reproductive Medicine (ASRM). (2013). Practice Committees of the American Society for Reproductive Medicine and Society for Assisted Reproductive Technology: Mature oocyte cryopreservation: A guideline. *Fertility and Sterility, 99*(1), 37–43.

Atkinson, B. J. (2013). Mindfulness training and the cultivation of secure, satisfying couple relationships. *Couple and Family Psychology: Research and Practice, 2*(2), 73–94.

Boivin, J., Bunting, L., Collins, J. A., & Nygren, K. G. (2007). International estimates of infertility prevalence and treatment-seeking: Potential need and demand for infertility medical care. *Human Reproduction, 22*(6), 1506–1512.

Boivin, J., & Gameiro, S. (2015). Evolution of psychology and counseling in infertility. *Fertility and Sterility, 104*(2), 251–259.

Boivin, J., Takefman, J., & Braverman, A. (2011). The fertility quality of life (FertiQoL) tool: Development and general psychometric properties. *Human Reproduction, 26*(8), 2084–2091.

Boivin, J., & Takefman, J. (1995). Stress levels across stages of in vitro fertilization in subsequently pregnant and nonpregnant women. *Fertility and Sterility, 64*(4), 802–810.

Brady, M. (2003). Preventing sexually transmitted infection and unintended pregnancy, and safeguarding fertility: Triple protection needs of young women. *Reproductive Health Matters, 11*(22), 134–141.

Bunting, L., Tsibulsky, I., & Boivin, J. (2013). Fertility knowledge and beliefs about fertility treatment: Findings from the international fertility decision-making study. *Human Reproduction, 28*(2), 385–397.

Bunting, L., & Boivin, J. (2010). Development and preliminary validation of the fertility status awareness tool: FertiSTAT. *Human Reproduction, 25*(7), 1722–1733.

Centers for Disease Control and Prevention, American Society for Reproductive Medicine, Society for Assisted Reproductive Technology. (2014a). *2012 assisted reproductive technology fertility clinic success rates report*. Atlanta, GA: US Department of Health and Human Services.

Centers for Disease Control and Prevention, American Society for Reproductive Medicine, Society for Assisted Reproductive Technology. (2014b). *National public health action plan for the detection, prevention, and management of infertility*. Atlanta, GA: Centers for Disease Control and Prevention.

Centers for Disease Control and Prevention. (2017). *Infertility: Frequently asked questions*. Retrieved from https://www.cdc.gov/reproductivehealth/infertility/index.htm.

Chan, C. H. Y., Chan, T. H. Y., Peterson, B. D., Lampic, C., & Tam, M. Y. J. (2015). Intentions and attitudes towards parenthood and fertility awareness among Chinese university students in Hong Kong: A comparison with Western samples. *Human Reproduction, 30*(2), 364–372.

Covington, S. N. (Ed.). (2015). *Fertility counseling: Clinical guide and case studies*. Cambridge University Press.

Daniluk, J. C. (2001). "If We Had It to Do Over Again ...": Couples' reflections on their experiences of infertility treatments. *The Family Journal, 9*(2), 122–133.

Davis, D. M., & Hayes, J. A. (2011). What are the benefits of mindfulness? A practice review of psychotherapy-related research. *Psychotherapy, 48*(2), 198–208.

Devine, K., Mumford, S. L., Goldman, K. N., Hodes-Wertz, B., Druckenmiller, S., Propst, A. M., & Noyes, N. (2015). Baby budgeting: Oocyte cryopreservation in women delaying reproduction can reduce cost per live birth. *Fertility and Sterility, 103*(6), 1446–1453.

Domar, A. D. (2015). Creating a collaborative model of mental health counseling for the future. *Fertility and Sterility, 104*(2), 277–280.

Domar, A. D., Clapp, D., Slawsby, E. A., Dusek, J., Kessel, B., & Freizinger, M. (2000). Impact of group psychological interventions on pregnancy rates in infertile women. *Fertility and Sterility, 73*(4), 805–811.

European Society for Human Reproduction and Embryology (ESHRE) Psychology and Counseling Guidelines Development Group. (2015). *Routine psychosocial care in infertility and medically assisted reproduction—a guide for fertility staff*. https://www.eshre.eu/Guidelines-and-Legal/Guidelines/Psychosocial-care-guideline.aspx.

Ferraretti, A. P., Goossens, V., Kupka, M., Bhattacharya, S., de Mouzon, J., Castilla, J. A., ... Nyboe Andersen, A. (2013). Assisted reproductive technology in Europe, 2009: Results generated from European registers by ESHRE. *Human Reproduction, 28*(9), 2318–2331.

Frederiksen, Y., Farver-Vestergaard, I., Skovgård, N. G., Ingerslev, H. J., & Zachariae, R. (2015). Efficacy of psychosocial interventions for psychological and pregnancy outcomes in infertile women and men: A systematic review and meta-analysis. *British Medical Journal Open, 5*(1), e006592.

Frederiksen, Y., O'Toole, M. S., Mehlsen, M. Y., Hauge, B., Elbaek, H. O., Zachariae, R., & Ingerslev, H. J. (2017). The effect of expressive writing intervention for infertile couples: A randomized controlled trial. *Human Reproduction, 32*(2), 391–402.

Fulford, B., Bunting, L., Tsibulsky, I., & Boivin, J. (2013). The role of knowledge and perceived susceptibility in intentions to optimize fertility: Findings from the International Fertility Decision-Making Study (IFDMS). *Human Reproduction, 28*(12), 3253–3262.

Galhardo, A., Cunha, M., & Pinto-Gouveia, J. (2013). Mindfulness-based program for infertility: Efficacy study. *Fertility and Sterility, 100*(4), 1059–1067.

Gameiro, S., Boivin, J., Peronace, L., & Verhaak, C. (2012). Why do patients discontinue fertility treatment? A systematic review of reasons and predictors of discontinuation in fertility treatment. *Human Reproduction Update, 18*(6), 652–669.

Garcia, D., Vassena, R., Prat, A., & Vernaeve, V. (2017). Poor knowledge of age-related fertility decline and assisted reproduction among healthcare professionals. *Reproductive Biomedicine Online, 34*, 32–37.

Germer, C. (2009). *The mindful path to self-compassion: Freeing yourself from destructive thoughts and emotions*. Guilford Press.

Greil, A. L., Slauson-Blevins, K., & McQuillan, J. (2010). The experience of infertility: A review of recent literature. *Sociology of Health & Illness, 32*(1), 140–162.
Harwood, K. (2015). On the ethics of social egg freezing and fertility preservation for nonmedical reasons. *Medicoleg Bioeth, 5,* 59–67.
Hashiloni-Dolev, Y., Kaplan, A., & Shkedi-Rafid, S. (2011). The fertility myth: Israeli students' knowledge regarding age-related fertility decline and late pregnancies in an era of assisted reproduction technology. *Human Reproduction, 26*(11), 3045–3053.
Hodes-Wertz, B., Druckenmiller, S., Smith, M., & Noyes, N. (2013). What do reproductive-age women who undergo oocyte cryopreservation think about the process as a means to preserve fertility? *Fertility and Sterility, 100*(5), 1343–1349.
Hutchinson, E. (2015). *A life course perspective. In dimensions of human behavior: The changing life course.* Sage.
Inhorn, M., & Patrizio, P. (2015). Infertility around the globe: New thinking on gender, reproductive technologies and global movements in the 21st century. *Human Reproduction, 21*(4), 411–426.
Kelly-Weeder, S., & Cox, C. (2006). The impact of lifestyle risk factors on female infertility. *Women and Health, 44*(4), 1–23.
Klock, S. C. (2015). When treatment appears futile: The role of the mental health professional and end-of-treatment counseling. *Fertility and Sterility, 104*(2), 267–270.
Kudesia, R., Chernyak, C., & McAvey, B. (2017). Low fertility awareness in U.S. reproductive-aged women and medical trainees: Creation and validation of the FIT-KS. *Fertility and Sterility, 108,* 711–717.
Lallemant, C., Vassard, D., Nyboe Andersen, A., Schmidt, L., & Macklon, N. (2016). Medical and social egg freezing: Internet-based survey of knowledge and attitudes among women in Denmark and the UK. *Acta Obstetricia et Gynecologica Scandinavica, 95*(12), 1402–1410.
Lamb, J., Huddleston, H., Purcell, K., Modan, A., Farsani, T., Dingeldein, M., … Fujiomoto, V. (2009). Asian ethnicity is associated with decreased pregnancy rates following intrauterine insemination. *Reproductive Biomedicine Online, 19*(2), 252–256.
Lampic, C., Svanberg, A. S., Karlström, P., & Tydén, T. (2006). Fertility awareness, intentions concerning childbearing, and attitudes towards parenthood among female and male academics. *Human Reproduction, 21*(2), 558–564.
Lancastle, D., & Boivin, J. (2008). A feasibility study of a brief coping intervention (PRCI) for the waiting period before a pregnancy test during fertility treatment. *Human Reproduction, 23*(10), 2299–2307.
Lazarus, R. S., & Folkman, S. (1984). *Stress, coping and appraisal.* New York: Springer.
Loftus, J., & Andriot, A. (2012). "That's what makes a woman": Infertility and coping with a failed life course transition. *Sociological Spectrum, 32*(3), 226–243.
Lundsberg, L., Pal, L., Gariepy, A., Xu, X., Chu, M., & Illuzzi, J. (2014). Knowledge, attitudes, and practices regarding conception and fertility: A population-based survey among reproductive-age United States women. *Fertility and Sterility, 101*(3), 767–774.
Martins, M.V., Basto-Pereira, M., Pedro, J., Peterson, B., Almeida, V., Schmidt, L., & Costa, M. E. (2016). Male psychological adaptation to unsuccessful medically assisted reproduction treatments: A systematic review. *Human Reproduction Update*, 22(4), 466–478.
Matthews, R., & Matthews, A. M. (1986). Infertility and involuntary childlessness: The transition to nonparenthood. *Journal of Marriage and the Family, 48,* 641–649.
McQuillan, J., Greil, A., White, L., & Jacob, M. (2003). Frustrated fertility: Infertility and psychological distress among women. *Journal of Marriage and Family, 65,* 1007–1018.
McGoldrick, M., Garcia Preto, N., & Carter, B. (2016). The life cycle in its changing context: Individual, family, and social perspectives. *The expanding family life cycle: Individual, family, and social perspectives* (pp. 1–44). Boston, MA: Pearson.
Mertes, H. (2015). Does company-sponsored egg freezing promote or confine women's reproductive autonomy? *Journal of Assisted Reproduction and Genetics, 32*(8), 1205–1209.
Mertes, H., & Pennings, G. (2011). Social egg freezing: For better, not for worse. *Reproductive Biomedicine Online, 23*(7), 824–829.

Mesen, T. B., Mersereau, J. E., Kane, J. B., & Steiner, A. Z. (2015). Optimal timing for elective egg freezing. *Fertility and Sterility, 103*(6), 1551–1556.

Mills, M., Rindfuss, R. R., McDonald, P., & Te Velde, E. (2011). Why do people postpone parenthood? Reasons and social policy incentives. *Human Reproduction Update, 17*(6), 848–860.

Morgan, S. P. (2003). Is low fertility a twenty-first-century demographic crisis? *Demography, 40*(4), 589–603.

Nielsen, H. S., Schmidt, L., Nyboe Andersen, A., Birch Petersen, K., Gyrd-Hansen, D., Jensen, T.K., … Knudsen, L. B. (2016). *Forebyggelse af nedsat frugtbarhed.* Retried from Vidensråd for Forebyggelse: http://www.vidensraad.dk/rapporter.

Noyes, N., Knopman, J. M., Melzer, K., Fino, M. E., Friedman, B., & Westphal, L. M. (2011). Oocyte cryopreservation as a fertility preservation measure for cancer patients. *Reproductive Biomedicine Online, 23*(3), 323–333.

O'Brien, Y., Martyn, F., Glover, L. E., & Wingfield, M. B. (2017). What women want? A scoping survey on women's knowledge, attitudes and behaviours towards ovarian reserve testing and egg freezing. *European Journal of Obstetrics & Gynecology and Reproductive Biology, 217,* 71–76.

Ockhuijsen, H., van den Hoogen, A., Eijkemans, M., Macklon, N., & Boivin, J. (2014a). Clarifying the benefits of the positive reappraisal coping intervention for women waiting for the outcomes of IVF. *Human Reproduction, 29*(12), 2712–2718.

Ockhuijsen, H., van den Hoogen, A., Eijkemans, M., Macklon, N., & Bovin, J. (2014b). The impact of a self-administered coping intervention on emotional well-being in women awaiting the outcome of IVF treatment: A randomized controlled trial. *Human Reproduction, 29*(7), 1459–1470.

Ockhuijsen, H. D., van Smeden, M., van den Hoogen, A., & Boivin, J. (2017). Validation study of the SCREENIVF: An instrument to screen women or men on risk for emotional maladjustment before the start of a fertility treatment. *Fertility and Sterility, 107*(6), 1370–1379.

Pascual-Leone, A., & Greenberg, L. S. (2007). Emotional processing in experiential therapy: Why the only way out is through. *Journal of Consulting and Clinical Psychology, 75*(6), 875.

Peterson, B. D. (2015). Fertility counseling for couples. In S. N. Covington (Ed.), *Fertility counseling: Clinical guide and case studies* (pp. 60–73). Cambridge, UK: Cambridge University Press.

Peterson, B. (2017). A validated measure for fertility awareness: An essential step toward informed reproductive decision-making. *Fertility and Sterility, 108*(4), 606–607.

Peterson, B. D., & Eifert, G. (2011). Using acceptance and commitment therapy to treat infertility stress. *Cognitive and Behavioral Practice, 18,* 577–587.

Peterson, B. D., Newton, C. R., & Rosen, K. H. (2003). Examining congruence between partners' perceived infertility-related stress and its relationship to marital adjustment and depression in infertile couples. *Family Process, 42*(1), 59–70.

Peterson, B. D., Newton, C. R., Rosen, K. H., & Schulman, R. S. (2006a). Coping processes of couples experiencing infertility. *Family Relations, 55*(2), 227–239.

Peterson, B. D., Newton, C. R., Rosen, K. H., & Skaggs, G. E. (2006b). Gender differences in how men and women who are referred for IVF cope with infertility stress. *Human Reproduction, 21*(9), 2443–2449.

Peterson, B. D., Pirritano, M., Christensen, U., & Schmidt, L. (2008). The impact of partner coping in couples experiencing infertility. *Human Reproduction, 23*(5), 1128–1137.

Peterson, B. D., Pirritano, M., Christensen, U., Boivin, J., Block, J., & Schmidt, L. (2009). The longitudinal impact of partner coping in couples following 5 years of unsuccessful fertility treatments. *Human Reproduction, 24*(7), 1656–1664.

Peterson, B. D., Pirritano, M., Tucker, L., & Lampic, C. (2012). Fertility awareness and parenting attitudes among American male and female undergraduate university students. *Human Reproduction, 27*(5), 1375–1382.

Petok, W. D. (2015). Infertility counseling (or the lack thereof) of the forgotten male partner. *Fertility and Sterility, 104*(2), 260–266.

Potdar, N., Gelbaya, T. A., & Nardo, L. G. (2014). Oocyte vitrification in the 21st century and post-warming fertility outcomes: A systematic review and meta-analysis. *Reproductive Biomedicine Online, 29*(2), 159–176.

Quinn, M., & Fujimoto, V. (2016). Racial and ethnic disparities in assisted reproductive technology access and outcomes. *Fertility and Sterility, 105*(5), 1119–1123.

Remennick, L. (2000). Childless in the land of imperative motherhood: Stigma and coping among infertile Israeli women. *Sex Roles, 43,* 821–841.

Revelli, A., Razzano, A., Delle Piane, L., Casano, S., & Benedetto, C. (2016). Awareness of the effects of postponing motherhood among hospital gynecologists: Is their knowledge sufficient to offer appropriate help to patients? *Journal of Assisted Reproduction and Genetics, 33*(2), 215–220.

Schmidt, L. (2006). Infertility and assisted reproduction in Denmark. *Danish Medical Bulletin, 53*(4), 390–417.

Schmidt, L., Sobotka, T., Bentzen, J. G., & Nyboe Andersen, A. (2012). Demographic and medical consequences of the postponement of parenthood. *Human Reproduction Update, 18*(1), 29–43.

Seifer, D., Frazier, L., & Grainger, D. (2008). Disparity in assisted reproductive technologies outcomes in black women compared with white women. *Fertility and Sterility, 90*(5), 1701–1710.

Shargh, N.A., Bakhshani, N.M., Mohebbi, M.D., Mahmudian, K., Ahovan, M., Mokhtari, M., & Gangali, A. (2016). The effectiveness of mindfulness-based cognitive group therapy on marital satisfaction and general health in woman with infertility. *Global Journal of Health Science, 8*(3), 230–235.

Smallwood, S., & Chamberlain, J. (2005). Replacement fertility, what has it been and what does it mean? *Population Trends, 119*(Spring), 16–27.

Stoop, D., Cobo, A., & Silber, S. (2014). Fertility preservation for age-related fertility decline. *The Lancet, 384*(9950), 1311–1319.

Van Voorhis, B. J. (2007). In vitro fertilization. *New England Journal of Medicine, 356*(4), 379–386.

Verhaak, C. M., Lintsen, A. M. E., Evers, A. W. M., & Braat, D. D. M. (2010). Who is at risk of emotional problems and how do you know? Screening of women going for IVF treatment. *Human Reproduction, 25*(5), 1234–1240.

Volmer, L., Rösner, S., Toth, B., Strowitzki, T., & Wischmann, T. (2017). Infertile partners' coping strategies are interrelated–implications for targeted psychological counseling. *Geburtshilfe und Frauenheilkunde, 77*(01), 52–58.

Will, E., Maslow, B., Kaye, L., & Nulsen, J. (2017). Increasing awareness of age-related fertility and elective fertility preservation among medical students and house staff: A pre- and post-intervention analysis. *Fertility and Sterility, 107,* 1200–1205.

Wyndham, N., Figueira, P. G. M., & Patrizio, P. (2012). A persistent misperception: Assisted reproductive technology can reverse the "aged biological clock". *Fertility and Sterility, 97*(5), 1044–1047.

Yu, L., Peterson, B., Inhorn, M., Boehm, J., & Patrizio, P. (2016). Knowledge, attitudes and intentions towards fertility awareness and oocyte cryopreservation among obstetrics and gynecology resident physicians. *Human Reproduction, 31,* 403–411.

Zegers-Hochschild, F., Adamson, G.D., Dyer, S., Racowsky, C., de Mouzon, J., Sokol, R., … van der Poel, S. (2017). The international glossary on infertility and fertility care, *Human Reproduction*, 32(9), 1786–1801.

Chapter 3
In Pursuit of Parenthood: The Highs and Lows of Fertility Treatment

Vera Skvirsky and Orit Taubman – Ben-Ari

3.1 Introduction

> We start out with so many expectations. Our own, our parents, those of our society. Sometimes the hardest thing is to be in a position where we recognize the distance between our expectations and reality…I remember that I stopped taking the pill the day after Ronny proposed. I really wanted to get pregnant even before the wedding. I hoped and waited every month to see the two stripes on the stick, maybe because something inside me knew that it probably wasn't going to be so easy…But it didn't happen…Not even the month after the wedding, the month after that, or the month after that…I wanted to hold our little boy or girl in my arms, I wanted to stop hurting, I wanted to start my own business, I wanted to feel I was using my abilities to get ahead…But the treatments put everything on hold. During that period I sometimes felt I couldn't have expectations about anything, because nothing was in my hands. (www.retters.co.il)

Procreation is widely perceived to be a natural developmental stage in the human life course (e.g., Erikson, 1963). This perception informs what most people think about becoming parents: it is a natural event that will happen when they are ready to undertake the role, while or after the achievement of other basic needs, such as finding a soulmate or satisfying career goals. But reality sometimes plots a different course for us. Nowadays, more and more people are dealing with infertility, defined as "the failure to achieve a successful pregnancy after 12 months or more of appropriate, unprotected intercourse or therapeutic donor insemination" (Practice Committee of the American Society for Reproductive Medicine, 2013, p. 63). Indeed, studies estimate that in 2010, 48.5 million couples worldwide were unable to have a child after five years of active attempts (Mascarenhas, Flaxman, Boerma, Vanderpoel, & Stevens, 2012), a 9% prevalence of infertility (of 12 months), and 56% of the couples seeking medical care (Boivin, Bunting, Collins, & Nygren, 2007).

V. Skvirsky (✉) · O. Taubman – Ben-Ari
The Louis and Gabi Weisfeld School of Social Work, Bar Ilan University, Ramat Gan, Israel
e-mail: verask@gmail.com

O. Taubman – Ben-Ari
e-mail: taubman@biu.ac.il

O. Taubman – Ben-Ari (ed.), *Pathways and Barriers to Parenthood*,
https://doi.org/10.1007/978-3-030-24864-2_3

Difficulties in the natural capacity to produce offspring often comes as an unpleasant surprise and typically arouses psychological distress. It is associated with the inability to achieve the desired social role of becoming a parent (Greil, Slauson-Blevins, & McQuillan, 2010, see also Morse & Steger, Chap. 1 in this volume), damages the sense of symbolic immortality leading to heightened levels of death anxiety (Yaakobi, Mikulincer, & Shaver, 2014, see also Solomon, Chap. 11 in this volume), and is considered a prolonged life crisis with elements of a chronically stressful situation (Greil, Schmidt, & Peterson, 2014). In a qualitative study, women described their perception of infertility and its treatment as "a struggle, a loss, a failure, a stressor, a painful experience, and an emotional roller coaster" (Berger, Paul, & Henshaw, 2013, p. 59). Elsewhere, they have reported greater experience of difficulties related to higher distress and lower well-being (Benyamini, Gozlan, & Kokia, 2005). A qualitative study of male infertility showed that men also reported feeling ignored, stigmatized and isolated (Arya & Dibb, 2016). However, most studies indicate that infertility is more distressing for women than for men, and that the experience and coping strategies of the two genders are different (Greil et al., 2010, 2014; Ying, Wu, & Loke, 2015). Moreover, infertility affects not only the individuals in the couple, but also the couple's psychological well-being as a unit (Ying et al., 2015, see also Peterson & Place, Chap. 2 in this volume).

The stress and potential damage to the mental health of people coping with infertility impact their quality of life (Rooney & Domar, 2016). Furthermore, studies have consistently found that stress and psychological burden are among the most frequent reasons given for the decision to discontinue treatment (Galst, 2018; Gameiro, Boivin, Peronace, & Verhaak, 2012; Greil et al., 2014). The current chapter describes individuals' experience of infertility at different stages in their journey to parenthood (at the beginning of treatment, during pregnancy, and after the birth), and considers diverse contributors to a variety of outcomes, both negative and positive.

3.2 Acknowledging a Fertility Problem and Beginning the Treatment Process

> There comes that moment when you realize you're a fertility patient…the moment the whole meaning falls on you. You lose part of your naiveté at that moment…It caught me unprepared. I couldn't stop crying. At that moment I understood that I was starting on a path whose end no one could see for sure. Nothing was certain. Fertility treatment didn't guarantee pregnancy, and pregnancy didn't guarantee children…Even though I had dozens of moments of optimism and strength later on, I remember that moment in the parked car and the fear and helplessness I felt…As a fertility patient I understand you can never know. Until you hold a healthy baby in your arms, anything can happen. (www.retters.co.il)

A couple who comes to their first consultation with a fertility specialist has already experienced a failure to conceive for at least a year. This means two things: first, that they acknowledge the problem (Olafsdottir, Wikland, & Möller, 2012); and secondly, that they have a "baseline" level of frustration and stress even before the beginning of the demanding series of examinations and medical procedures ahead of them (Domar, & Gross, 2012; Fassino, Piero, Boggio, Piccioni, & Garzaro, 2002). Although the findings of a study conducted in Scotland indicate higher psychological distress among women as the number of infertility clinic appointments increases (Souter, Hopton, Penney, & Templeton, 2002), the very beginning of treatment is a uniquely stressful event. While only a few studies thus far have examined this initial stage, research interest in it has recently been growing. For example, in 2016, Casu and Gremigni developed the Infertility-Related Stress Scale, administering it to participants recruited at the time of their initial infertility consultation. The results showed that patients with above-threshold levels of anxiety and depression reported higher infertility-related stress in both intrapersonal (e.g., mental health) and interpersonal (e.g., work performance) domains, particularly in the former.

A number of studies have related to the mental and physical health of men and women at the start of this complicated process. For example, a Portuguese study compared three groups: infertile couples attending their first medical appointment at an infertility medical center; those at the beginning of ART (Assisted Reproductive Technologies) treatments (during the hormonal simulation phase); and presumed fertile couples (childless and not pregnant or trying to get pregnant at the time of the study), and found more similarities than differences between infertile and presumed fertile couples (Moura-Ramos, Gameiro, Soares, Santos, & Canavarro, 2010). However, the infertile group presented higher levels of infertility global stress than did ART couples, and 20% of infertile women scored above the norms in depression, compared to 16.5% in the ART and 13.6% in the presumed fertile groups. Similarly, an Italian study found that anxiety and depression levels were higher for infertile couples at the time of their first contact with a specialist in obstetrics and gynecology than in fertile couples (Fassino et al., 2002). And in a Swedish study, women after an initial fertility clinic visit reported a considerably increased prevalence of anxiety symptoms than pregnant women, regardless of whether the latter had conceived naturally or with the aid of ART (Joelsson et al., 2017).

Gender may also play a role here, although the nature of its association with psychological and physical well-being following the first consultation for infertility is not entirely clear. Whereas some studies show that women score higher than men on depression and psychophysical condition (e.g., Casu & Gremigni 2016; Valoriani et al., 2016), others have found no significant gender differences (Moura-Ramos et al., 2010). Moreover, in 55% of cases in which men scored above the cut-off point on a depression questionnaire, their partners did as well (Valoriani et al., 2016).

Psychological distress at this point in time may affect the decision of whether or not to pursue treatment. In the Netherlands, for example, almost half of the patients left before starting any form of actual treatment, with one of their main reasons being emotional distress (Brandes et al., 2009). Elsewhere as well, patients who do not pursue treatment have been found to have higher baseline depression scores than those who choose to embark on the treatment process (Eisenberg et al., 2010).

Nevertheless, the first consultation also has the potential to positively impact psychological distress and anxiety by providing more reliable information. A study carried out in the U.S. indicates a modest improvement in women's knowledge of reproductive anatomy, ART, and fertility factors after the initial infertility visit (Childress et al., 2015). In addition, patients' positive and negative appraisals of treatment changed over time: negative appraisals (threat and loss), as well as anxiety scores, decreased, while positive appraisals (challenge) increased. A similar decline in state anxiety scores over time was found following consecutive referrals to an infertility clinic (Edelmann & Connolly, 2000). Moreover, women showed a greater reduction in anxiety over time than did men, regardless of the diagnosis. Thus, the initial consultation may help reduce stress and anxiety levels, which, in turn, may impact the decision to pursue treatment.

A series of Israeli studies examined contributors to the perceived stress, mental health, and life satisfaction of women after their initial consultation with a fertility specialist, and found that higher levels of personal resources were associated with greater positive outcomes in mental health. More specifically, higher hope, a positive resource characterized both by a cognitive element, whereby mental capabilities are used to find solutions for achieving desired goals, and by an affective element expressed in the emotional response to the success (or failure) of such efforts (Snyder, 2002), was associated with greater well-being (Ben Shlomo, Skvirsky, Taubman – Ben-Ari, Azuri, & Horowitz, 2017). Higher rumination (self-consciousness motivated by a sense of threat, loss, or injustice; Trapnell & Campbell, 1999) was associated with greater distress (Ben Shlomo, Skvirsky et al., 2017); higher attachment anxiety, considered a sign of difficulties in emotional regulation, was associated with less life satisfaction, higher perception of stress, and more negative emotions, whereas higher avoidant attachment was associated with more negative emotions (Ben Shlomo et al., 2019; Skvirsky, Taubman – Ben-Ari, Ben Shlomo, Azuri, & Horowitz, 2019); higher perception of meaning in life was related to lower levels of perceived stress (Skvirsky et al., 2019); higher levels of self-mastery (the extent that an individual feels control over their life) were related to lower perception of stress (Ben Shlomo, Pascal, Taubman – Ben-Ari, Azuri, & Horowitz, 2017); and higher levels of self-mastery and lower levels of stress were associated with greater life satisfaction (Ben Shlomo, Pascal, et al., 2017).

Interpersonal resources have also been shown to play a role in coping with fertility issues. Numerous studies have revealed the significance of the couple relationship (Greil et al., 2010; see also Peterson & Place, Chap. 2 in this volume), while others indicate the importance of family support (High & Steuber, 2014; Vasaard, Lund, Pinborg, Boivin, & Schmidt, 2012). This suggests another potential interpersonal resource, the perceived support a woman receives from her mother, a unique figure in her life, and the quality of the relationship between the two women (Bojczyk, Lehan, McWey, Melson, & Kaufman, 2011).

> Dear Mom…it hurts, my whole body hurts…Mom, my heart and soul hurt…The doctor keeps giving me another invasive examination, another shot I'm no longer afraid of. It's become routine…My stomach hurts from all the needles stuck into it and the serum shot into it raising a glimmer of hope that maybe this month will be my month. Mom, I'm scared it won't work.

> It hurts me to see you cry off on the side and try to encourage me with words that just infuriate me, that hurt me and put pressure on me and make me feel guilty and feel that I'm unworthy in my own eyes and in yours.
>
> Dear beloved Mom, I know you want the best for me and that you simply don't know how to cope, how to help and support me in this process I'm going through…I don't always know how to cope with my infertility either…But what I do know for certain is that I need you, Mom. I need your sensitivity, your pampering, your understanding and acceptance…[I need you to] respect me and understand…and most of all – don't tell me to relax. Mom, I need you so much. Just be there for me, soft and embracing…hug me like you used to. (www.medabrotimahut.co.il/2011/01/)

Despite its importance, the mother-daughter relationship has received very little attention in infertility research. The few studies conducted in the context of infertility indicate the importance of this relationship at the beginning of treatment. Thus, women's self-disclosure to the mother was related to lower levels of perceived stress (Skvirsky et al., 2019); higher perceived mother's support in the form of active engagement (including the woman in discussions of her condition, taking an interest in her feelings, and displaying behaviors that support problem-solving; Buunk, Berkhuysen, Sanderman, Nieuwland, & Ranchor, 1996; Coyne & Smith, 1994) has been linked to women's greater well-being and lower distress; higher mothers' overprotection was associated with greater psychological distress (Skvirsky, Taubman – Ben-Ari, Ben Shlomo, Azuri, & Horowitz, 2018); and a more supportive, close, and warm relationship with the mother was associated with higher positive emotions (Ben Shlomo et al., 2019).

One highly significant variable that cannot be ignored in any discussion of infertility is the woman's age at the start of fertility treatment. From the medical standpoint, there is a decrease in fertility and ovarian functioning and an increase in the length of time required to conceive among women in their mid-30 s, with 35 considered the cut-off point at which the decline in fertility becomes sharper (Liu et al., 2012). It is rather surprising, therefore, that research appears to indicate an association between older age and better mental health. Psychological distress has been shown to be higher among younger women (Souter et al., 2002), and an examination of women 11–17 years after fertility treatment indicated that those who were older at the time of their first consultation reported better mental health at the time of the study (Gameiro et al., 2014). In recent studies conducted in Israel, younger women (below the age of 35) also reported more psychological distress and negative affect at the beginning of fertility treatment than older women (Ben Shlomo et al., 2019; Ben Shlomo, Skvirsky et al., 2017), and women's younger age also contributed to higher perceived stress (Skvirsky et al., 2019). Moreover, these studies show that internal resources mediate between age and mental health. Thus, older women were found to display less of a tendency for rumination, which, in turn, was associated with better mental health, and also reported more hope, which, in turn, was associated with higher well-being (Ben Shlomo, Skvirsky et al., 2017). In addition, a moderation effect was found for mothers' support, indicating that younger women are more dependent on suitable mother's support to enhance their mental health than women aged 35 and over (Skvirsky et al., 2018). These findings suggest that age brings with it greater maturity, in the form of more secure personal resources and less dependence on environmental support. Perhaps more importantly, they show that age plays a role not only in a woman's physiological ability to conceive, but also in her psychological well-being, and that the two roles are not necessarily parallel. Moreover, there appear to be gender differences in respect to the link between age and mental health, although specific findings in this regard are inconsistent. For example, one study found that infertility-related stress was significantly higher in women, regardless of age, than in men (Casu & Gremigni, 2016), while another indicated that men, but not women, showed an increased risk of experiencing non-somatic signs of depression with increasing age (Valoriani et al., 2016).

Other background variables that have been examined in respect to mental health at the start of fertility treatment have not produced significant results. No significant associations were found, for instance, between psychological distress and duration of infertility, the presence of existing children, or the cause of infertility (Souter et al., 2002). Similarly, no significant relations were found between the cause or type of infertility (primary, i.e., no previous pregnancy or secondary, i.e., previous pregnancies regardless of outcomes) and psychological and physical well-being (Valoriani et al., 2016), or perceived stress (Skvirsky et al., 2019), at the time of the first ART consultation. However, when looking deeper into the type of infertility, it was found that women with secondary infertility without children were less satisfied with life than both women with secondary infertility with children and women with primary infertility (Ben Shlomo et al., 2019). However, the fact that at this point, individuals without a history of infertility may still be unaware of the origins of their problem may explain some of these results.

3.3 Fertility Treatment: Between Hope and Frustration

> During the treatments I try very hard not to brood over the negative and be optimistic and strong. It's important to me that when I look back on it I'll feel that along with the difficulty, it was also a good experience. That I learned and developed and the treatments helped me to find my strong points and accentuate them. On the whole, I've succeeded, and I'm still succeeding, in seeing the good that derives from this period. And yet, you can't ignore the difficulty, the pain. (http://www.retters.co.il)

A substantial body of literature relates to the implications of the fertility treatment that follows the initial consultation and diagnosis. On the whole, research indicates that fertility treatment is associated with elevated levels of distress (see also Peterson & Place, Chap. 2 in this volume). A longitudinal study conducted in the U.S. (Greil, McQuillan, Lowry, & Shreffler, 2011), for example, reported that treatment caused women fertility-specific distress over and above that aroused by infertility itself. Similarly, a review of gender differences in emotional reactions to IVF (in vitro fertilization) concluded that women displayed elevated anxiety and depression levels prior to each treatment, which became even higher on the day of the treatment and during the waiting period before the pregnancy test. On the other hand, men only reported feeling a higher level of depression before the pregnancy test, with anxiety levels being generally stable throughout the treatment cycle (Ying, Wu, & Loke, 2016).

In light of the emotional burden that accompanies infertility and its treatment, below we consider the effect on successful outcomes of ART. In other words, we ask whether a history of treatment affects couples during the subsequent periods of pregnancy and parenthood.

3.4 Pregnancy Following Fertility Treatment: The Next Step in the Journey to Parenthood

Pregnancy is the hoped-for outcome of fertility treatment and the natural stage before becoming a parent. While couples may now enjoy the relief and satisfaction that come after the stressful period of treatments, they may also feel the mixed emotions characteristic of pregnancy in general, including anxiety, distress, and depression. Qualitative studies in the general population highlight feelings of uncertainty and vulnerability: fear of losing the baby; the lack of control or pain involved in labor; concerns about the relationship with the partner; and feelings of isolation, whether due to the sense that the pregnancy does not meet expectations or difficulty in sharing anxieties (Evans, Morrell, & Spiby, 2017; Rowe, & Fisher, 2015; Staneva, Bogossian, & Wittkowski, 2015). Pregnant women report higher levels of depression than their male partners, with maternal depression being a risk factor for the development of depressive symptoms in fathers and vise versa (Arnal-Remón, Moreno-Rosset, Ramírez-Uclés, & Antequera-Jurado, 2015; Sundström Poromaa, Comasco, Georgakis, & Skalkidou, 2017).

If pregnancy itself is such a complex emotional period, conceiving after experiencing infertility complications might be expected to accentuate the emotional upheaval. We might assume that given the effort it took, the pregnancy will be even more gratifying and joyful. Indeed, a study conducted in Israel shows that women who conceived by IVF experienced lower negative affect and more positive mood regarding self, baby, and spouse during pregnancy than did women who conceived naturally. Moreover, women who had undergone two to three IVF cycles had lower negative affect scores than women who had conceived after the first treatment cycle, and mood regarding spouse depended on whether or not he had been the sole source of the couple's infertility (Harf-Kashdaei, & Kaitz, 2007).

However, the opposite might also be true: the pregnancy may be experienced as especially stressful due to the anxieties and frustrations born in the treatment process. The results of a qualitative Italian study seem to confirm this possibility. Couples pregnant with their first child via ART were asked to tell their pregnancy story from the very first attempts to conceive, when they still believed they were fertile, through the diagnosis of infertility and treatment, and to the pregnancy itself (Smorti & Smorti, 2013). The authors identified four consecutive themes in the narratives of the infertility and pregnancy experiences: the first one is "doubt", when together with the desire for a child, the first doubts and worries arise, due to the failure to conceive spontaneously. The second: "final sentence" relates to the diagnostic evaluation and receiving the harsh news about infertility: "the sentence constitutes a break in their life and it is experienced like a crash into a terrible truth which is very difficult to accept" (p. 170). Acknowledging the news concerning infertility means for the couples that from now on, they will have to use fertility treatments to achieve pregnancy. The next phase comprises of struggle and victory, which includes a struggle characterized by self-blame, a sense of responsibility and the desire for control during the treatments. When the pregnancy is finally achieved, couples report feeling the nightmare is over and the dream is beginning, and experience a feeling that they have won a struggle that has been achieved together. However, this is followed by a final phase, the "monitoring" of the pregnancy, which is characterized by worries, fear, and stress for women, whereas men tend to heave a sigh of relief with the conception, and then respond to the pregnancy as they would to a "normal" one.

In another qualitative study conducted in England among pregnant primiparous women and their male partners who had conceived with the help of fertility treatment (French, Sharp, & Turner, 2015), all the participants described the treatment as emotionally, physically, and mentally demanding, even when pregnancy had already been achieved. As for the pregnancy itself, many of the themes in the prospective parents' narratives dealt with anxiety, including fear of losing the baby, with both women and men describing the effort to avoid focusing too much on birth and parenthood for fear of "jinxing" it. The participants, and especially the women, expressed difficulty adjusting to pregnancy and planning for parenthood, including a sense of numbness and low mood in the early weeks. Moreover, the authors identified a "self-silencing" theme, whereby many women who felt low or ambivalent in the wake of the pregnancy had trouble expressing these feelings to others for fear of appearing ungrateful for the fact that they were finally pregnant. Some men were unable to express their feelings to friends and family who had conceived naturally because they felt different. Moreover, a quantitative Portuguese study (Gameiro, Moura-Ramos, Canavarro, & Soares, 2010) found that in the 24th week of pregnancy, primiparous women and their partners who conceived through ART perceived the pregnancy to be more demanding and riskier, but also more rewarding, than counterparts who conceived spontaneously. All these findings paint a picture of pregnancy after fertility treatment as a unique and complex experience for both women and men.

A systematic review (Hammarberg, Fisher, & Wynter, 2008) found consistent evidence that marital satisfaction, emotional well-being, and self-regard during pregnancy are similar in ART groups and comparison groups, although anxiety about the survival of the fetus appears to be higher. The finding of greater pregnancy-specific anxiety after treatment has been corroborated in a number of recent studies (McMahon et al., 2013; Stevenson, Trotter, Bergh, & Sloane, 2016), as well as in a review (Gourounti, 2016). On the other hand, it has been found that women after ART display lower state and trait anxiety (McMahon et al., 2013), or the same level of general anxiety (Joelsson et al., 2017), compared to counterparts who conceived spontaneously. Gourounti (2016), however, concludes that findings concerning general anxiety levels during pregnancy after ART are inconclusive. The qualitative part of a mixed method study among women who conceived via IVF (Stevenson et al., 2016) may help explain these inconsistencies as it indicates the complex nature of anxiety. Here, three themes emerged regarding pregnancy-related anxiety. The most common was anxiety over the health of the fetus, followed by worries about the woman's own health and safety, and concerns regarding her ability to perform the role of mother (as a first-time mother or due to multiple gestation).

Findings regarding depression are also inconclusive. Some studies indicate that women who conceive after IVF have either the same (e.g., Gambadauro, Iliadis, Bränn, & Skalkidou, 2017; Joelsson et al., 2017; Monti et al., 2015) or less (e.g., McMahon et al., 2013), depressive symptomatology than women who conceive naturally, a conclusion also reached in Gourounti's (2016) review. However, an Italian study (Monti, Agostini, Fagandini, La Sala, & Blickstein, 2009) reported that women who became pregnant via ART exhibited higher depression than women who conceived naturally.

Research has also examined the connection between ART and quality of life. Gourounti (2016) concludes that women who conceived with the help of IVF display poorer quality of life than those who conceived naturally. For example, findings obtained in Canada (Vinturache et al., 2015) and Italy (De Pascalis et al., 2012) show that women who conceived via fertility treatment report poorer physical health during pregnancy than women who conceived spontaneously. The Italian study also indicates that women scored lower on most dimensions of quality of life than men, regardless of the method of conception, and that ART couples had lower social quality of life and showed a decrease in this dimension from the second to the third trimester that was not observed among non-ART couples (De Pascalis et al., 2012).

A recent review concludes that no major detrimental emotional impact on pregnancy has been found following fertility treatment (Galst, 2018). This suggests that when IVF results in pregnancy, the negative emotions vanish, that is, that treatment-induced stress is related primarily to the threat of failure (Verhaak et al., 2007). But this may not be the whole picture. The following conclusion drawn from a qualitative study (Dornelles, MacCallum, Lopes, Piccinini, & Passos, 2016) may more accurately describe women's experience of pregnancy resulting from ART. The authors state: "The experience of pregnancy following ART is interwoven with mixed feelings, such as happiness, a sense of triumph, but also regret and fears. Having infertility and its treatment as a background gives pregnancy a different start which may affect the way it is experienced" (p. 126).

Moreover, in accordance with the findings for age at the start of fertility treatment, older maternal age of women following ART or a spontaneous pregnancy has been associated with lower depression and anxiety symptoms, lower maternal-fetal attachment, as well as greater resilience, during the third trimester of pregnancy (McMahon, Boivin, Gibson, Hammarberg et al., 2011). Nevertheless, the researchers contend that personality and context factors (such as the quality of the relationship with the intimate partner) are more important than age or mode of conception in predicting pregnancy mood (depression and anxiety symptoms) and pregnancy-specific adjustment. In other words, with ART conception setting the stage for a more complex experience of pregnancy, women conceiving through ART simultaneously experience more pregnancy-related anxiety and more intense feelings of attachment to the growing fetus (McMahon, Boivin, Gibson, Hammemberg et al., 2011).

3.5 The End of the Road: Early Parenthood Following Fertility Treatment

> I always have the feeling that motherhood after fertility treatment is a very different kind of motherhood because suddenly something in the process of bringing children into the world can not at all be taken for granted. All of a sudden we go from making plans to being controlled by the reality of life, and what we thought would happen in a certain way doesn't always happen. And then the boy or girl arrives in the world and we find ourselves asking questions, overwhelmed by the emotion of all the things we have gone through and the difficulties we were forced to undergo.
>
> I feel that after I gave birth it took me a very long time to bond with Arbel. Suddenly I had a huge sense of freedom, that I could live again after 4 and a half hard years. I learned that everyone feels different, but from what I've heard and seen from women about motherhood after treatment, they have either a very strong attachment or a very strong estrangement. I felt estranged. (http://www.retters.co.il)

Pregnancy follows immediately on the heels of the experience of fertility treatment. But what about parenthood? Do all the difficulties and negative emotions aroused by the attempt to become parents fade away as soon as the desired goal is achieved, or do they persist and affect parenthood as well?

Two recent qualitative studies, one in the U.S. and the other in Iran, address this issue. Both examined the experience of first-time mothers who conceived after fertility treatment. In the American study (Ladores & Aroian, 2015), mothers referred to the impact of infertility identity over time, which the authors term "lingering identity as infertile." This theme included topics such as anxiety during pregnancy, perceiving motherhood as surreal, and feeling unprepared for the role of mother. A second theme was gratitude for the gift of motherhood, an attitude that caused the women to place unrealistic expectations on themselves, resulting in feelings of guilt and shame when they were unable to tackle their new role with ease and grace. Consequently, they felt they had to keep silent and were incapable of disclosing their negative thoughts and emotions. Similarly, in the Iranian study (Mohammadi et al., 2015), the main theme that emerged was "super-mothering." The authors explain that most of the participants gave birth after a long wait and considerable emotional investment, anxiety, and difficulty. These experiences led them to aspire to be super-mothers, expressed in four sub-themes: over-care, over-protection, over-emotional investment, and over-expectations of themselves and others. The findings of these studies support Hammarberg et al.'s (2008) conclusion that following ART, parenthood might be idealized, hindering adjustment and the development of a confident parental identity.

Although qualitative studies point to the unique challenges of motherhood following ART, quantitative studies indicate more similarities than differences. A recent systematic review and meta-analysis found no increased risk for significant postpartum depressive symptoms after medically assisted conception, and no significant difference in such symptoms between women who used medically assisted conception and those with a spontaneous pregnancy (Gressier et al., 2015). The results of even more recent studies support these findings, indicating that conception by means of IVF is not associated with maternal depressive symptoms postpartum (Gambadauro et al., 2017), and that mothers who receive IVF treatment are not at increased risk of postnatal depression (Vikström, Sydsjö, Hammar, Bladh, & Josefsson, 2017) or postpartum psychosis (Vikström, Josefsson, Hammar, Bladh, & Sydsjö, 2017).

However, contradictory findings have also been reported. It was found that only women who had undergone previous ART treatments (before their current pregnancy) showed a substantial increase in depression scores at 15 days postpartum, compared to their scores during pregnancy, whereas women with no previous ART attempts exhibited no similar change (Monti et al., 2015). On the other hand, a cross-sectional study conducted in the Netherlands indicated that a higher number of treatment cycles was associated with lower risk for mother's decline in mental health (Jongbloed-Pereboom et al., 2012).

Interestingly, in a qualitative Australian study of men who became fathers after IVF, the majority of participants reported that the difficulties associated with fertility and conception did not impact their experience of parenthood. Rather, they indicated that once the pregnancy had been achieved and the child was born, fertility issues had no further relevance (Bracks-Zalloua, McMahon, & Gibson, 2011). These findings echo Smorti and Smorti's (2013) claim that after the conception, men respond as they would to a "normal" pregnancy. In addition, a quantitative study found no difference in life satisfaction between new first-time fathers by mode of conception (Taubman – Ben-Ari, Skvirsky, Bar Shua, & Horowitz, 2017). Thus, there appear to be gender differences in the experience of parenthood following fertility treatment.

As noted above, age plays a crucial role in women's physiological ability to conceive (Liu et al., 2012). According to an Australian study (McMahon, Boivin, Gibson, Fisher et al., 2011), older age also increases the likelihood of cesarean section, prior miscarriages, and terminations at an older gestational age. Nonetheless, no indication of increased prevalence of postpartum depression has been found in older first time mothers, nor in first time mothers conceiving through ART irrespective of age (McMahon, Boibin, Gibson, Fisher et al., 2011). Nor did age play a role in adjustment to parenthood (psychological, relationship, and parenting stress) among first time parents conceiving through IVF (Bracks-Zalloua, Gibson, & McMahon, 2010).

The literature also points to other factors that may impact the postpartum mental health of both parents, such as singleton versus twin/multiple birth. Interestingly, it was found that twin/multiple parenthood, but not ART, negatively affected the mental health (depression, stress, anxiety) of new mothers and fathers (van den Akker, Postavaru, & Purewal, 2016; Vilska et al., 2009). In contrast, results of another study indicate that parents of twins conceived after infertility treatments showed higher anxiety at mid-pregnancy, as well as higher anxiety and depression at 3 months post-partum than parents of singletons also conceived after treatments (Tendais & Figueiredo, 2016).

Studies of adjustment to parenthood have also examined other domains, including quality of marital relations (Gameiro et al., 2010; Taubman – Ben-Ari et al., 2017) and parenting stress (Flykt et al., 2011; Gameiro et al., 2010; Taubman – Ben-Ari, Skvirsky, Bar Shua, & Horowitz, 2018), neither of which was found to differ between parents conceiving through ART or spontaneously. However, a gender difference was found, with Portuguese fathers, but not mothers, who conceived through ART perceiving themselves to be more competent than fathers who conceived spontaneously (Gameiro et al., 2010).

In addition, there is a growing trend in recent years to explore the potential positive or beneficial outcomes of stressful situations, and particularly the possibility of experiencing personal growth. In this vein, a number of Israeli studies have examined the personal growth of new mothers and fathers in the transition to parenthood (see also Taubman – Ben-Ari, Chap. 16 in this volume). Interestingly enough, despite the stressful path taken by those forced to undergo fertility treatment, the mode of conception was not found to contribute to personal growth (Noy, Taubman – Ben-Ari, & Kuint, 2015; Spielman, & Taubman – Ben-Ari, 2009; Taubman – Ben-Ari et al., 2018; Taubman – Ben-Ari, & Spielman, 2014).

3.6 A Long Journey

We have sought here to paint the complex picture of the experience of infertility that emerges from the empirical literature, adopting a developmental perspective. We have examined the different phases in the journey to parenthood, from early attempts to conceive through the period after the birth of a child. Though quite rare, longitudinal studies from pregnancy to parenthood shed light on the complexity of the experience and provide a more in-depth understanding of the process, the context, and the connections between variables over time. One trend that has been identified, for example, is that whereas couples who have undergone fertility treatment may perceive the ultimate pregnancy as more threatening and risky than couples conceiving spontaneously, no differences are found in respect to their response to parenthood. Moreover, a longitudinal design showed that only ART parents reported a decrease in psychological quality of life over time (Gameiro et al., 2010). Other studies portray pregnancy as a period in which women following ART feel better psychologically than those who conceived spontaneously, although once again, differences disappear when embarking on parenthood (Vinturache et al., 2015).

Recent studies go beyond the traditional approach of longitudinal designs, using trajectory analysis to identify changes in variables over time. For example, a study conducted in Portugal (Tendais & Figueiredo, 2016) examined the effects of mode of conception, type of pregnancy, and parent gender on anxiety and depression levels at each trimester of pregnancy, childbirth, and 3 months postpartum, as well as the effects of these factors on the trajectories of anxiety and depressive symptoms over time. The findings reveal differences between parents in the two conception groups, with those after fertility treatment displaying an increase in anxiety scores from pregnancy to postpartum, whereas no such change was found for parents conceiving spontaneously. Furthermore, the depression scores of women in the fertility treatment group increased over time, whereas those of women conceiving spontaneously decreased.

Another study that used trajectory analysis was conducted in Finland among first-time fathers (Vänskä et al., 2017), and aimed to identify their latent mental health trajectory classes from the pre- to postnatal period and their associations with early fathering experiences (i.e., parenting stress). The study reveals similar trajectory classes among fathers conceiving naturally and through ART, and these classes predicted similar fathering experiences in both groups in respect to early dyadic interaction and infant characteristics, although ART fathers reported a more negative experience in the parenting domain (resources and limitations one posits as a parent).

3.7 The Complexity of the Big Picture

> Yesterday I met with a friend who has begun treatment. She's at the very beginning, still doing the investigations and tests to determine where the problem is. The question that keeps nagging at her is: "Why is this happening to me?" I also asked myself the same question at the beginning of the road. We all do, don't we? There's no answer, and as time passes I understand that, unfortunately, each of us has a different difficulty to bear in life. Some have financial difficulties, some have difficulties with love. I have a difficulty with children. That's my difficulty and I've learned to accept it without asking questions. I've learned to accept it and try to make the best, sweetest lemonade possible from my lemon. Because at the end of the day it doesn't matter what obstacle we have to overcome. What matters is how we cope with it. (http://www.retters.co.il)

Becoming a parent after experiencing infertility differs from the normative path to parenthood, and thus demands special attention. In our attempt to describe the unique nature of this journey, we have not sought to systematically review all the existing literature on the topic, but rather to clarify just how complex the big picture is.

As we have seen, acknowledging infertility and its consequences is an intense and taxing experience from the very beginning. It is followed by the treatments themselves, which take a toll on both the individual and the couple level. A pregnancy achieved by ART similarly has unique aspects, and may be experienced as stressful and accompanied by anxiety and depression, but also as more rewarding. Once the child is born, although mothers who conceived via ART describe how infertility affected their perceptions and feelings in qualitative studies, most quantitative studies show no differences in the mental health or life satisfaction of parents by mode of conception.

Although considerable effort has been invested in exploring different aspects of the experience of infertility, the developmental outlook appears to be the approach most missing from the literature, with a small number of highly informative exceptions. The few longitudinal studies using trajectory analysis from pregnancy to postpartum provide deeper understanding of the complexity in the transition to parenthood. More research of this sort could also help us gain a better understanding of the dynamics which explain the balance that may already be achieved with pregnancy and appears to be typical of parenthood. Moreover, since the process leaves its mark even years after treatment (Ying et al., 2016), future studies might examine its consequences, both negative or positive, in the longer term as well.

This chapter sheds light on the importance of the initial infertility consultation. As the beginning of treatment was also found to be associated with the crucial decision of whether or not to pursue treatment, it is vital to relate to distress at this point in time. In respect to the periods of pregnancy and parenthood, research has focused particularly on the experiences and mental states of women. The findings regarding gender differences raise interesting questions for further studies, and highlight the importance of engaging both men and women in future research in order to gain a fuller picture of the experience of infertility. Dyadic studies would also provide insight into the dynamics between the couple and the interrelations between their coping strategies. In addition, the perspective of the extended family (parents, grandparents, siblings), not to mention the social surroundings such as friends and colleagues, has rarely been taken into consideration. These individuals, too, may be experiencing difficulties at second-hand, and may develop fears and worries being helpless figures in this experience. Expanding our knowledge of the social network would deepen our understanding of both the context in which the couple functions and the unique experience of these additional agents in their life.

> Today (two and a half years after I gave birth), whenever I go to a wedding and dance the night away, I feel a small sense of victory in my heart. Anyone who knows me knows I've always liked to party. I've always liked to dance and do crazy things. Then the treatments started. And I come home and there's a friend's wedding and I don't know – Maybe I'm pregnant? Maybe not? During that time I felt that my mind was always focused on me. I'm careful not to drink. Not to eat sushi or raw fish. Not to dance too much so I don't accidentally get elbowed. Not to jump around too much because it might not be good for my uterus. Not to let anyone pick me up so they don't accidentally drop me. Not to get shoved. I'm always being careful.
>
> And then I go to the bathroom and the bleeding starts…and at those times I feel a little cheated. I did everything - everything!! – to make sure it worked, and now again it didn't happen.
>
> And what about the next time? I'll be careful again. Maybe that's what brought the bad luck?
>
> So many thoughts. So many decisions around the simplest question in the world – to dance at a wedding or not?
>
> It's like even when you're happy, no one knows what's really going on inside. No one imagines the fears and anxiety. Because being a fertility patient is forever. It's every moment and every minute. Not just when they're extracting eggs or injecting them. (http://www.retters.co.il)

References

Arnal-Remón, B., Moreno-Rosset, C., Ramírez-Uclés, I., & Antequera-Jurado, R. (2015). Assessing depression, anxiety and couple psychological well-being in pregnancy: A preliminary study. *Journal of Reproductive and Infant Psychology, 33*(2), 128–139.

Arya, S. T., & Dibb, B. (2016). The experience of infertility treatment: The male perspective. *Human Fertility, 19*(4), 242–248.

Ben Shlomo, S., Pascal, M., Taubman – Ben-Ari, O., Azuri, Y., & Horowitz, E. (2017). Life satisfaction of women in early stages of fertility treatment. *Women & Health, 57*(5), 566–582.

Ben Shlomo, S., Skvirsky, V., Taubman – Ben-Ari, O., Azuri, Y., & Horowitz, E. (2017). Mental health of women entering fertility treatment: What role do age and internal resources play? *Stress & Health, 33*(4), 470–476.

Ben Shlomo, S., Taubman – Ben-Ari, O., Skvirsky, V., Azuri, J., Weissman, A., & Horowitz, E. (2019). Subjective well-being of women at the beginning of fertility treatment. *Journal of Reproductive and Infant Psychology.*

Benyamini, Y., Gozlan, M., & Kokia, E. (2005). Variability in the difficulties experienced by women undergoing infertility treatments. *Fertility and Sterility, 83*(2), 275–283.

Berger, R., Paul, M. S., & Henshaw, L. A. (2013). Women's experience of infertility: A multi-systemic perspective. *Journal of International Women's Studies, 14*(1), 54–68.

Boivin, J., Bunting, L., Collins, J. A., & Nygren, K. G. (2007). International estimates of infertility prevalence and treatment-seeking: Potential need and demand for infertility medical care. *Human Reproduction, 22*(6), 1506–1512.

Bojczyk, K. E., Lehan, T. J., McWey, L. M., Melson, G. F., & Kaufman, D. R. (2011). Mothers' and their adult daughters' perceptions of their relationship. *Journal of Family Issues, 32*(4), 452–481.

Bracks-Zalloua, P., Gibson, F., & McMahon, C. (2010). Age and gender differences in relationship and psychological adjustment to parenthood in couples conceiving through In-Vitro Fertilisation (IVF). *The Educational and Developmental Psychologist, 27*(2), 90–103.

Bracks-Zalloua, P., McMahon, C., & Gibson, F. (2011). IVF-conceiving fathers' experiences of early parenthood. *Journal of Relationships Research, 2,* 1–9.

Brandes, M., van der Steen, J. O. M., Bokdam, S. B., Hamilton, C. J. C. M., de Bruin, J. P., Nelen, W. L. D. M., & Kremer, J. A. M. (2009). When and why do subfertile couples discontinue their fertility care? A longitudinal cohort study in a secondary care subfertility population. *Human Reproduction, 24*(12), 3127–3135.

Buunk, A. P., Berkhuysen, M. A., Sanderman, R., Nieuwland, W., & Ranchor, A. V. (1996). *Actieve betrokkenheid, beschermend bufferen en overbescherming. Meetinstrument voor de rol van de partner bij hartrevalidatie.* [Active engagement, protective buffering, and overprotection. Assessment of the spouse's role in heart revalidation.] *Gedrag & Gezondheid, 24,* 304–313.

Casu, G., & Gremigni, P. (2016). Screening for infertility-related stress at the time of initial infertility consultation: Psychometric properties of a brief measure. *Journal of Advanced Nursing, 72*(3), 693–706.

Childress, K. J., Lawson, A. K., Ghant, M. S., Mendoza, G., Cardozo, E. R., Confino, E., & Marsh, E. E. (2015). First contact: The intersection of demographics, knowledge, and appraisal of treatment at the initial infertility visit. *Fertility and Sterility, 104*(1), 180–187.

Coyne, J. C., & Smith, D. A. F. (1994). Couples coping with a myocardial infarction: Contextual perspective on patient self-efficacy. *Journal of Family Psychology, 8*(1), 43–54.

De Pascalis, L., Agostini, F., Monti, F., Paterlini, M., Fagandini, P., & La Sala, G. B. (2012). A comparison of quality of life following spontaneous conception and assisted reproduction. *International Journal of Gynecology and Obstetrics, 118*(3), 216–219.

Domar, A., & Gross, J. (2012). Stress and ART. In E. S. Ginsburg & C. Racowsky (Eds.), *In vitro fertilization: A comprehensive guide* (pp. 201–209). New York: Springer.

Dornelles, L. M. N., MacCallum, F., Lopes, R. C. S., Piccinini, C. A., & Passos, E. P. (2016). The experience of pregnancy resulting from Assisted Reproductive Technology (ART) treatment: A qualitative Brazilian study. *Women and Birth, 29*(2), 123–127.

Edelmann, R. J., & Connolly, K. J. (2000). Gender differences in response to infertility and infertility investigations: Real or illusory. *British Journal of Health Psychology, 5*(4), 365–375.

Eisenberg, M. L., Smith, J. F., Millstein, S. G., Nachtigall, R. D., Adler, N. E., Pasch, L. A., & Katz, P. P. (2010). Predictors of not pursuing infertility treatment after an infertility diagnosis: Examination of a prospective U.S. cohort. *Fertility and Sterility, 94*(6), 2369–2371.

Erikson, E. H. (1963). *Childhood and society* (2nd ed.). New York: Norton.

Evans, K., Morrell, C. J., & Spiby, H. (2017). Women's views on anxiety in pregnancy and the use of anxiety instruments: A qualitative study. *Journal of Reproductive and Infant Psychology, 35*(1), 77–90.

Fassino, S., Piero, A., Boggio, S., Piccioni, V., & Garzaro, L. (2002). Anxiety, depression and anger suppression in infertile couples: A controlled study. *Human Reproduction, 17*(11), 2986–2994.

Flykt, M., Lindblom, J., Punamäki, R.-L., Poikkeus, P., Repokari, L., Unkila-Kallio, L., … Tulppala, M. (2011). Prenatal expectations in transition to parenthood: Former infertility and family dynamic considerations. *Couple and Family Psychology: Research and Practice, 1*(S), 31–44.

French, L. R. M., Sharp, D. J., & Turner, K. M. (2015). Antenatal needs of couples following fertility treatment: A qualitative study in primary care. *British Journal of General Practice, 65*(638), e570–e577.

Galst, J. P. (2018). The elusive connection between stress and infertility: A research review with clinical implications. *Journal of Psychotherapy Integration, 28*(1), 1–13.

Gambadauro, P., Iliadis, S., Bränn, E., & Skalkidou, A. (2017). Conception by means of in vitro fertilization is not associated with maternal depressive symptoms during pregnancy or postpartum. *Fertility and Sterility, 108*(2), 325–332.

Gameiro, S., Boivin, J., Peronace, L., & Verhaak, C. M. (2012). Why do patients discontinue fertility treatment? A systematic review of reasons and predictors of discontinuation in fertility treatment. *Human Reproduction Update, 18*(6), 652–669.

Gameiro, S., Moura-Ramos, M., Canavarro, M. C., & Soares, I. (2010). Psychosocial adjustment during the transition to parenthood of Portuguese couples who conceived spontaneously or through assisted reproductive technologies. *Research in Nursing & Health, 33*(3), 207–220.

Gameiro, S., van den Belt-Dusebout, A. W., Bleiker, E., Braat, D., van Leeuwen, F. E., & Verhaak, C. M. (2014). Do children make you happier? Sustained child-wish and mental health in women 11–17 years after fertility treatment. *Human Reproduction, 29*(10), 2238–2246.

Gourounti, K. (2016). Psychological stress and adjustment in pregnancy following assisted reproductive technology and spontaneous conception: A systematic review. *Women and Health, 56*(1), 98–118.

Greil, A. L., McQuillan, J., Lowry, M., & Shreffler, K. M. (2011). Infertility treatment and fertility-specific distress: A longitudinal analysis of a population-based sample of U.S. women. *Social Science & Medicine, 73*(1), 87–94.

Greil, A. L., Schmidt, L., & Peterson, B. (2014). Understanding and treating the psychosocial consequences of infertility. In A. Wenzel (Ed.), *The Oxford handbook of perinatal psychology*. Oxford, UK: Oxford University Press.

Greil, A. L., Slauson-Blevins, K., & McQuillan, J. (2010). The experience of infertility: A review of recent literature. *Sociology of Health & Illness, 32*(1), 140–162.

Gressier, F., Letranchant, A., Cazas, O., Sutter-Dallay, A. L., Falissard, B., & Hardy, P. (2015). Post-partum depressive symptoms and medically assisted conception: A systematic review and meta-analysis. *Human Reproduction, 30*(11), 2575–2586.

Hammarberg, K., Fisher, J. R., & Wynter, K. H. (2008). Psychological and social aspects of pregnancy, childbirth and early parenting after assisted conception: A systematic review. *Human Reproduction Update, 14*(5), 395–414.

Harf-Kashdaei, E., & Kaitz, M. (2007). Antenatal moods regarding self, baby, and spouse among women who conceived by in vitro fertilization. *Fertility and Sterility, 87*(6), 1306–1313.

High, A. C., & Steuber, K. R. (2014). An examination of support (in)adequacy: Types, sources, and consequences of social support among infertile women. *Communication Monographs, 81*(2), 157–178.

Joelsson, L. S., Tydén, T., Wanggren, K., Georgakis, M. K., Stern, J., Berglund, A., & Skalkidou, A. (2017). Anxiety and depression symptoms among sub-fertile women, women pregnant after infertility treatment, and naturally pregnant women. *European Psychiatry, 45*, 212–219.

Jongbloed-Pereboom, M., Middelburg, K. J., Heineman, M. J., Bos, A. F., Haadsma, M. L., & Hadders-Algra, M. (2012). The impact of IVF/ICSI on parental well-being and anxiety 1 year after childbirth. *Human Reproduction, 27*(8), 2389–2395.

Ladores, S., & Aroian, K. (2015). The early postpartum experience of previously infertile mothers. *Journal of Obstetric, Gynecologic, and Neonatal Nursing, 44*(3), 370–379.

Liu, K., Case, A., Cheung, A.P., Sierra, S., AlAsiri, S., Carranza-Mamane, B., … Wong, B.C. (2012). Advanced reproductive age and fertility. *International Journal of Gynecology and Obstetrics, 117*, 95–102.

Mascarenhas, M. N., Flaxman, S. R., Boerma, T., Vanderpoel, S., & Stevens, G. A. (2012). National, regional, and global trends in infertility prevalence since 1990: A systematic analysis of 277 Health Surveys. *PLOS Medicine, 9*(12), e1001356.

McMahon, C. A., Boivin, J., Gibson, F. L., Fisher, J., Hammarberg, K., Wynter, K., & Saunders, D. (2011). Older first-time mothers and early postpartum depression: A prospective cohort study of women conceiving spontaneously or with assisted reproductive technologies. *Fertility and Sterility, 96*(5), 1218–1224.

McMahon, C. A., Boivin, J., Gibson, F. L., Hammarberg, K., Wynter, K., Saunders, D., & Fisher, J. (2011). Age at first birth, mode of conception and psychological wellbeing in pregnancy: Findings from the parental age and transition to parenthood Australia (PATPA) study. *Human Reproduction, 26*(6), 1389–1398.

McMahon, C. A., Boivin, J., Gibson, F. L., Hammarberg, K., Wynter, K., Saunders, D., & Fisher, J. (2013). Pregnancy-specific anxiety, ART conception and infant temperament at 4 months postpartum. *Human Reproduction, 28*(4), 997–1005.

Mohammadi, N., Shamshiri, M., Mohammadpour, A., Vehviläinen-Julkunen, K., Abbasi, M., & Sadeghi, T. (2015). 'Super-mothers': The meaning of mothering after assisted reproductive technology. *Journal of Reproductive and Infant Psychology, 33*(1), 42–53.

Monti, F., Agostini, F., Fagandini, P., La Sala, G. B., & Blickstein, I. (2009). Depressive symptoms during late pregnancy and early parenthood following assisted reproductive technology. *Fertility and Sterility, 91*(3), 851–857.

Monti, F., Agostini, F., Paterlini, M., Andrei, F., De Pascalis, L., Palomba, S., & La Sala, G. B. (2015). Effects of assisted reproductive technology and of women's quality of life on depressive symptoms in the early postpartum period: A prospective case control study. *Gynecological Endocrinology, 31*(5), 374–378.

Moura-Ramos, M., Gameiro, S., Soares, I., Santos, T. A., & Canavarro, M. C. (2010). Psychosocial adjustment infertility: A comparison study of infertile couples, couples undergoing assisted reproductive technologies and presumed fertile couples. *Psicologia, Saúde & Doenças, 11*(2), 299–319.

Noy, A., Taubman – Ben-Ari, O., & Kuint, J. (2015). Well-being and personal growth in mothers of full-term and pre-term singletons and twins. *Stress & Health, 31*(5), 365–372.

Olafsdottir, H. S., Wikland, M., & Möller, A. (2012). Nordic couples' decision-making processes in anticipation of contacting a fertility clinic. *Journal of Reproductive and Infant Psychology, 30*(2), 180–192.

Practice Committee of the American Society for Reproductive Medicine. (2013). Definitions of infertility and recurrent pregnancy loss: A committee opinion. *Fertility and Sterility, 99*(1), 63.

Rooney, K. L., & Domar, A. D. (2016). The impact of stress on fertility treatment. *Current Opinion in Obstetrics and Gynecology, 28*(3), 198–201.

Rowe, H., & Fisher, J. (2015). Do contemporary social and health discourses arouse peripartum anxiety? A qualitative investigation of women's accounts. *Women's Studies International Forum, 51*, 56–65.

Skvirsky, V., Taubman – Ben-Ari, O., Ben Shlomo, S., Azuri, J., & Horowitz, E. (2019). Contributors to women's perceived stress at the start of assisted reproductive technology. *The Journal of Psychology; Interdisciplinary and Applied, 153*(1), 23–36.

Skvirsky, V., Taubman – Ben-Ari, O., Ben Shlomo, S., Azuri, J., & Horowitz, E. (2018). Are mothers a source of support for women entering fertility treatment? *Health Care for Women International, 39*(7), 719–733.

Smorti, M., & Smorti, A. (2013). Medical successes and couples' psychological problems in assisted reproduction treatment: A narrative based medicine approach. *The Journal of Maternal-Fetal & Neonatal Medicine, 26*(2), 169–172.

Snyder, C. R. (2002). Hope theory: Rainbows in the mind. *Psychological Inquiry, 13*(4), 249–275.

Souter, V. L., Hopton, J. L., Penney, G. C., & Templeton, A. A. (2002). Survey of psychological health in women with infertility. *Journal of Psychosomatic Obstetrics & Gynecology, 23*(1), 41–49.

Spielman, V., & Taubman – Ben-Ari, O. (2009). Parental self-efficacy and stress-related growth in the transition to parenthood: A comparison between parents of pre- and full-term babies. *Health and Social Work, 34*(3), 201–212.

Staneva, A. A., Bogossian, F., & Wittkowski, A. (2015). The experience of psychological distress, depression, and anxiety during pregnancy: A meta-synthesis of qualitative research. *Midwifery, 31*(6), 563–573.

Stevenson, E. L., Trotter, K. J., Bergh, C., & Sloane, R. (2016). Pregnancy-related anxiety in women who conceive via in vitro fertilization: A mixed methods approach. *The Journal of Perinatal Education, 25*(3), 193–200.

Sundström Poromaa, I., Comasco, E., Georgakis, M. K., & Skalkidou, A. (2017). Sex differences in depression during pregnancy and the postpartum period. *Journal of Neuroscience Research, 95*(1–2), 719–730.

Taubman – Ben-Ari, O., Skvirsky, V., Bar Shua, E., & Horowitz, E. (2017). Satisfaction in life among fathers following fertility treatment. *Journal of Reproductive and Infant Psychology, 35*(4), 334–341.

Taubman – Ben-Ari, O., Skvirsky, V., Bar Shua, E., & Horowitz, E. (2018). Personal growth of new fathers following assisted reproductive technology or spontaneous pregnancy. *Parenting: Science and Practice, 18*(3), 190–199.

Taubman – Ben-Ari, O., & Spielman, V. (2014). Personal growth following the first child's birth: A comparison of parents of pre- and full-term babies. *Social Work Research, 38*(2), 91–106.

Tendais, I., & Figueiredo, B. (2016). Parents' anxiety and depression symptoms after successful infertility treatment and spontaneous conception: Does singleton/twin pregnancy matter? *Human Reproduction, 31*(10), 2303–2312.

Trapnell, P. D., & Campbell, J. D. (1999). Private self-consciousness and the five-factor model of personality: Distinguishing rumination from reflection. *Journal of Personality and Social Psychology, 76*(2), 284–304.

Valoriani, V., Lotti, F., Lari, D., Miccinesi, G., Vaiani, S., Vanni, C., … Noci, I. (2016). Differences in psychophysical well-being and signs of depression in couples undergoing their first consultation for assisted reproduction technology (ART): An Italian pilot study. *European Journal of Obstetrics & Gynecology and Reproductive Biology, 197*, 179–185.

van den Akker, O., Postavaru, G. I., & Purewal, S. (2016). Maternal psychosocial consequences of twins and multiple births following assisted and natural conception: A meta-analysis. *Reproductive BioMedicine Online, 33*(1), 1–14.

Vänskä, M., Punamäki, R. L., Tolvanen, A., Lindblom, J., Flykt, M., Unkila-Kallio, L., … Tiitinen, A. (2017). Paternal mental health trajectory classes and early fathering experiences: Prospective study on a normative and formerly infertile sample. *International Journal of Behavioral Development, 41*(5), 570–580.

Vasaard, D., Lund, R., Pinborg, A., Boivin, J., & Schmidt, L. (2012). The impact of social relations among men and women in fertility treatment on the decision to terminate treatment. *Human Reproduction, 27*(12), 3502–3512.

Verhaak, C. M., Smeenk, J. M., Evers, A. W., Kremer, J. A., Kraaimaat, F. W., & Braat, D. D. (2007). Women's emotional adjustment to IVF: A systematic review of 25 years of research. *Human Reproduction Update, 13*(1), 27–36.
Vikström, J., Josefsson, A., Hammar, M., Bladh, M., & Sydsjö, G. (2017a). Risk of postpartum psychosis after IVF treatment: A nationwide case-control study. *Human Reproduction, 32*(1), 139–146.
Vikström, J., Sydsjö, G., Hammar, M., Bladh, M., & Josefsson, A. (2017b). Risk of postnatal depression or suicide after in vitro fertilisation treatment: A nationwide case–control study. *BJOG; An International Journal of Obstetrics & Gynaecology, 124*(3), 435–442.
Vilska, S., Unkila-Kallio, L., Punamäki, R.L., Poikkeus, P., Repokari, L., Sinkkonen, J., … Tulppala, M. (2009). Mental health of mothers and fathers of twins conceived via assisted reproduction treatment: A 1-year prospective study. *Human Reproduction, 24*(2), 367–377.
Vinturache, A., Stephenson, N., McDonald, S., Wu, M., Bayrampour, H., & Tough, S. (2015). Health-related quality of life in pregnancy and postpartum among women with assisted conception in Canada. *Fertility and Sterility, 104*(1), 188–195.e1.
Yaakobi, E., Mikulincer, M., & Shaver, P. R. (2014). Parenthood as a terror management mechanism: The moderating role of attachment orientations. *Personality and Social Psychology Bulletin, 40*(6), 762–774.
Ying, L. Y., Wu, L. H., & Loke, A. Y. (2015). Gender differences in experiences with and adjustments to infertility: A literature review. *International Journal of Nursing Studies, 52*(10), 1640–1652.
Ying, L., Wu, L. H., & Loke, A. Y. (2016). Gender differences in emotional reactions to in vitro fertilization treatment: A systematic review. *Journal of Assisted Reproduction and Genetics, 33*(2), 167–179.

Chapter 4
Fertility Problems and Fertility Care in Sub-Saharan Africa: The Case of Kenya

Henny M. W. Bos, Floor B. van Rooij, Tammary Esho, Wanjiru Ndegwa, Aida Bilajbegovic, Benjamin Kioko, Luca Koppen, S. Kemunto Migiro, Solomon Mwendah and Trudie Gerrits

H. M. W. Bos (✉) · F. B. van Rooij
Research Institute of Child Development and Education, University of Amsterdam, Amsterdam, The Netherlands
e-mail: h.m.w.bos@uva.nl

F. B. van Rooij
e-mail: f.b.vanrooij@uva.nl

T. Esho · B. Kioko · S. Kemunto Migiro · S. Mwendah
Department of Community and Public Health, Technical University of Kenya, Nairobi, Kenya
e-mail: etamarry@gmail.com

B. Kioko
e-mail: benjaminkioko81@gmail.com

S. Kemunto Migiro
e-mail: kmigiro@gmail.com

S. Mwendah
e-mail: mwenda.solomon11@gmail.com

W. Ndegwa
Footsteps for Fertility Foundation, Nairobi, Kenya
e-mail: wndegwa@gmail.com

A. Bilajbegovic · L. Koppen · T. Gerrits
Amsterdam Institute for Social Science Research,
University of Amsterdam, Amsterdam, The Netherlands
e-mail: aida.bilajbegovic@student.uva.nl

L. Koppen
e-mail: lucakoppen@gmail.com

T. Gerrits
e-mail: G.J.E.Gerrits@uva.nl

O. Taubman – Ben-Ari (ed.), *Pathways and Barriers to Parenthood*,
https://doi.org/10.1007/978-3-030-24864-2_4

4.1 Introduction

Although having children is important for the majority of people across the world, providing fertility care to involuntarily childless people is not a priority for many governments, and certainly not in sub-Saharan African countries. Reasons given for the neglect of fertility problems and treatment possibilities in these countries are concerns about the growing population size, scarcity of health care resources and infrastructure, and the heavy burden of other life-threatening diseases such as HIV/AIDS or higher priority health outcomes such as maternal mortality (Inhorn, 2009; Ombelet, 2012; Van Balen & Gerrits, 2001). Governments and NGO's are giving more priority to reproductive health programs in support of contraception and safe abortions. This is especially problematic as previous studies show that in highly pro-natalist settings the personal and social consequences of having fertility problems might have a devastating impact on the people involved (Daar & Merali, 2002; Inhorn & Patrizio, 2015).

Approximately eight to twelve percent of all reproductive-aged women and men worldwide are affected by infertility (e.g., Inhorn & Patrizio, 2015). It is estimated that around the world tens of millions of couples are dealing with primary infertility, which is the inability to conceive after 12 months of regular unprotected intercourse (Greil, McQuillan, Shreffler, Johnson, & Slauson-Blevins, 2011) and even more people are confronted with secondary infertility, which is the inability to conceive following a prior pregnancy (Inhorn & Patrizio, 2015). However, the prevalence of women and men who are confronted with primary or secondary fertility problems varies around the world. Infertility rates are especially high in Central and South Asia, the Middle East and sub-Saharan Africa (Inhorn & Patrizio, 2015). In sub-Saharan Africa, the prevalence of secondary infertility is much higher than primary infertility (e.g., Nachtigall, 2006), mainly due to poor maternity care and high rates of unsafe abortions (Inhorn & Patrizio, 2015). The high prevalence rates of fertility problems are also related to higher rates of sexually transmitted infections (STIs), and other infectious diseases such as lepromatous leprosy and malaria (Larsen, 1996; Saporta & Yuksel, 1994). In non-Western settings where parenthood is culturally mandatory (e.g., Donkor, 2008; Dyer, 2007) involuntary childlessness is also related to sexual risk behaviour as a result of attempts to conceive extra-maritally, and therefore infertility also increases the chance of being infected with STIs and HIV/AIDS (e.g., Inhorn, 2009; Inhorn & Patrizio, 2015).

Although at international fora and in various declarations, for example from the World Health Organisation (WHO, 2017), infertility is recognized as a major health concern especially in resource poor areas, it has led to few activities to address this issue in these countries (Ombelet, 2012). For example, few initiatives have been undertaken to inform and support people who are dealing with fertility problems or to prevent infertility (Ombelet, 2012). Also, diagnostic examinations are seldom offered in the public health system and treatments like in vitro fertilization (IVF) are only done in private clinics. Due to the limited availability and/or inaccessibility of proper information, diagnostics and treatments (Gerrits & Shaw, 2010; Ndegwa, 2014), many couples will remain involuntarily childless.

Not being able to have children is for most people a major life problem (See also, Peterson & Place, Chap. 2; Skvirsky & Taubman – Ben-Ari, Chap. 3 in this volume). A considerable body of research, mostly conducted in Western countries, has shown that involuntary childlessness has strong psychological and psychosomatic consequences in terms of, for example, depression, anxiety, lowered self-esteem, feelings of blame and guilt, and reduced sexual interest. Infertility has also been associated with increased risk of gender-based violence (Dyer, 2007; Van Balen & Bos, 2009). For only a small minority of involuntarily childless women and men in the Western world, these effects on their psychological wellbeing are at a clinical level (Greil, 1997), and in the West most involuntarily childless people are not excluded from being involved in the activities of their friends' and relatives' children (Wirtberg, Moller, Hogstrom, Tronstad, & Lalos, 2007). The limited quantitative research in sub-Saharan Africa, however, shows that in many countries involuntarily childless couples face severe negative psychosocial consequences. Childless women are frequently stigmatized, isolated, ostracized, disinherited and neglected by the entire family and even the local community (Daar & Merali, 2002; Van Balen & Bos, 2009). Research in Ghana, however, found that more highly educated infertile women felt less stigmatized than less educated infertile women (Donkor & Sandall, 2007).

4.2 Kenya and Infertility

In Kenya, a country of 38.6 million people, the prevalence of primary infertility is about 2%, while about 30% of all women and men of reproductive age are affected by secondary infertility (Ministry of Health Kenya, 2007). Although the few existing studies about the prevalence of infertility show that Kenya is grossly affected by the problem, little is known about how people who have to deal with fertility problems are experiencing their situation. The few studies that have focused on people's experiences with fertility problems in Kenya found that, as in many other low and middle income countries, women are traditionally blamed for infertility (Kamau, 2011; Kimani & Olenja, 2001). In this chapter we present findings from a research project carried out in Kenya in 2016. The aim of the project was to generate new insights regarding fertility problems and fertility care in Nairobi, Kenya.

4.3 Our Study

An interdisciplinary team from the Netherlands (University of Amsterdam) and Kenya (Technical University of Kenya) carried out the study, consisting of researchers from the fields of child development and education, public health and medical anthropology. The study was funded with a small grant from Share-Net International, which is the Knowledge Platform for Sexual and Reproductive Health and Rights (SRHR) initiated and funded by the Dutch Ministry of Foreign Affairs. A similar study has been undertaken in Ghana. Ethical clearance and research permits were received from Institutional Review Boards (IRBs) at the University of Amsterdam, the National Commission of Science and Technology in Kenya, and the Kenyatta National Hospital from the University of Nairobi.

The study consisted of a quantitative component (a paper-pencil questionnaire) and a qualitative component (individual interviews and focus group discussions). The questionnaire study was conducted with patients facing fertility problems who were recruited from one private clinic and one government hospital in Nairobi. In addition, participants were recruited when they attended a patient support group meeting in Nairobi. A total of 75 women (and 2 men, but due to the limited number of male participants they were omitted from further analyses) facing fertility problems who were seeking help from health providers completed a paper-pencil questionnaire (further referred to as questionnaire), most of them on the spot when they visited a clinic or the patient support group meeting. Almost all questions that were used in the questionnaire were based on standardized instruments that have been used in Western and non-Western countries.

For the qualitative component, in-depth interviews were held with 21 individuals (20 women and 1 man) and 3 male-female couples. The participants were recruited from 2 private clinics, 1 government hospital, 2 churches in Nairobi or when they attended patient support group meetings in Nairobi. The participants were recruited when visiting these places and the criteria for participation was 'anybody that is trying or tried to conceive and faces or faced fertility problems'. The participants chose the place for the interviews. Most interviews took place either at participants' homes or at a clinic. Qualitative data were also collected by means of two focus group discussions in which a total of 19 women participated. The focus groups were held at one of the private clinics, selected because the private clinic participated in their organization. In addition, interviews were conducted with several key informants (3 gynecologists, 2 NGO founders, one person from the ministry of health, 4 pastors, etc.), who were working with people who have to deal with fertility problems. All interviews were recorded and transcribed for analyses.

The majority (93.3%) of the 75 women (mean age 34.0 years old, $SD = 4.99$) who completed the questionnaire had a partner and most of them (88%) also lived together with their partner (average period: 6 years) in Nairobi. All women who filled in the questionnaire had a job and most of them were working in the commercial sector, which meant they were not from the poorest socio-economic groups in Nairobi. Most of the women ($n = 55$) were struggling to get pregnant from their current partner for the first time. A minority ($n = 20$) of the participants with a partner had got pregnant from their current partner. However, 9 of these 20 did not give birth to a child and the remaining 11 of these 20 women were seeking help because they were having problems with getting pregnant for a second time. Two (of the 75) women had a child in a previous relationship and 12 (of the 75) women reported that their current partner had a child from a previous relationship. Sixty-four (85.3%) of the 75 women reported they knew whether the fertility problems had to do with them (81.3%), with their partner (7.8%) or with both of them (10.9%).

For the qualitative sample, the people who were interviewed or who participated in the focus groups were on average 37.2 years old ($SD = 6.22$) and all participants lived in Nairobi. Most of them were living with a partner and reported primary fertility problems.

4.4 The Absence of Male Participants

Finding male participants for a study on fertility problems is a well-known problem, both in Western and non-Western contexts (Becker, 2000; Sandelowski, 1993). The fact that it was very hard to recruit male participants for the current study, both for the questionnaires and the interviews, could be explained by the fact that people were recruited during their visit to a clinic, and most of the time these are women who seek help in medical centres on their own, or as one of the gynecologists who was interviewed said:

> Men, even if they have a problem, they would not come and it's very difficult to investigate men in this country, because of the belief that if they are able to perform sexuality then they are not fertile. They don't seem to understand that, actually, that (if) you are sexually able (this) does not mean that the sperms are normal. So, there is a disconnection on that issue. So, they refuse to come for checking, yeah. So, you find that almost it is very rare that you find the couple coming, the man and the wife, no, it's the women who will come (…).

The fact that we could find only a few men to participate in our study reflects what is called the "gendered medicalization of fertility problems" (Bell, 2014; Mumtaz, Shahid, & Levay, 2013).

In developing countries, the predominant perception is that infertility and fertility problems do not affect men and that women are the cause of infertility (Hörbst, 2010). One of the few male participants who was interviewed told us: "*To my opinion, women are pointed at, because most of the time they are seen as the ones with the problem*" (man, 42 years old). This is even the case when a medical check has already shown that there are no problems with the fertility of the wife and that the husband should be checked (Hörbst, 2010).

4.5 Knowledge of Fertility Problems

We assessed the knowledge of the 75 women who filled out the questionnaire about specific risk factors for lower fertility. This was done with the Fertility Knowledge Questionnaire, developed by a research team from Cardiff University, UK (Fulford, Bunting, Tsibulsky, & Boivin, 2013), which consists of 13 statements about knowledge on indicators for: reduced fertility (e.g. smoking, weight, history of STIs and mumps after puberty); misconceptions about fertility (e.g. woman fertile even without periods); and basic facts about infertility and its treatment (e.g., recommended time limit for referral to a specialist). Participants could answer whether a statement was true, false or that they did not know the answer. A correct answer was assigned one point and an incorrect, do not know or missing answer with zero points. Points were summed, divided by the total number of questions and multiplied by 100 to produce a percentage 'correct fertility knowledge' score with a range of zero to 100%.

Table 4.1 shows for each statement of the fertility knowledge instrument the percentage of correct answers in our study. We found in our study among the 75 Kenyan women a 'correct fertility knowledge' score of 55.0%. We compared this score with scores measured using the same instrument in a multi-country study by Bunting, Tsibulsky, and Boivin (2013). Bunting et al. (2013) investigated fertility knowledge in 79 countries (Kenya was not included). They used the 2010 Human Development Index (HDI) to categorize the countries' levels of socio-economic development. The HDI is compiled by the United Nations Development Programme (UNDP, http://hdr.undp.org/en/statistics/) and combines life expectancy, educational attainment and income as a reference for social and economic development, and ranks countries into four categories of development (very high, high, medium and low). Based on the HDI, Bunting et al. (2013) categorized 32 countries (for example, the U.K. and U.S.A) as (Very) High Human Development (VHHD) countries, and 47 countries (for example, India and Brazil) as Medium or Low Human Development countries (MLHD). The overall fertility knowledge score that Bunting et al. (2013) found in the 32 VHHD countries was 64.3%, compared to 44.9% for the 47 MLHD countries (overall score for all countries: 56.9%). In our study the average fertility knowledge score was similar to this overall knowledge score, and relatively high compared to the MLHD group (Kenya is a MLHD country according to the HDI). Nevertheless, within the Kenyan group, the level of knowledge differed widely by question, with 8 (61.5%) of the 13 statements scoring less than 50% correct answers (Table 4.1). Many key informants who were interviewed stated that the little knowledge people have about infertility is due to the fact that (in)fertility is a taboo subject. In effect, the issue is silenced in the public arena. People in Kenya do not openly talk about issues related to (in)fertility, which contributes to their limited knowledge about the subject. In addition, access to information about infertility and fertility treatment is very limited in Kenya.

One of the interviewed gynecologists also referred to the low levels of fertility knowledge among his patients: "*People are not aware of how their body works*". He linked this to the limited attention given to sexuality and reproduction in the curriculum of schools in Kenya, and stated that as a result people are not aware of the implications of STIs on someone's fertility.

4.6 The Need to Have Children

Conceiving a child after you are married is very important for women in Kenya (Kamau, 2011) and this was also found in the answers of the women on the questions

Table 4.1 Fertility knowledge

	Correct answer	Percentage of women answering correctly
A woman is less fertile after the age of 36 years old	True	45.3
A couple would be classified as infertile if they did not achieve a pregnancy after one year of regular sexual intercourse without using contraception	True	26.7
Smoking decreases female fertility	True	82.7
Smoking decreases male fertility	True	86.7
If you have a healthy lifestyle you are fertile	False	45.3
About one in ten couples are infertile	True	29.3
If a man produces sperm he is fertile	False	81.3
These days, a woman in her forties has a similar chance of getting pregnant as a woman in her thirties	False	33.3
If a man has had mumps after puberty he is more likely to later have a fertility problem	True	44.0
A woman who never menstruates is still fertile	False	40.0
If a woman is overweight by more than 13 kilos (28 lb) then she may not be able to get pregnant	True	38.7
If a man can achieve an erection then it is an indication that he is fertile	False	84.0
People who have had a sexually transmitted disease are likely to have reduced fertility	True	77.3

that were related to their need to become a parent, measured in the questionnaire with the Need for Parenthood subscale of the Fertility Problem Inventory, developed by Newton, Sherrad, and Glavac (1999), see Table (4.2). Combining the answer categories "agree" and "strongly agree", our study found that almost all participants, for example, reported that as long as they could remember they wanted to become a mother (94.4%), and that they saw this as a more important goal in their life than having a career (91.3%). Almost all participants also reported that they felt that they were born to become a mother (90.0%), that their marriage needs a child (84.5%), that they will do everything to have a child (80.8%), and that conceiving a child is one of the most important things in a couple's relationship (79.2%).

While these figures may reflect the women's views and wishes, some of the interviewed women also recognized the societal pressure affecting their 'choice'. As one of the participants mentioned:

> Okay, (…) in Kenya (…) when you get married, it is expected that you have children. Not having a kid is not something you decide, it is something that the society already decided for you (…) it is something that you just follow. (woman, 35 years old)

For almost all participants who filled in the questionnaire it was also very hard to accept that they would live a life without having children (Table 4.2). This was measured with the Rejection of Childfree Lifestyle subscale of the Fertility Problem Inventory (Newton et al., 1999). For example, only a minority (1.4%) reported to "agree" or "strongly agree" with the statement that there is a certain freedom regarding not having children that appeals to them, or "agree" or "strongly agree" that they see a number of advantages if they did not have children (4.3%).

The socialization of women and societal pressure to become a mother and women's strong rejection of a childfree lifestyle, was well illustrated by one of the interviewees: "*The society prepared you as a girl (…) that one day you get married, you get kids of your own*" (woman, 33 years old). This woman also told us that she—as a young girl—had to take care of her younger cousins (she had to bath and dress them) because, as her mother used to say "*One day you will have kids of your own*". However, not all interviewed women linked womanhood to being a mother: "*Being a women is not about having kids but it is about being courageous*" (woman, 33 years old).

4.7 Rejections from Society Because of not Having a Child

One of the interviewed gynecologists confirmed that women in Kenya who do not conceive are experiencing a lot of social pressure from Kenyan society: "*If you can't have a family, you are deficient, you are not hundred percent, you have a problem*". This was also reflected in the quantitative results when we investigated the experiences of stigmatization due to being childless and/or having fertility problems (measured the Perceived Stigma Scale developed by Donkor and Sandall in 2007 and consisting of 3 items) with answer categories 0 "does not apply to me" and 1

Table 4.2 Need of having children and rejection of child free lifestyle (percentages)

	Strongly disagree	Disagree	Somewhat disagree	Somewhat agree	Agree	Strongly agree
Need of having children						
I will do just everything to have a child	4.1	1.4	6.8	6.8	24.7	56.2
I have often felt that I was born to be a parent	0.0	1.4	0.0	8.6	32.9	57.1
As long as I can remember, I've wanted to be a parent	1.4	0.0	0.0	4.2	31.0	63.4
Pregnancy and childbirth are the two most important events in a couple's relationship	1.4	5.6	4.2	9.7	29.2	50.0
My marriage needs a child	1.4	2.8	5.6	5.6	32.4	52.1
Being a parent is a more important goal than having a satisfying career/job	1.4	1.4	2.9	2.9	21.7	69.6
Rejection on child free lifestyle						
I could visualize a happy life together, without a child (or another child)	40.8	8.5	2.8	18.3	15.5	14.1
We could have a long and happy relationship without a child (or another child)	59.7	12.5	1.4	8.3	11.1	6.9
Having a child (or another child) is not necessary for my happiness	67.1	4.3	8.6	10.0	7.1	2.9
Not having a child would allow me to make time to do other satisfying things	68.1	18.8	5.8	1.4	0.0	5.8
There is a certain freedom without having children that appeals to me	76.8	15.9	0.0	5.8	0.0	1.4
Couples without children are just as happy as those with children	63.4	12.7	8.5	7.0	4.2	4.2

(continued)

Table 4.2 (continued)

	Strongly disagree	Disagree	Somewhat disagree	Somewhat agree	Agree	Strongly agree
I could see a number of advantages if we didn't have children	77.1	14.3	2.9	1.4	1.4	2.9
A future without a child (or another child) would frighten me	7.6	4.5	9.1	4.5	30.3	43.9
I feel emptiness because cf our fertility problems	2.9	5.9	1.5	10.3	30.9	48.5
Having a child (or another child)is not the major focus of my life	62.0	9.9	7.0	11.3	5.6	4.2

"yes, does apply to me"). About three-quarters of the women reported that other people treat them as inferior and look down upon them (74.3%) or that they felt that because of their situation (being childless or having fertility problems) people felt uncomfortable with them (74.3%). Almost two-thirds of the women (63.5%) reported that because of their childlessness or fertility problems other people in their environment avoided them. We also computed a sum score based on these three aspects of stigmatization which revealed that on average the participants reported a 2.12 out of 3.00 ($SD = 1.26$) on this stigmatization scale, with a majority (62.2%) reporting a "yes" on all three items.

One of the women who participated in the focus groups shared her experiences about stigmatization by saying that in her village it was very common for women to send other people's children out for groceries but when she would ask someone else's child to do this for her, people would tell her that she should first get her own child before she can ask other people's children to do things for her. This was for her a very painful experience. Another woman also experienced something similar:

> If another mother has a baby, other women are able to go there and hold that baby, but because I have no baby, I am not allowed to go there and hold the baby. (woman, 34 years old)

Other women told us that they were not allowed to touch other people's children in their community, because the mothers were afraid that they [the participants] would cause bad luck to the children. Sometimes the women even experienced violence from other people in their community, they were segregated from the community or experienced other insulting and insensitive comments from people in the community in which they are living:

> Yeah, people in the community say you're useless, you're useless in bed. They hit you, they started talking: 'you can, you are doing work, but work for nothing', things like that. In fact, when they see my husband coming from the shopping, they tell like 'Why you need shopping when you have nobody to feed? You are tired, but you're doing work for what'. Yeah, things like that. (woman, 42 years old)

One of the participants told us in an interview that her in-laws made a lot of comments about her inability to conceive. The in-laws told her that she wasted the resources of their son, which was very painful for her to be confronted with.

Not all participants, however, experienced such negative attitudes from people around them. Also from other studies carried out in non-Western countries it is known that in particular women and men from higher socio-economic backgrounds seemed to be able to protect themselves and their partners from negative familial and communal attitudes (e.g., Donkor & Sandall, 2007). One example in our study was a well-educated woman who had been able to protect herself from negative attitudes related to childlessness by being and portraying herself as a "businesswoman". As she had always been a woman who had found her study and career important and had also been seen as such by family and friends, they rarely asked her any questions about the absence of children in her marriage.

4.8 Fertility-Related Quality of Life

The agonizing experiences of having fertility problems and being rejected by other people had consequences for participants' perceived quality of life. All interviewees referred to the grief they were feeling because of their impaired fertility. Some interviewed women told us that because they were not able to conceive a child they did not feel complete or—in the words of one of our participants—"*without a baby you cannot be called a woman*" (woman, 41 years old). One of the few men that participated in the interviews argued that the feeling of not being complete when you are not able to conceive a child is not exclusive for women and according to him in Kenya manhood is also largely dependent on parenthood:

> Well … for men, for those who are married, there is the idea that you cannot have problems with getting children, because then you are not a man. […]As a man you cannot stand in front of people and talk when you do not have children, […] because 'who are you'?. You are nothing. (man, 48 years old)

In the questionnaire we included the Fertility Quality of Life questionnaire (FertiQoL; Boivin, Takefman, & Braverman, 2011) to assess the impact of fertility problems on social, emotional, mind-body and relational domains. Based on the participants' responses, the raw scores were calculated and the scaled scores were computed in accordance with instructions available at http://sites.cardiff.ac.uk/fertiqol/scoring. For each domain the score can be between 0 and 100, with a higher score meaning a higher level of quality of life.

The earlier quotes, showing the feelings of isolation from the community, are reflected in the participants' mean scores for the social domain of quality of life, or the extent to which the participants' social interactions were affected by fertility problems. The minimum and maximum reported scores for this social domain of quality of life were 8.33 (low quality of life) and 100 (high quality of life). On average the women scored on this social domain 48.16. ($SD = 18.85$). For the emotional dimension, reflecting the impact of negative emotions such as jealousy, resentment, sadness and depression on quality of life, the minimum and maximum reported scores were 12.50 and 100 respectively, and on average the score was 42.44 ($SD = 20.38$). The mind-body domain shows the impact of fertility problems on physical health (e.g., fatigue, pain), cognitions (e.g., concentration) and behaviour (e.g., disrupted daily activities, delayed life plans). The minimum reported score on this scale was 12.50 and the maximum was 100, with an average score of 49.06 ($SD = 22.70$). The relational domain of quality of life is about the impact of fertility problems on the marriage or partnership (e.g., sexuality, communication, commitment) and the reported scores for this aspect were between 20.83 and 83.33 with an average score of 51.97 ($SD = 14.50$). The wide range of impacts which fertility problems had on the relational domain of quality of life were also reflected in the interviews. One of the interviewees, for example, referring to the impact that not being able to conceive has on her relationship with her partner, stated:

> At this moment (…) I don't feel close, close together, because I feel so tired, there is a problem that is supposed to be tackled, that is supposed to be managed. But we are finding ourselves in a different direction. I am on my own side, euhm, we no longer go for out, we no longer go for coffee, we lead a normal life, yeah, work, home, work, home, work, home. (woman, 35 years old)

On the other hand, there were also participants who told us that the whole situation of dealing with fertility problems had strengthened their relationship with their partner, which is also reported in the literature on infertility in Western countries (Gerrits, 2016), as illustrated by one of the participants who told us:

> I think the relationship has become more closer, the time we are supposed to do the [pregnancy] test he is always on my toes: are you okay, do you need something? He wants to take me out, he just want to keep me happy. (woman, 34 years old)

4.9 Loneliness Versus Support and Sharing

Many participants expressed in the interviews their feelings of being alone in their experience of fertility problems, especially at the beginning of these problems. In one of the interviews, a woman described her first reaction when her gynecologists told her that she had damaged fallopian tubes:

> It was bad, I cried a lot, like, for two months I spent my days crying, my nights crying. It was so bad. I even had to take some alcohol to calm me down, because I was alone, completely, like, alone. (woman, 34 years old)

An aspect that contributes to this loneliness is, according to many interviewees, the fact that people are not expected to talk about their fertility problems. Interviewees noted that in Kenya, issues related to sexuality and reproduction are seen as matters only discussed with the partner. One of the interviewed women mentioned that women and men are sometimes "counseled" by the church when they get married that "*you do not move bedroom matters to the public*" (woman, 35 years old). In the questionnaire we also found that 92.0% of the participants reported that they had not asked a friend or a relative for advice regarding their conception problems.

The fact that having fertility problems is a "silenced" topic in Kenya means people feel extremely lonely, do not have a lot of support, and are also unaware of other people facing similar challenges. This silence might also contribute to people in general having less knowledge about (in)fertility, as mentioned by a woman in one of the focus groups: "*the limited information about infertility is partly due to the fact that people do not share their stories*".

Following a clinic or hospital visit, however, this silence could change. More than three-quarter (78.2%) of the questionnaire participants mentioned that they sometimes or (quite) often asked other childless people for advice. As all participants were recruited with the help of clinics or patient support groups, it is obvious that they had met other people with fertility problems in the clinic. Interviewees also pointed to the importance of participating in a support group (as some of them did), to decrease the feeling of being alone, to find hope and also as a safe place to share one's feelings and get information from other people in a similar situation:

> I feel very comfortable, because we are sharing problems. You see, you are not the only one, there are other people. Even when you see that someone is pregnant, you see that there is hope. Even though she may have not gone through the IVF, but you see there is hope. There is support, they can't abuse you, no, because you have met each other through this [support group], you talk, you share and pass information, I think that is good. (woman, 42 years old)

4.10 Fertility Treatment: Considerations and Experiences

Many factors might influence people's decision making about using medical treatment such as IVF (Boivin, Bunting, Collins, & Nygren, 2007). The questionnaire also included 27 statements to assess these factors. The statements are based on the "Treatment Uptake" instrument developed by Bunting and Boivin (2007) based on a literature review. Participants were asked to indicate the degree of importance they gave to each statement when they were considering using fertility treatment (see Table 4.3). When we combine the answer categories "very important" and "extremely important" the most frequently mentioned considerations were: (1) The success rate of fertility treatment (97.1%), (2) The opportunity of identifying why I could not get pregnant (97.1%), (3) Whether we could get fertility treatment where we live (92.9%), (4) How easy it is (or not) to get medical advice or treatment (92.2%), (5) The idea that we had tried everything to have a baby (91.0%), and (6) Whether health insurance could cover the cost of the fertility treatment (89.4%).

In the interviews, participants told us how hard it was to find information about causes of infertility and that it was also very difficult to find their way to a gynecologist who provided fertility treatment, or in the words of one of the interviewed women: "*It was not easy to find information out there about where IVF is done in Kenya*" (woman, 33 years old). One of the gynecologists also explained that due to the limited access to information about infertility and fertility treatment, people facing fertility problems postpone seeking help in the biomedical realm. This can lead to poorer treatment results, because women are often too old by the time they reach a gynecologist who provides assisted reproductive technology (ART) services. This gynecologist also emphasized the importance of educating people about visiting a doctor when they have not conceived after one year.

In the questionnaire we also asked people to respond to the statement that fertility treatment is too expensive and 85.5% did (strongly) agree with this statement. In Kenya there are 7 private fertility clinics (located in Eldoret, Mombasa and Nairobi)

Table 4.3 Considerations for treatment (percentages)

	Not important at all	Somewhat important	Moderately important	Very important	Extremely important
The success rate of fertility treatment	0.0	1.4	1.4	25.7	71.4
The opportunity of identifying why I could not get pregnant	1.4	0.0	1.4	24.6	72.5
My feelings about adoption	32.8	7.5	13.4	14.9	31.3
My partner's feelings about adoption	26.2	10.8	15.4	15.4	32.3
Our ability to pay for fertility medical advice or treatment	16.4	3.3	6.6	23.0	50.8
My beliefs and attitudes towards fertility treatment	29.9	10.4	1.5	25.4	32.8
My partner's beliefs and attitudes towards fertility treatment	32.3	6.2	4.6	26.2	30.8
Whether our health insurance covers the cost of fertility treatment	4.5	4.5	1.5	19.7	69.7
The idea that we had tried everything to have a baby	1.5	3.0	4.5	20.9	70.1
How easy it was to get medical advice or treatment	1.6	1.6	4.7	29.7	62.5
Whether we could have a happy future without having children	9.4	4.7	3.1	21.9	60.9
Fear that nothing could be done to help us have a baby	10.6	6.1	4.5	21.2	57.6

(continued)

Table 4.3 (continued)

	Not important at all	Somewhat important	Moderately important	Very important	Extremely important
Whether close family/friends could accept a child born as a result of fertility treatment	19.1	4.4	2.9	16.2	57.4
Whether I could accept a child born as a result of fertility treatment	12.9	2.9	1.4	15.7	67.1
Whether my partner could accept a child born as a result of fertility treatment	11.8	2.9	13.2	13.2	57.4
My religious or moral beliefs about fertility treatment	36.4	7.6	7.6	21.2	27.3
My partner's religious or moral beliefs about fertility treatment	32.8	10.3	5.2	29.3	22.4
The potential negative emotional effects of the fertility treatment	11.5	37.7	11.5	13.1	26.2
The referral or waiting time for the fertility treatment	7.4	7.4	13.2	14.7	57.4
The potential negative physical effects of a fertility treatment	4.5	33.3	16.7	16.7	28.8
Whether we could get fertility treatment where we live	4.3	1.4	1.4	20.0	72.9
Fear for being refused for treatment because of my (or my partner's) age, fertility history, lifestyle or because I (or my partner) already had a child	29.3	4.5	4.5	20.9	46.3

(continued)

Table 4.3 (continued)

	Not important at all	Somewhat important	Moderately important	Very important	Extremely important
Whether fertility treatment would be a strain on my relationship with my partner	39.4	4.5	12.1	21.2	22.7
Confidence that I could be satisfied putting my energy into other life goals	23.9	13.0	10.9	17.4	34.8
My partner's age	19.4	8.1	3.2	19.4	50.0
The reputation of the fertility clinic and its practitioners	9.4	6.3	6.3	17.2	60.9
My age	16.9	1.5	6.2	21.5	53.8

and they are providing about 1000 IVF cycles per year (Ndegwa, 2014). The costs of an IVF are indeed high, namely 4500 US dollar for one cycle (Ndegwa, 2014). The high costs of ART services, for example an IVF cycle, mean that the majority of people in Kenya, who are dealing with fertility problems, are not able to afford ART services, creating huge access inequalities to appropriate fertility care (see also: Gerrits, 2012; Inhorn & Birenbaum-Carmeli, 2008; Inhorn & Patrizio, 2015). In the literature this is described as 'stratified reproduction' (Colen, 1995, p. 5). Almost all interviewees told us that they had to borrow money to pay for fertility treatments such as IVF or Intrauterine Insemination (IUI). The CEO of an organization for education on reproductive health that was interviewed linked more affordable infertility treatment to de-stigmatization of fertility problems in Kenya:

> So, for me, I want, I want a stigma free country on infertility. On how we are going to get a stigma free country is when we have cheaper, easily available treatment of infertility, because today if, if I cannot get a baby, you're talking about me, second year I don't get, the third, the fifth, the tenth, eleventh year, what will happen? The stigma will still be there. But, for example, today you talk about me and say "Cecilia doesn't get a baby, he [the husband] needs to get out of that marriage" and then the second year I get a baby, what is that? It means that people will shut up, because there will be a solution for, for infertility.

This is exactly what Inhorn and Patrizio (2015) underlined as well: more affordable and accessible ARTs in developing countries are not only needed to treat fertility problems, but effective ARTs also decrease the (gendered) stigmatization of infertility.

In the interviews, people also shared the feeling that medical professionals are more preoccupied with earning money than with providing good health care and giving adequate information. One of the interviewees who underwent several IVFs and IUIs and still was not pregnant, found out later, when she went to another doctor, that the IVFs and IUIs could never have been effective because there was a septum in her uterus and she said:

> It did not even bother them to put me through a single test before starting the procedures. The consequences are always for the patient and never for the doctors. It are the doctors who are going home with the money. (woman, 44 years old)

This is of concern because people starting the whole treatment procedure do so based on trust in the doctor's knowledge, especially given the biomedical complexity of infertility and fertility treatment and the limited access to information about these topics in Kenya. In the words of one of the interviewees "*I did not consult any other doctor, because I just thought, yeah my doctor said I do this … so, I do this.*" (woman, 26 years old)

Notwithstanding the many complaints, participants also had positive experiences with medical professionals. One of the interviewed women, for example, visited another clinic after several bad experiences with the first clinic. She got the address of the second clinic from a personal contact; this clinic was more specialized in infertility and its treatment and there she was diagnosed with blockages to the fallopian tubes, which, according to the interviewee, needed to be removed before IVF could take place. In the second clinic she felt well informed, as the doctor took time to explain her medical condition and for the first time she felt "*this doctor is not just after the money.*" (woman, 33 years old)

4.11 Conclusion and Recommendations

Our study on infertility and fertility care in Kenya showed the various consequences of fertility problems and the difficulties people experienced with finding the right information and accessing fertility care. These findings are in line with findings in other sub-Saharan countries (Gerrits & Shaw, 2010). It should be noted that the participants mainly consisted of women living in Nairobi, and the majority of women who filled in the questionnaire were working in the commercial sector and did not belong to a low SES group. So there is still scarce information about women of low SES or women living in rural areas who face fertility problems, and very little is known about Kenyan men. The experiences of people living in rural areas might be different and are presumably likely to be worse compared to those who are living in large cities such as Nairobi.

Our study showed that knowledge regarding fertility varied widely among our research group and was on average limited on several topics. People were especially unaware of declining fertility with age, and the declining chance of getting pregnant when overweight, and had misconceptions about all sperm being fertile, and being fertile when not menstruating, as well as how many people face infertility. As also suggested by one of the interviewed gynecologists, informing people in Kenya through education in schools, clinics and other locations (such as churches) about (in)fertility and risk factors associated with impaired fertility, and also educating people about seeking medical advice on time, may improve their chances of fertility (see also Bunting et al., 2013). Several studies on other diseases have shown that increasing knowledge of signs, symptoms and preventable causes does reduce risk, reduce delay in seeking help, and improve health outcomes (Grunfeld, Hunter, Ramirez, & Richards, 2003; Oliveria et al., 1999). Bunting et al. (2013) emphasized that one could expect similar benefits from increasing fertility knowledge, although the high costs involved in fertility treatments may strongly reduce these benefits. Education might also lead to destigmatization of infertility (see also Gerrits et al., 2017).

Holmström and Röing (2010) emphasize that medical professionals should provide correct information to their patients about the success rates and possibilities of ARTs, so that their patients can make well informed and empowered decisions in their steps to undergo fertility treatment (or not). In our study, we found that according to the interviewees, professionals did not always provide appropriate information because they presumably also had a business to run (the private clinic). Elsewhere, two Sri Lankan IVF clinicians have drawn attention to the challenges practitioners in private IVF clinics (including they themselves) are facing (Palihawadana &

Seneviratne, 2015). On the one hand, they have an obligation to inform their patients realistically about the availability of ART facilities and the range of possible solutions for infertility problems; on the other hand, they have to advertise and promote themselves in the media, as 'any private sector enterprise' that can resolve people's infertility problems (Gerrits, 2015, Palihawadana & Seneviratne, 2015). According to Franklin and Roberts (2006) the money-making focus may affect the trust that people have in the medical ART world. However, we should also mention that our participants also reported positive stories about some private clinics which do inform their patients very well and really want to help them.

In Kenya, like in many sub-Saharan countries, motherhood is considered imperative for womanhood. In our study, for example, this was reflected in the answers that most women gave about it often not being a choice to have a child but a "decision" made for women by society. Like in other studies in non-Western countries (see for an overview: Van Balen & Bos, 2009), we found that many women reported feelings of grief, incompleteness, loneliness and low scores on instruments measuring quality of life. To deal with these feelings some participants did mention the importance of patient support networks (see, for example, Peterson & Place, Chap. 2 in this volume). Many researchers have emphasized the importance of support groups for patients with particular health issues, such as HIV/AIDS, in sub-Saharan African context (Gillett & Parr 2010; Moyer, Igonya, Both, Hardon, & Cherutich, 2013). Little is known about the importance of support groups for people with fertility problems in these contexts, while they are known to play an important role in many Western countries (e.g., Van Uden-Kraan, Drossaert, Taal, Seydel, & Van de Laar, 2009) and lately have been set up in a number of Sub-Saharan African countries such as in Ghana (Gerrits, 2015, 2016).

Globally, ARTs have brought a solution for many infertile people and they are generally seen as highly desirable (Gerrits, 2015). It is therefore not surprising that ARTs are also seen as a welcome opportunity in a context in which there are a lot of socio-cultural and psychological consequences for unwanted childlessness, especially for women. Franklin (1997) described ART as a "technology of hope" when these technologies were initially introduced in Western contexts. Franklin (1997) also argued that this (gendered) medicalization of infertility can change from what users might experience as something to increase their reproductive agency into something which adds a new kind of pressure or obligation on women (and men) to use. In line with this we argue that it is not only important to make ART more accessible, but efforts should also be made to destigmatize infertility and unwanted childlessness, because only then childless couples will not be isolated and discriminated against (Ombelet, 2011). On the other hand, the use of ART can also be seen as a way for people to cope with societal pressure and negative attitudes around them (Bochow, 2015) and in itself may have a destigmatizing effect (Inhorn & Patrizaio, 2015).

Our study also showed that access to diagnostic information and treatment was very important for the participants; however, the access to these 'technologies of hope' is limited because of the costs and availability. In Kenya ARTs are only available in the private sector, and thus are very expensive, and so only accessible to some couples, and sometimes only after borrowing a large amount of money. Not surprisingly almost all participants (even while most of them belonged to higher income groups) agreed with the statement that fertility treatment is too expensive. This leads to what the literature labels as 'stratified reproduction' (Colen, 1995). This 'stratified reproduction' is in contrast with international statements which have been made since 1948. In 1948 the United Nations (UN) Universal Declaration of Human Rights stated that: "Men and women of full age, without any limitation due to race, nationality or religion, have the right to marry and to raise a family". This statement was followed by a statement at the UN International Conference on Population and Development (ICPD) in Cairo in 1994: "Reproductive health therefore implies that people have the capability to reproduce and the freedom to decide if, when and how often to do so …. And to have information and the means to do so …" (UN, 1998), and then in 2004 at the World Health Assembly: "the provision of high-quality services for family-planning, including infertility services" was once more confirmed (World Health Organization, 2004). These statements underline the right to have access to fertility treatments when couples are unable to have children (Ombelet, 2011). The 'stratified reproduction' resulting from unequal access to ARTs in Kenya (like in many other countries) contrasts with these international statements, and one of the remaining questions is "why would citizens of developing countries not have the right to have at least one child, especially if we succeed to simplify care and make them [ARTs] affordable for a much larger part of the population?" (Ombelet, 2011, p. 260).

Several initiatives have been undertaken in the last couple of years to simplify diagnostic procedures for fertility problems, to use less expensive ovarian stimulation medication and to use IVF procedures that are more affordable, but still safe and effective (Frydam & Ranoux, 2008; Ombelet, 2011, 2014; Ombelet, Cooke, Dyer, Serour, & Devroey, 2008). The project undertaken by the Belgian non-profit organization the Walking Egg (tWE) is an example of such an initiative. One of the main goals of the Walking Egg is to make infertility care universally available and accessible (Ombelet, 2011; Ombelet & Campo, 2007). As part of the Walking Egg initiative, a new simplified method of IVF culturing was developed, called tWE lab method (for more technical information see the tWE lab system: Klerkx et al., 2014). Studies carried out at the IVF unit in Genk (Belgium) showed that the outcomes of this more affordable culture method were identical with those from a conventional IVF method (Ombelet, 2014; Van Blerkom et al., 2014), while the costs of this tWE lab method are between 10 and 15% of the costs of a conventional IVF (Klerck et al., 2014).

Nevertheless, it will take time until more people have access to fertility care; and even when they have access to fertility care, this will not always result in a pregnancy and a child. According to the Centres for Disease Control and Prevention (CDC, 2011), the success rate of a single IVF using a woman's own ova is 30–40% for women below 35 years. The rate then decreases steadily thereafter to around 10% by the age of 43 years. Therefore, we contend—following the gynecologist Willem Ombelet—that it is important to not only focus on broadening access to

ARTs, but also on preventing infertility, for example by preventing sexually transmitted infections and infections resulting from unhygienic maternity care and unsafe abortion practices, and challenging existing negative attitudes regarding unwanted childlessness (Ombelet, 2011).

References

Becker, G. (2000). *The elusive embryo. How women and men approach new reproductive technologies*. Berkeley and London: University of California Press.

Bell, A. V. (2014). *Misconception: Social class and infertility in America*. New Brunswick: Rutgers University Press.

Bochow, A. (2015). Ethics, identities and agency: ART, elites and HIV/AIDS in Botswana. In K. Hampshire & B. Simpson (Eds.), *Assisted reproductive technologies in the third phase: Global encounters and emerging moral worlds* (pp. 135–151). Oxford & New York: Berghahn Books.

Boivin, J., Bunting, L., Collins, J. A., & Nygren, K. G. (2007). International estimates of infertility prevalence and treatment-seeking: Potential need and demand for infertility medical care. *Human Reproduction, 22,* 1506–1512.

Boivin, J., Takefman, J., & Braverman, A. (2011). The fertility quality of life (FertiQoL) tool: Development and general psychometric properties. *Fertility and Sterility, 96*(8), 409–415.

Bunting, L., & Boivin, J. (2007). Decision-making about seeking medical advice in an internet sample of women trying to get pregnant. *Human Reproduction, 22*(6), 1662–1668.

Bunting, L., Tsibulsky, I., & Boivin, J. (2013). Fertility knowledge and beliefs about fertility treatment: Findings from the international fertility decision-making study. *Human Reproduction, 28*(2), 385–397.

CDC, (2011). *Assisted reproductive technologies. Fertility clinic success rates report.* Atlanta: National Center for Chronic Disease Prevention and Health Promotion. Division of Reproductive Health.

Colen, S. (1995). Like a mother to them: Stratified reproduction and West Indian childcare workers and employers in New York. In F. Ginsburg & R. Rapp (Eds.), *Conceiving the new world order: The global politics of reproduction* (pp. 78–102). Berkeley: University of California Press.

Daar, A. S., & Merali, Z. (2002). In: Infertility and social suffering: The case of ART in developing countries. In E. Vayena, P. J. Rowe, & P. D. Griffin (Eds.), *Current practices and controversies in assisted reproduction* (pp. 15–21). Geneva: World Health Organization.

Donkor, E. S. (2008). Socio-cultural perceptions of infertility in Ghana. *Africa Journal of Nursing and Midwifery, 10*(1), 22–34.

Donkor, E. S., & Sandall, J. (2007). The impact of perceived stigma and mediating social factors on infertility-related stress among women seeking infertility treatment in Southern Ghana. *Social Science and Medicine, 65*(8), 1683–1694.

Dyer, S. J. (2007). The value of children in African countries–insights from studies on infertility. *Journal of Psychosomatic Obstetrics & Gynecology, 28*(2), 69–77.

Franklin, S. (1997). Embodied progress: A cultural account of assisted conception. London & New York: Routledge.

Franklin, S., & Roberts, C. (2006). *Born and made: An ethnography of preimplantation genetic diagnosis*. Princeton: Princeton University Press.

Frydman, R., & Ranoux, C. (2008). INVO: A simple, low cost effective assisted reproductive technology. *Human Reproduction, 1,* 85–89.

Fulford, B., Bunting, L., Tsibulsky, I., & Boivin, J. (2013). The role of knowledge and perceived susceptibility in intentions to optimize fertility: Findings from the International Fertility Decision-Making Study (IFDMS). *Human Reproduction, 28*(12), 3253–3262.

Gerrits, T. (2012). Biomedical infertility care in low resource countries: Barriers and access: Introduction. *Facts, Views & Vision in Obstetrics, Gynaecology and Reproductive Health, Monograph*, 1–6.

Gerrits, T. (2015). ARTs in resource-poor areas: Practices, experiences, challenges and theoretical debates. In K. Hampshire & B. Simpson (Eds.), *Assisted reproductive technologies in the third phase: Global encounters and emerging moral worlds* (pp. 94–104). Oxford: Berghahn Books.

Gerrits, T. (2016). *Patient-centered IVF: Bioethics and care in a Dutch clinic*. New York: Berghahn Books.

Gerrits, T., & Shaw, M. (2010). Biomedical infertility care in sub-Saharan Africa: A social science review of current practices, experiences and view points. *Facts, Views & Vision in Obstetrics, Gynaecology and Reproductive Health, 2*(3), 194–207.

Gerrits, T., Van Rooij, F., Esho, T., Ndegwa W., Goossens, J., Bilajbegovic, A., … Bos, H. M. W. (2017). Infertility in the Global South: Raising awareness and generating insights for policy and practice. *Facts, Views, & Vision in Obstetrics, Gynaecology and Reproductive Health, 9*(1), 39–44.

Gillett, H. J., & Parr, J. (2010). Disclosure among HIV-positive women: The role of HIV/AIDS support groups in rural Kenya. *African Journal of AIDS Research, 9*(4), 337–344.

Greil, A. L. (1997). Infertility and psychological distress: A critical review of the literature. *Social Science and Medicine, 45*(11), 1679–1704.

Greil, A. L., McQuillan, J., Shreffler, K. M., Johnson, K. M., & Slauson-Blevins, K. S. (2011). Race-ethnicity and medical services for infertility: Stratified reproduction in a population-based sample of US women. *Journal of Health and Social Behavior, 52*(4), 493–509.

Grunfeld, E. A., Hunter, M. S., Ramirez, A. J., & Richards, M. A. (2003). Perceptions of breast cancer across the lifespan. *Journal of Psychosomatic Research, 54*(2), 141–146.

Holmström, I., & Röing, M. (2010). The relation between patient-centeredness and patient empowerment: A discussion on concepts. *Patient Education and Counseling, 79*(2), 167–172.

Hörbst, V. (2010). Male perspectives on infertility and assisted reproductive technologies (ART) in sub-Saharan contexts. *Facts, Views & Vision in Obstetrics, Gynaecology and Reproductive Health, Monograph*, 22–27.

Inhorn, M. C. (2009). Right to assisted reproductive technology: Overcoming infertility in low-resource countries. *International Journal of Gynecology & Obstetrics, 106*(2), 172–174.

Inhorn, M. C., & Birenbaum-Carmeli, D. (2008). Assisted reproductive technologies and culture change. *Annual Review of Anthropology, 37*, 177–196.

Inhorn, M. C., & Patrizio, P. (2015). Infertility around the globe: New thinking on gender, reproductive technologies and global movements in the 21st century. *Human Reproduction Update, 21*(4), 411–426.

Kamau, P. M. (2011). *The experiences of infertility among married Kenyan women*. Kalamazoo: Western Michigan University.

Kimani, V., & Olenja, J. (2001). Infertility: Cultural dimensions and impact on women in selected communities in Kenya. *African Anthropologist, 8*(2), 200–216.

Klerkx, E., Janssen, M., Van der Auweral, I., Campol, R., Goossens, J., Vereecke, A., & Ombelet, W. (2014). Simplified IVF laboratory method. *Facts, Views & Vision in Obstetrics, Gynaecology and Reproductive Health, Monograph*, 4–5.

Larsen, U. (1996). Childlessness, subfertility, and infertility in Tanzania. *Studies in Family Planning, 27*(1), 18–28.

Ministry of Health Kenya. (2007). *Desk review: Infertility in Kenya*. Nairobi, Kenya: Ministry of Health, Division of Reproductive Health.

Moyer, E., Igonya, E. K., Both, R., Hardon, A., & Cherutich, P. (2013). The duty to disclose in Kenyan health facilities: A qualitative investigation of HIV disclosure in everyday practice. *SAHARA: Journal of Social Aspects of HIV/AIDS Research Alliance, 10*(Supplement 1), 60–72.

Mumtaz, Z., Shahid, U., & Levay, A. (2013). Understanding the impact of gendered roles on the experiences of infertility amongst men and women in Punjab. *Reproductive Health, 10*(3), 3–13.

Nachtigall, R. D. (2006). International disparities in access to infertility services. *Fertility and Sterility, 85*(4), 871–875.

Ndegwa, S. W. (2014). Affordable ART in Kenya: The only hope for involuntary childlessness. *Facts, Views & Vision in Obstetrics, Gynaecology and Reproductive Health, Monograph*, 21–22.

Newton, C. R., Sherrard, M. A., & Glavac, I. (1999). The fertility problem inventory: Measuring perceived infertility related stress. *Fertility and Sterility, 72*(1), 54–62.

Oliveria, S. A., Christos, P. J., Halpern, A. C., Fine, J. A., Barnhill, R. L., & Berwick, M. (1999). Patient knowledge, awareness, and delay in seeking medical attention for malignant melanoma. *Journal of Clinical Epidemiology, 52*(11), 1111–1116.

Ombelet, W. (2011). Global access to infertility care in developing countries: A case of human rights, equity and social justice. *Facts, Views & Vision in Obstetrics, Gynaecology and Reproductive Health, 3*(4), 257–266.

Ombelet, W. (2012). Global access to infertility care in developing countries: A case of human rights, equity and social justice. *Facts, Views & Vision in Gynaecology, 3*, 7–16.

Ombelet, W. (2014). Is global access to infertility care realistic? The Walking Egg Project. *Reproductive Biomedicine Online, 28*(3), 267–272.

Ombelet, W., & Campo, R. (2007). Affordable IVF for developing countries. *Reproductive Biomedicine Online, 15*(3), 257–265.

Ombelet, W., Cooke, I., Dyer, S., Serour, G., & Devroey, P. (2008). Infertility and the provision of infertility medical services in developing countries. *Human Reproduction Update, 14*(6), 605–621.

Palihawadana, T. S., & Seneviratne, H. R. (2015). Practitioner perspective: A view from Sri Lanka. In K. Hampshire & B. Simpson (Eds.), *Assisted reproductive technologies in the third phase: Global encounters and emerging moral worlds* (pp. 171–180). Oxford, US: Berghahn Books.

Sandelowski, M. (1993). *With child in mind. Studies of the personal encounter with infertility*. Philadelphia: University of Pennsylvania Press.

Saporta, L., & Yuksel, A. (1994). Androgenic status in patients with lepromatous leprosy. *BJU International, 74*(2), 221–224.

United Nations. (1948). *The Universal declarations of human rights*. New York: United Nations.

United Nations. (1998). *International conference on population and development*. New York: United Nations.

Van Balen, F., & Bos, H. (2009). The social and cultural consequences of being childless in poor-resource areas. *Facts, Views, & Vision in Obstetrics, Gynaecology and Reproductive Health, 1*(2), 106–121.

Van Balen, F., & Gerrits, T. (2001). Quality of infertility care in poor-resource areas and the introduction of new reproductive technologies. *Human Reproduction, 16*(2), 215–219.

Van Blerkom, J., Ombelet, W., Klerkx, E., Janssen, M., Dhont, N., Nargund, G., & Campo, R. (2014). First births with a simplified culture system for clinical IVF and embryo transfer. *Reproductive Biomedicine Online, 28*(3), 310–320.

Van Uden-Kraan, C. F., Drossaert, C. H., Taal, E., Seydel, E. R., & van de Laar, M. A. (2009). Participation in online patient support groups endorses patients' empowerment. *Patient Education and Counseling, 74*(1), 61–69.

Wirtberg, I., Moller, A., Hogstrom, L., Tronstad, S.-E., & Lalos, A. (2007). Life 20 years after unsuccessful infertility treatment. *Human Reproduction, 22*(2), 598–604.

WHO. (2004). *World Health Assembly*. See: www.who.int/mediacentre/releases/2004Assembly.

WHO. (2017). *Sexual health and its linkages to reproductive health: An operational approach*. Geneva: World Health Organization.

Chapter 5
Fertility Treatment Through the Eyes of the Media: Words, Metaphors, and Images in Israeli Media Coverage of Fertility and Fertility Treatment

Shirley Ben Shlomo and Oneg Kabizon-Pery

5.1 Introduction

The first child conceived through in vitro fertilization (IVF) was born in 1978. Media coverage of the event sparked a heated public debate over the potential implications of technological intervention in the context of fertility and birth (Michelle, 2007). In the last three decades, assisted reproductive technology (ART) has developed so rapidly (Shalev & Lemish, 2011) that resulting births are no longer breaking news. Instead, media reference to fertility treatment and its implications has become more mature, and is often characterized by a critical attitude.

The discourse in the various media outlets not only reflects the dominant values in society, but also shapes public opinion (Bassan & Michaelsen, 2013; Sangster & Lawson, 2014), as well as social and cultural attitudes and beliefs (Graham & Rich, 2014). It does so by framing subjects on the public agenda as positive, neutral, or negative (Sangster & Lawson, 2014), thereby imposing a particular meaning on a situation, event, or issue. This power may also be used manipulatively to serve the needs of certain social "players" or institutions (Jaworski, 2009), and influence the attitudes and choices of individuals regarding the existing social agenda accordingly (van den Akker, Fronek, Blyth, & Frith, 2016).

In respect to ART, there is a mutual dependency between the media on the one hand, and reproductive policy and the social attitudes associated with it on the other (Bassan & Michaelsen, 2013; Sangster & Lawson, 2014). The media appears to be a key factor in the individual's perceptions, as it both reflects accepted values and norms (Piotrow, Kincaid, Rimon, & Rinehart, 1997) and furthers the construction and internalization of stereotypical perceptions (Graham & Rich, 2014). Thus, the

S. Ben Shlomo (✉) · O. Kabizon-Pery
The Louis and Gabi Weisfeld School of Social Work, Bar Ilan University, Ramat Gan, Israel
e-mail: Shirley.Ben@biu.ac.il

O. Kabizon-Pery
e-mail: onegkabizon@gmail.com

O. Taubman – Ben-Ari (ed.), *Pathways and Barriers to Parenthood*,
https://doi.org/10.1007/978-3-030-24864-2_5

individual's decision of whether or not to embark on ART may be influenced both by the sociocultural context and by the way in which the procedure is framed and presented to the public in the media (Shalev & Lemish, 2012).

5.2 Functionalist Representation of Reproductive Culture and Policy

The functionalist approach depicts society as a collection of institutions and systems that operate harmoniously and in coordination with one another. The media is considered one of the major social institutions working to preserve the social order, its function being to maintain the existing status quo and reassure the public by providing information, correlating and interpreting it, transmitting cultural norms and values, and mobilizing to promote society's interest (McQuail, 2010).

As long as the media and the nation are speaking the same language, the message conveyed to the public is clear. For example, a study conducted in a gynecological center in Iran, a pronatalist country, sought to identify the factors promoting hope among 23 women who had experienced failed cycles of fertility treatment. The main factors emerging from interviews with these women were spiritual strength, family support, and knowledge acquired through various media outlets. Thus, the information provided by the media regarding ART and its implications influenced the women's sense of hope and their decision to continue the medical procedure (Mosalanejad, Parandavar, Gholami, & Abdollahifard, 2014), in line with the national culture.

A similar study conducted in England (Peddie, van Teijlingen, & Bhattacharya, 2005) interviewed 25 women after several failed IVF cycles, but in this case they had chosen not to continue treatment. It was found that most of the participants began ART with unrealistic expectations, and were highly vulnerable to pressure from society in general, and the media in particular. According to the authors, many couples embark on ART with very high expectations, despite the fact that only 20–25% of the initial cycles of IVF end in childbirth. The majority of women in the study stated that it was their own decision to discontinue the procedures, although they had consulted with friends and relatives. Some were desperate for additional information that would justify putting an end to the demanding treatment cycles, but nevertheless looked on the Internet for data on the success rate of the latest technologies before making the final decision.

Like the women in the Iranian study (Mosalanejad et al., 2014), the English women referred to the media as a major factor in deciding whether or not to continue treatment, as well as a source of pressure, as it gave the impression that having children was a social obligation. They noted that news coverage repeatedly highlighted the latest developments and breakthroughs in ART, reporting that they had enabled many couples to obtain the desired goal. Thus, for example, the participants were presented with descriptions of couples who had conceived "against all odds," women who had become pregnant after only the third cycle of IVF, and those who had conceived after they had adopted a child. Such reports, which appear regularly in the media, were found to highly increase the pressure to continue fertility treatment in the attempt to become pregnant (Peddie et al., 2005).

In Israel, as well, the media appears to apply pressure on women to commit to treatment at any cost. An analysis of news coverage (Shalev & Lemish, 2012) revealed a trend in the media to convey the message that "the sacred end justifies the means." Women willing to undergo treatment, no matter how difficult, are represented as inspiring and praiseworthy. The overriding aim is to become pregnant, and the more women strive and suffer to do so, the more positive, glowing, and even heroic the coverage they receive. What is more, the media portrays ART as a type of disciplinary regime, and encourages women to dedicate themselves to it. Furthermore, at the time of the study, news coverage appeared to frame infertility as a deviation from the social norm, that is, a physical problem that demanded a cure. The "cure" proposed was ART, whose accessibility and effectiveness are, in fact, a source of national pride in Israel (Shalev & Lemish, 2012).

Internalization and application of the message conveyed in the Israeli media can be seen in the results of a study by Birenbaum-Carmeli and Dirnfeld (2008), who examined 137 Israeli women undergoing IVF treatments. The majority of participants expressed considerable optimism regarding the ultimate success of the procedure, a high level of commitment to treatment, and a willingness to undergo as many treatment cycles as necessary.

A Canadian study (Sangster & Lawson, 2014) revealed a similar activist approach in the local media. The analysis of 157 print news items containing the word "infertility" showed that the majority painted an alarming picture, adhered to a biomedical perspective, and employed a language promoting the semantics of words such as "suffering," "frustration," "effort," "struggle," "failure," and "victims." According to the authors, as a result of this framing, media consumers may acquire only a partial understanding of fertility problems and how they can be dealt with, and will find it hard to define infertility in a way that does not favor medical intervention.

In some cases, the media expresses appreciation for women's willingness to undergo ART even when the procedures are unsuccessful. An Australian study (Graham & Rich, 2014), for instance, examined the representation of childless women in 327 news items and found that they were the object of sympathy as long as they wished to be mothers and did everything possible to achieve that aim. The women who met these criteria included both those with heartbreaking stories of the emotional, physical, and economic difficulties entailed in the fertility treatment they underwent, and those who had missed the opportunity to have children during their fertile years and were now sad and regretful. Their depiction, peppered with words like "heartbreak" and "loss," promoted the perception of childless women as vulnerable and deserving of pity. In the view of the authors, this framing reflects the assumption that all women want children, and represents the views of those working to further legislation regarding ART, surrogacy, and adoption. At the same time, technological developments now allow women to conceive at an older age, and social changes encourage young women to develop their independence and shape their lives as they wish (Shaw & Giles, 2009). These processes have also influenced the view of fertility and parenthood in the media.

5.3 Fertility Age: The Role of the Media in Shaping Public Perceptions

Medical research tends to emphasize the significance of women's chronological age for fertility, indicating that once women have reached their mid-30s, physiological changes in the female body lead to a decrease in fertility and ovarian function and a rise in the length of time required to conceive. More specifically, 35 is considered the cut-off point at which the decline in fertility becomes sharper (Liu et al., 2012). Nevertheless, recent decades have seen a steady rise in the age of first-time mothers throughout the world, a trend enabled by technological developments (Carolan, 2005; Hashiloni-Dolev, Kaplan, & Shkedi-Rafid, 2011; Shalev & Lemish, 2012). Moreover, mothers in their forties and fifties are receiving growing attention in the popular media, as evidenced by a TV documentary entitled *Pregnant at 70*, about women around the world who became pregnant late in life, which was broadcast on the American channel TLC (Sterling, 2013).

This global media trend is also reflected in Israel, a country in which every woman is entitled to fertility treatments up to the age of 45 or until the birth of two live babies. A study by Shalev and Lemish (2012) found that from 1995 to 2003, late parenthood was represented in the Israeli media as a promising and positive strategy, and the doctors who helped make it possible were portrayed in glowing terms as heroes positioning the country at the forefront of ART. In addition, during that period, media coverage largely framed fertility treatment late in life as a normative and legitimate option, ignoring the risks involved. According to Marxist media theory (McQuail, 2010), this type of framing is designed to preserve the dominance of the medical elite, pharmaceutical companies, and other economic interests. From this point of view, by means of supposedly documentary TV programs and press interviews that present only half-truths, the mind of the public is distracted from the real story.

Indeed, the media often encourages late motherhood by not telling the whole story. Thus, for instance, although every detail of celebrities' lives is aired in the international media, it is extremely rare for any of them to admit to having fertility problems. One example is the actress Halle Berry, who became pregnant in her late forties. The press release issued by her publicist stated that she had conceived spontaneously. Similarly, the singers Jennifer Lopez and Mariah Carey claimed to have conceived naturally although they were also both in their late forties (Carey later offered a different version). Such stories are liable to stifle the discourse regarding the difficulties and risks that might arise during fertility treatment in general, and at an older age in particular, and are therefore potentially misleading (Edge, 2014). A number of celebrities, however, have spoken openly about medical procedures they underwent in order to conceive, thereby opening a window for their fans to a more accurate and comprehensive understanding of ART. The actress Nicole Kidman and her husband, country singer Keith Urban, for instance, have one biological child, two adopted children, and one child born to a surrogate mother (Scherman, Misca, Rotabi, & Selman, 2016).

Although reality shows are generally looked down upon as being of poor quality and not truly reflecting reality, the stories they tell typically have a strong effect on viewers (Lewis, 2004). Lately, series documenting the daily lives of celebrities have become particularly popular. Those following the lives of young couples often include episodes that deal with fertility and pregnancy concerns, such as ectopic pregnancy. Furthermore, the process of fertility treatment has recently been shown on programs such as *Guiliana and Bill*, *Khloe and Lamar*, *Keeping Up with the Kardashians*, and others. These celebrities do not hesitate to bring TV crews with them to their meetings with fertility specialists, and even into the treatment room. Viewers have consequently been exposed to the whole procedure, including positive and negative results and miscarriages. Such documentaries, with their great psychological power, thus fulfill the potential to present a different version of acceptable social norms regarding fertility. Revealing the full picture of ART aids in informing the viewers about all aspects of the process, including the emotional and psychological implications (Edge, 2014).

Although health systems worldwide regard 35 as the point at which pregnancy entails greater risk for both the mother and the infant, there is no accepted definition of the age considered too late to have children. One possible cut-off point is 45, as a pregnancy occurring at age 45 or over is defined as "post-menopausal" (Hashiloni-Dolev et al., 2011). The age at which a woman is able to conceive also impacts the state's willingness to fund fertility treatments. For example, in Israel fertility treatments are fully funded women up to age 45 until the birth of two live infants.

An analysis of items in the Canadian press (Sangster & Lawson, 2014) revealed that according to the media, the leading cause of fertility problems is the decision to delay having children (other causes mentioned include medical condition, obesity, sexually transmitted diseases, drug abuse, and stress), and that ART is the optimal way to deal with infertility. Similarly, a study of how the British media frames post-menopausal mothers found that most of the news coverage referred to these older women as "delaying" or "postponing" motherhood, or "putting it on ice" (Shaw & Giles, 2009). The authors argue that these semantics imply an optimal age for giving birth. The regular use of the word "delay" in the specific context of older mothers suggests a negative, critical attitude. In the Israeli media as well, delayed conception is presented as potentially incurring punishment in the form of fertility problems, with the way to atone for this sin being altruistic devotion to treatment (Shalev & Lemish, 2012).

In some cases, the media does not make do with issuing warnings of the risks of postponing conception, but also adopts a didactic role, actually admonishing women. Graham and Rich's (2014) study of the popular Australian media found that it reprimands women who choose to delay motherhood for whatever reason, presenting them as selfish. This framing calls on women to stop being complacent and understand that ART can not always fix the ravages of time. In order to prove this point, the Australian media frequently reveals the "truth" about fertility treatment by reporting statistics and statements from specialists concerning the failure rate of attempts to achieve pregnancy at an older age. Items of this sort are written in a threatening tone and use words such as "fear," "urgent," and "implications" meant to serve as a warning. Similarly, in nearby New Zealand, the local media often refers to the high cost of ART (particularly IVF) and its limited success rate (Michelle, 2007).

As noted above, the age of first-time mothers is rising steadily. Nevertheless, in recent years the media throughout the world has not only been cautioning against the small chance of conceiving at a later age, whether spontaneously or with the aid of ART, but has also tended to frame older mothers negatively.

5.4 The Media as a Critical Mirror of Women's Fertility Choices

Women who become mothers at an older age are often framed in the media as irresponsible, selfish career women unworthy of social approval (Graham & Rich, 2014; Greil, McQuillan, & Slauson-Blevins, 2011; Lahad & Madsen, 2016; Shalev & Lemish, 2012; Shaw & Giles, 2009). They are criticized for choosing education and career at the expense of missing the optimal age for pregnancy, a decision for which they are termed "misguided and selfish," women who "want to have it all," and so on (Shaw & Giles, 2009). In the eyes of the media in the US and other industrialized nations, the typical patient in a fertility clinic is a middle-aged white woman who chose to put off having children in order to focus on her career (Greil et al., 2011). The Israeli media similarly frames older mothers as women focused on themselves, their career, and their liberal, hedonistic lifestyle (Shalev & Lemish, 2012), and one of the major themes of the framing of childless women in the Australian press is their depiction as career women who chose career over motherhood (Graham & Rich, 2014).

Moreover, in many parts of the world older motherhood is seen as a deviation from the natural order, and in recent years the media appears to be reflecting and reinforcing this common perception (Greil et al., 2011; Lahad & Madsen, 2016; Shaw & Giles, 2009). One example is the widespread coverage of the pregnancy of Patricia Rashbrook, an Englishwoman who gave birth at the age of 62, which predominantly adopted a judgmental tone. Many of the items questioned whether it was natural for a women to perform maternal functions, such as nursing an infant, at such an advanced age (Shaw & Giles, 2009).

In addition, the media raises questions as to an older mother's ability to raise her child properly. A recent study conducted in Denmark (Lahad & Madsen, 2016) found that media framing of 40+ mothers was generally cautionary. Furthermore, the women were often labeled ridiculous, and doubt was expressed regarding their right to ART. Thus, for example, the public television station, run by the government, produced numerous programs in which professionals discussed the capability of older women to set boundaries or discipline their children, and many items in the popular press quoted a senior gynecologist who declared that the children would be orphaned before the age of 18. Similar claims appeared in the media items in Britain, which alleged that the children of older mothers would probably be miserable (Shaw & Giles, 2009).

The British media also linked late motherhood to quality time and leisure (Shaw & Giles, 2009). This theme, which includes reference to the connection between freezing eggs and lifestyle, portrays older mothers as spoiled. At the same time, however, the texts often describe the challenges and difficulties of raising children, resulting in an ambivalent framing whereby mothers enjoy childrearing when it occurs at the optimal age, but it is a form of punishment if it does not come at the natural time. This is a rhetorical device similarly aimed at presenting late motherhood as a violation of the natural order.

5.5 The Political Relationship Between Feminism and Pronatalism Through the Eyes of the Media

On the whole, the political relationship between feminism and pronatalism is ambivalent, as feminism encourages combining career and motherhood (Brown & Ferree, 2005). Nonetheless, older women are often depicted in the media as representatives of the '60s generation, which was intent on bending the natural order to its own will. The prevalent discourse suggests that women from that generation are continuing to violate the laws of nature by means of ART. Furthermore, the media cautions that this selfish attitude comes at a cost: older mothers will be judged and condemned by their children once they grow up (Shaw & Giles, 2009). In the Australian press, women who choose not to have children because of their feminist views are depicted not as strong and independent, but as the victims of feminism. The media thus promotes the perception that believing that career can be a substitute for motherhood is a dangerous and objectionable feminist fallacy (Graham & Rich, 2014).

5.6 Anti-ART Media Campaigns

As noted above, the media can influence individuals' perceptions and opinions of ART (Sangster & Lawson, 2014) and its effectiveness (Shalev & Lemish, 2012), optimal timing (Graham & Rich, 2014; Shaw & Giles, 2009), and so on. Exploiting this power, various entities have launched large-scale media campaigns cautioning against fertility treatment.

In 2001, the American Society for Reproductive Medicine launched a campaign aimed at conveying the message that delaying conception is the wrong choice, and derives from the mistaken belief that ART makes it possible to put off having children. The campaign included large posters in public places, such as buses and shopping malls, that warned against the limitations of ART and stressed that age was a major factor in infertility (Sterling, 2013). As hoped, the campaign attracted considerable media attention, which helped the organization to spread its message.

Fourteen years later, in Autumn, 2015, the city of Copenhagen launched a similar, controversial, campaign that encouraged its citizens to have children earlier in life. Denmark, a welfare state with a liberal gender policy, takes pride in being family-oriented and particularly in allowing for a balance between working hours and family time. Nevertheless, as described above, in recent years the popular media has been increasingly critical of older mothers, an attitude reinforced by the city's "Count Your Eggs" campaign. Developed in collaboration with local fertility clinics and the Copenhagen University Hospital, it consisted of posters, postcards in cafes and parks, and a prominent posting on the city's Facebook page. The dominant message was that the chances of becoming pregnant are twice as high at 25 than at 35. In addition, the campaign offered examples of the advantages of being a young mother, such as having more energy to cope with the children's needs, and contained slogans including: Don't Wait for the Perfect Moment; Don't Compromise Your Maternal Needs; and You *Can* Be Pregnant and a Student (Lahad & Madsen, 2016).

Another anti-ART campaign presented the issue from a different perspective. The "Born" campaign in Poland in late 2007 was launched in the wake of the minister of health's announcement that IVF treatments would be subsidized as part of the public health service. His statement raised a media storm that ultimately prevented implementation of this measure. The controversy induced the Catholic Church to initiate a massive campaign presenting ART as unethical and the "test-tube babies" born with its help as unnatural monsters, much like Frankenstein. Analysis of the campaign in the media (Radkowska-Walkowicz, 2012) revealed that it attributed "monstrosity" to IVF children from four main perspectives: physical (possible deformity); psychological (survivor syndrome, identity crisis); social (loneliness, uncertain place in family relations); and ethical (a life burdened by the death of many embryos).

5.7 Surrogacy in the Media

The formal definition of ART also includes surrogacy (Zegers-Hochschild et al., 2009). Surrogacy is employed when pregnancy is impossible, either for medical or social reasons. The procedure can use IVF to create an embryo from the ovum and sperm of the parents or donors, or artificial insemination to fertilize the surrogate's eggs (van den Akker, Camara, & Hunt, 2016). This complex issue, which often engenders problematic situations, has received extensive media coverage which differs from the coverage given other types of fertility treatment.

Among other things, the media framing of reports on surrogacy sheds light on changes in policy (Crawshaw, Blyth, & van den Akker, 2012). An excellent example can be found in the international media storm surrounding the story of Baby Gammy.

In August, 2014, twins were born to a surrogate mother in Thailand as a result of a commercial surrogacy contract. The intended parents abandoned one of the infants, apparently because he was diagnosed with Down's Syndrome, taking only his healthy sister back home to Australia. The story of the abandoned baby, named Gammy, went global, becoming the subject of over 2000 items in the media around the world in just a few days. Shortly afterward, an International Forum on Intercountry Adoption and Global Surrogacy was convened to debate the options for international regulation of globalized commercial surrogacy (Scherman et al., 2016).

Many industrialized countries permit only altruistic surrogacy for which there is no financial restitution (Bassan & Michaelsen, 2013). A recent study (van den Akker, Camara et al., 2016) examined the framing of this type of surrogacy in 99 items published in the press in Britain and other countries between 1984 and 2014. The most extensive coverage of the subject appeared in 2000–2004 and again in 2008–2014. It was found that the framing was largely negative, with the majority of headlines, as well as the texts, using phrases representing warnings ("moral mine field") and high vulnerability ("The Ministry of Health and Social Security claims that most babies of surrogate mothers are born in secrecy"). Furthermore, a link was found between the nature of the framing of the news item and the style of the paper in which it was published. Thus, the tabloid press highlighted the social aspects, only occasionally relating to legal issues, while papers identified with the middle class or quality journalism focused primarily on the legal ramifications of altruistic surrogacy and implications for the couples seeking to become parents in this manner.

5.8 The Media Framing of Reproductive Tourism

The term "reproductive tourism" refers to travel to another country for ART, such as IVF, sperm or egg donations, surrogacy, and genetic diagnosis, and for international adoption (Bassan & Michaelsen, 2013). The most common practice is for people from an industrialized country to go to one that is less developed for high-quality fertility treatment at an affordable price. The combination of lenient legislation and relatively poor economic status has led to a thriving industry in reproductive tourism in a number of developing countries. India, where commercial surrogacy was legal until recently, is a prominent example (Bassan & Michaelsen, 2013). Indeed, it is estimated that 5000 babies have been born to surrogate mothers in this country. In the wake of statistics like these, the issue of intercountry surrogacy and its consequences have become a subject of controversy and criticism in the media (Sandoval, 2016), particularly regarding concern for the protection and wellbeing of the surrogate mothers (Bassan & Michaelsen, 2013).

A recent study of 46 Internet ads published by egg donor agencies (Keehn, Howell, Sauer, & Klitzman, 2015) found that the donors are often depicted as women excited to be able to exercise their noble and altruistic right to help other women become mothers. The clients are said to have the opportunity to choose the best genes for their child from an "egg brochure" detailing the characteristics of the donor. Despite this supposed altruism, the agencies are clearly motivated by commercial considerations. The procedure is generally presented as safe, thereby diverting attention away from the risks involved. Furthermore, the line between objective medical information and marketing texts is blurred. The authors of the study therefore identify a need to regulate egg donations by formulating and putting in place a code of ethics.

In view of legislation in Israel (discussed in greater detail below), the ART procedures undergone by Israelis in other countries consist mainly of egg donations and surrogacy (Bassan & Michaelsen, 2013). In the summer of 2009, a group of doctors and patients from Israeli fertility clinics traveled to Romania to retrieve eggs from local women. Most of the media reports of the trip used words like "selling eggs" and "illegal trade" that expressed concern over the practice. A year later, in June, 2010, the Knesset (the Israeli parliament) passed the Egg Donation in Israel Act, which made it legal for women who had not themselves undergone fertility treatment to donate their eggs. Previously, the majority of women undergoing treatment chose to freeze their eggs for their own later use so as to avoid further painful procedures. As a result of the new law, the decision to go abroad for an egg donation now depends on supply and demand. However, as the local supply is very low, and the law limits surrogacy to infertile heterosexual couples, many Israelis continue to consider undergoing these procedures elsewhere (Bassan & Michaelsen, 2013).

In light of this situation, Bassan and Michaelsen (2013) examined the attitude of the Israeli and German media to couples who choose to undergo ART procedures outside their own country. Analysis of the use of the term "reproductive tourism" in the popular media in the two countries revealed that its meaning was dependent on the target audience. Two opposing attitudes were expressed. The first, representing the critics, employed "tourism" as an economic term. The second, representing the suppliers of the service, employed "tourism" to refer to the effort saved by potential clients should they choose to take advantage of the service. Thus, although the two attitudes promote different values, they make use of the same term, whether the aim is to generate social change, such as making the service legal and accessible for the entire population, or to normalize and trivialize it. The authors conclude that in both Israel and Germany, the media does not use the word "tourism" to portray travel to another country in this context as a pleasure trip, but to symbolize and criticize the economic aspects of the international reproductive industry. The couples who go abroad for ART treatments do not employ the term themselves, and it is likely that they would be offended by being labelled "reproductive tourists."

5.9 Reproductive Policy in Israel

Israel is an excellent arena for the study of all matters relating to fertility treatment (Birenbaum-Carmeli & Dirnfeld, 2008; Shalev & Lemish, 2012), including its representation in the media, due primarily to its unique reproductive policy. Although the infertility rate is no higher in Israel than in other Western countries (Shalev & Lemish, 2012), the state almost fully subsidizes IVF until the birth of two children for any heterosexual couple or single mother (Bassan & Michaelsen, 2013; Birenbaum-Carmeli & Dirnfeld, 2008). These treatments are part of the basic services dispensed by law by the country's Health Maintenance Organizations (HMOs), which provide health insurance to all citizens.

This unusual policy is grounded in history, religion, and politics (Shalev & Lemish, 2012). In terms of history, one of the most telling factors is the national trauma of the Holocaust. When the State of Israel was established immediately after the attempt to exterminate the whole of the Jewish people and the virtually inconceivable loss of six million Jews, there was a sense of urgency to create new life to replace that which had been taken away (Shalev & Lemish, 2012). Having children and raising a family was perceived to be the best response to the Nazi atrocities. A further element underlying reproductive policy in Israel is Jewish tradition. The Biblical injunction to "be fruitful and multiply" (Genesis 1:28) is one of the most deeply rooted religious commandments in Israeli society, and defines a high birth rate as a major objective of the Jewish people. Furthermore, Jewish tradition is an integral part of the country's politics, of which one factor influencing reproductive policy is the constant threat to Israel's existence. This has given rise to a "demographic race" aimed at preserving and ensuring a Jewish majority in the country (Bassan & Michaelsen, 2013; Birenbaum-Carmeli & Dirnfeld, 2008; Shalev & Lemish, 2012).

The Zionist pronatalist ideology, whereby a high birth rate is a means of guaranteeing the continuation of the Jewish people and political survival of Israel, frames giving birth as a national mission entrusted to the bodies of Jewish women (Birenbaum-Carmeli & Dirnfeld, 2008), and motherhood as a public gender responsibility (Shalev & Lemish, 2012). In order to encourage this ideology, since the establishment of the state, mothers have been entitled to government benefits including a generous maternity grant, awards to mothers of large families, legal protection for the employment rights of mothers, tax benefits, and so on (Birenbaum-Carmeli & Dirnfeld, 2008).

Not only is the generous subsidization of ART in Israel unusual, but the relevant legislation is also unique. Israel is the only country in the world to have a surrogacy law that gives the government control and regulation of surrogacy contracts via a public committee (Hashiloni-Dolev, 2006). In addition, as noted above, a law regarding egg donations was enacted in 2010 stipulating that the government will subsidize ART for women up to the age of 45 using their own eggs, and up to the age of 54 using donor eggs (Shalev & Lemish, 2012). Given these circumstances, which directly encourage women to give birth by making ART readily accessible and offering benefits to mothers, Israel holds the world record for fertility treatments administered. The number of treatment cycles and fertility clinics per capita is higher than anywhere else in the West (Shalev & Lemish, 2012), making Israeli women the greatest consumers of ART (particularly IVF) worldwide (Birenbaum-Carmeli & Dirnfeld, 2008).

5.10 ART in the Israeli Media

The review of the literature reveals that most of the media coverage of ART in Israel has been positive. The results of the study by Shalev and Lemish (2012) show that the Israeli media consistently contributed to the encouragement of fertility treatment and framed infertility as a temporary condition. The decision not to undergo treatment was framed as anomalous, and the absence of coverage of women who made this choice defined it as negligible. Moreover, the study indicated that while delaying childbirth was presented as a major cause of infertility, late pregnancies were framed as an admirable choice. Women who gave birth late in life were represented as mature, stable, and ready for motherhood, and the doctors who made it possible as heroes.

These results are reflected in a study conducted among 410 Israeli BA students (Hashiloni-Dolev et al., 2011), which found that most of them had misconceptions about the chances of conceiving at a later age (after 35) and of genetic motherhood at a very late age. Only 11% of the participants knew that it was unlikely for a woman in her mid-forties to become pregnant naturally and genetically, and that it required the use of eggs retrieved at an earlier age and then frozen. It is reasonable to assume that the optimistic attitude of the students derived, at least in part, from the extensive media coverage of such women, which largely refrained from reporting the difficulties and implications of the procedure. According to a study conducted several years earlier (Birenbaum-Carmeli & Dirnfeld, 2008), even women undergoing treatment themselves were lacking in information, perhaps also as a result of the voids in the media coverage. The only negative coverage was found in the study by Bassan and Michaelsen (2013) in regard to the metaphoric meaning of the term "reproductive tourism" (which was also given a positive meaning in certain cases) and the claim that it encouraged the objectification of women.

Thus, research shows that the large majority of media coverage in Israel frames ART in a positive light. This approach diverts attention away from the risks involved, promotes a pronatalist biomedical attitude, and limits criticism of the country's reproductive policy (Hashiloni-Dolev et al., 2011; Shalev & Lemish, 2012). Studies conducted in other countries have yielded different results. Some found that the media took on the role of responsible adult cautioning against misguided notions of ART (Graham & Rich, 2014; Michelle, 2007; Radkowska-Walkowicz, 2012; Sterling, 2013), reprimanding women who deliberately postpone motherhood (Graham & Rich, 2014; Greil et al., 2011; Shaw & Giles, 2009), and calling on women to give birth at a young age (Lahad & Madsen, 2016; Sterling, 2013).

It is important to note that, on the whole, the Israeli studies presented here are not as current as those conducted in other countries. It is possible that recent years have seen a change in the framing of ART in the Israeli media, bringing it more in line with that found elsewhere. To the best of our knowledge, no existing comprehensive study analyzed the representation of ART in the Israeli media in the last five years. The current study aimed to fill that gap.

5.11 The Current Study

The study adopted the critical discourse approach of Machin and Mayr (2012) in an effort to characterize the representation of the issue of fertility in general, and fertility treatment in particular, in the Israeli media in the past five years. Machin and Mayr suggest tools for examining the linguistic and visual semiotic choices in journalistic texts that convey ideological messages. According to the authors, the connotations aroused by the words in a text are of special importance. In particular, they point to words whose connotations relate to the business world, such as "innovation," "competition," and "strategy." The use of terms belonging to what they call "corporate-speak," a discourse associated in our mind with the glamorous world of successful corporations, often hides actual problems in reality, and thus their potential solution as well. This approach is in line with the Cognitive Metaphor Theory of Lakoff and Johnson (2003), whereby we tend to conceive of major concepts in one domain through their similarity to concepts in another domain. Thus, for example, we speak of economic "growth," a concept taken from the natural world, implying that, like nature, the economy is unpredictable and not controlled by human decisions. Other semiotic strategies include over wordiness, the sparsity or absence of words, structural contrasts, and the use of the words of experts and professionals to support the text.

5.11.1 Corpus and Procedure

Both the print and electronic data banks of major media organizations in Israel were searched for news items and articles from 2012–2017 dealing with fertility treatment. A total of 215 relevant items were found. Of these, 44 were excluded as they were copied from items published by the same organization in another media, and an additional four because they referred the reader to a video clip. The final corpus therefore consisted of 167 items, about half from the daily newspaper *Yedioth Ahronoth* (56 from the print version and 22 from the electronic version), 57 from the Mako Internet site belonging to the TV station Channel 2, 14 from the Nana10 site belonging to TV's Channel 10, and 18 from the daily paper *Israel Hayom*.

5.11.2 Method

Employing the principles of media discourse analysis described above, the researchers looked for both linguistic metaphors and expressions and visual images in the texts. Each of the researchers individually categorized the metaphors and images identified according to the domain to which they belong. A comparison was then conducted between the analyses to validate the division into categories.

5.11.3 Results

Five major themes emerged from the analysis of the linguistic expressions identified in the media items relating to fertility treatment. The first is *age and timing of treatment*, e.g., "a grandmother's baby"; "orphaned by age"; "she didn't find the time"; "risks of older age"; "late blessing." The second theme was a *positive attitude toward treatment*, e.g., "treatment of hope"; "sparks of hope"; "childless women succeeded in giving birth"; "a miracle happened"; "pride in the team effort." The third theme was allusions to the world of *Jewish religious law or Israeli culture*, e.g., "in sorrow thou shalt bring forth children"; "goodness for the good"; "to be a blond people in our land" (a play on the words of the national anthem "to be a free people in our land); "a man gets conception" (a play on the words of a popular song, "a man gets lost"). The fourth theme was reference to the *natural world*, e.g., "the global sperm crisis"; "wild sperm"; "it was like lightning struck"; "a cloud of silence"; "nature has its own laws"; "creating where nature decided not to create."

The fifth theme, found to be the most common, was *corporate-speak*, e.g., "Israel is a vault of frozen embryos"; "the uterus decided to take early retirement"; "a baby at a reasonable price"; "the cost of the pregnancy"; "the egg market"; "egg recession"; "baby bank"; "baby factory"; "they can change sorrow into a Lamborghini." Corporate-speak is also reflected in the words of Israeli celebrities. Thus, for example, in an interview with the actor Alon Neuman, he stated, "Israeli society conveys the sense that one or two kids isn't okay. You need more and more. It's like an obsession. Instead of looking at the kid, teaching him, you go straight on to the new one. It's like a cellphone. You haven't yet figured out all its features and you already want the new model."

The linguistic expressions were accompanied by visual images, with the most prominent being photos of couples, women, and doctors in white coats performing medical procedures. The most common image was a clock in one form or another: an hourglass, a clock on a pregnant belly, a woman holding a clock, and so on.

5.11.4 Discussion

This study of Israeli coverage of fertility issues in the past five years found that one of the main themes in the media in Israel, similar to elsewhere in the world, is the connection between a woman's age and her fertility. The issue is reflected both in linguistic expressions such as "she didn't find the time," and in visual images such as an hourglass. Another prominent message conveyed by the media is the lack of control associated with fertility treatment, which is expressed primarily in phrases taken from the natural world, such as "nature has its own laws." Moreover, the language indicates domains in which the individual has a certain degree of control, as opposed to those in which we are relatively defenseless against the forces of nature. The images of doctors in white coats holding medical instruments communicate a similar idea. As only the doctors have the necessary knowledge, authority rests solely in their hands, while their patients are generally presented as powerless.

The most significant finding of the study is the extensive use of corporate-speak. In the context of Israeli society, corporate-speak in reference to fertility treatment is highly relevant in view of the country's unique reproductive policy The use of words like "bank," "factory," "market," and "vault," taken from the business world, highlights the paternalistic attitude of the establishment to fertility and childbirth, along with the responsibility Israeli society takes on itself by adopting a pronatalist policy. The Israeli media thus displays a functionalist approach, cooperating with the establishment by the use of metaphors drawn from corporate-speak, references to Jewish religion and Israeli culture, and positive expressions implying hope. Moreover, it serves as a mouthpiece for the establishment by urging women not to put off having children and is critical of those who choose to start a family at an older age.

5.12 Conclusion and Recommendations

The first part of this chapter reviewed the way in which fertility and fertility treatment are presented by the media around the world. One of the most obvious conclusions to be drawn from this review is the link between the nature of a given society and local media coverage. As we have seen, the more a society encourages childbirth, the more functional the media coverage, whereas the more the society allows men and women to make their own decisions and does not take a stand in regard to their fertility, the more critical the coverage. In Israel, which is both a pronatalist and a liberal society, media coverage appears to be mixed. While it is largely functional, critical voices are also heard.

This chapter has sought to contribute to our understanding of how the media reflects social expectations in respect to fertility and fertility treatment. The mixed approach that emerged from a study of the Israeli media in recent years is in line with the growing trend in Israel to regard fertility and childbirth as personal issues rather than social norms. Future studies might compare media items in Israel with those elsewhere in the world in an attempt to identify the linguistic and visual discourse, as well as the connection between the media discourse and the public discourse, in different societies. Furthermore, it would be interesting to examine how public attitudes to fertility, pregnancy, and childbirth are influenced by the nature of media reports in a given society.

References

Bassan, S., & Michaelsen, M. A. (2013). Honeymoon, medical treatment or bibusiness? An analysis of the meanings of the term "reproductive tourism" in German and Israeli public media discourses. *Philosophy, Ethics, and Humanities in Medicine, 8,* 9.

Birenbaum-Carmeli, D., & Dirnfeld, M. (2008). In vitro fertilisation policy in Israel and women's perspectives: The more the better? *Reproductive Health Matters, 16*(31), 182–191.

Brown, J. A., & Ferree, M. M. (2005). Close your eyes and think of England: Pronatalism in the British print media. *Gender & Society, 19*(1), 5–24.

Carolan, M. (2005). 'Doing it properly': The experience of first mothering over 35 years. *Health Care for Women International, 26*(9), 764–787.

Crawshaw, M., Blyth, E., & van den Akker, O. (2012). The changing profile of surrogacy in the UK: Implications for national and international policy and practice. *Journal of Social Welfare Family Law, 34*(3), 267–277.

Edge, B. W. (2014). Infertility on E!: Assisted reproductive technologies and reality television. *Feminist Media Studies, 14*(5), 873–876.

Graham, M., & Rich, S. (2014). Representations of childless women in the Australian print media. *Feminist Media Studies, 14*(3), 500–518.

Greil, A., McQuillan, J., & Slauson-Blevins, K. (2011). The social construction of infertility. *Sociology Compass, 5*(8), 736–746.

Hashiloni-Dolev, Y. (2006). Genetic Counseling for Sex Chromosome Anomalies (SCAs) in Israel and Germany: Assessing medical risks according to the importance of fertility in two cultures. *Medical Anthropology Quarterly, 20*(4), 469–486.

Hashiloni-Dolev, Y., Kaplan, A., & Shkedi-Rafid, S. (2011). The fertility myth: Israeli students' knowledge regarding age-related fertility decline and late pregnancies in an era of assisted reproduction technology. *Human Reproduction, 26*(11), 3045–3053.

Jaworski, B. K. (2009). Reproductive justice and media framing: A case-study analysis of problematic frames in the popular media. *Sex Education, 9*(1), 105–121.

Keehn, J., Howell, E., Sauer, M. V., & Klitzman, R. (2015). How agencies market egg donation on the Internet: A qualitative study. *The Journal of Law, Medicine & Ethics, 43*(3), 610–618.

Lahad, K., & Madsen, K. H. (2016). "Like having new batteries installed!": Problematizing the category of the "40+ mother" in contemporary Danish media. *NORA-Nordic Journal of Feminist and Gender Research, 24*(3), 181–195.

Lakoff, G., & Johnson, M. (2003). *Metaphors we live by*. Chicago: University of Chicago Press.

Lewis, J. (2004). The meaning of real life. In L. Ouellette & S. Murray (Eds.), *Reality TV: Remaking Television Culture* (pp. 288–302). New York: NYU Press.

Liu, K., Case, A., Cheung, A. P., Sierra, S., Alasiri, S., Carranza-Mamane, B., … Wong, B. C. (2012). Advanced reproductive age and fertility. *International Journal of Gynecology and Obstetrics, 117,* 95–102.

Machin, D., & Mayr, A. (2012). *How to do critical discourse analysis*. London: Sage.

McQuail, D. (2010). *Mass communication theory* (6th ed.). Beverley Hills, CA: Sage.

Michelle, C. (2007). Human clones talk about their lives: Media representations of assisted reproductive and biogenetic technologies. *Media, Culture and Society, 29*(4), 639–663.

Mosalanejad, L., Parandavar, N., Gholami, M., & Abdollahifard, S. (2014). Increasing and decreasing factors of hope in infertile women with failure in infertility treatment: A phenomenology study. *Iranian Journal of Reproductive Medicine, 12*(2), 117–124.

Peddie, V. L., van Teijlingen, E., & Bhattacharya, S. (2005). A qualitative study of women's decision-making at the end of IVF treatment. *Human Reproduction, 20*(7), 1944–1951.

Piotrow, P. T., Kincaid, D. L., Rimon, J. G., & Rinehart, W. (1997). *Health Communication: Lessons from family planning and reproductive health.* Westport: Praeger.

Radkowska-Walkowicz, M. (2012). The creation of "monsters": The discourse of opposition to in vitro fertilization in Poland. *Reproductive Health Matters, 20*(40), 30–37.

Sangster, S. L., & Lawson, K. L. (2014). 'Falling down the rabbit hole': The construction of infertility by news media. *Journal of Reproductive and Infant Psychology, 32*(5), 486–496.
Sandoval, J. A. (2016). Labour pains: The birth of assisted reproductive technology policy in India. *Journal of Creative Communications, 11*(2), 119–134.
Scherman, R., Misca, G., Rotabi, K., & Selman, P. (2016). Global commercial surrogacy and international adoption: Parallels and differences. *Adoption & Fostering, 40*(1), 20–35.
Shalev, S., & Lemish, D. (2011). Women as consumers of reproductive technology: Media representation versus reality. *Journal of Interdisciplinary Feminist Thought, 5*(1), Article 2.
Shalev, S., & Lemish, D. (2012). "Dynamic Infertility": The contribution of news coverage of reproductive technologies to gender politics. *Feminist Media Studies, 12*(3), 371–388.
Shaw, R. L., & Giles, D. C. (2009). Motherhood on ice? A media framing analysis of older mothers in the UK news. *Psychology and Health, 24*(2), 221–236.
Sterling, E. W. (2013). *From no hope to fertile dreams: Procreative technologies, popular media, and the culture of infertility*. Dissertation, Georgia State University.
van den Akker, O., Camara, I., & Hunt, B. (2016a). 'Together… for only a moment': British newspaper constructions of altruistic non-commercial surrogate motherhood. *Journal of Reproductive and Infant Psychology, 34*(3), 271–281.
van den Akker, O., Fronek, P., Blyth, E., & Frith, L. (2016b). 'This neo-natal ménage à trois': British media framing of transnational surrogacy. *Journal of Reproductive and Infant Psychology, 34*(1), 15–27.
Zegers-Hochschild, F., Adamson, G.D., de Mouzon, J., Ishihara, O., Mansour, R., Nygren, K., … Van der Poel, S. (2009). The international committee for monitoring assisted reproductive technology (ICMART) and the world health organization (WHO) revised glossary on ART terminology. *Human Reproduction, 24*(11), 2683–2687.

Chapter 6
Health and Development of Children Born Following Assisted Reproductive Technology Treatments

Adel Farhi, Saralee Glasser and Liat Lerner-Geva

6.1 Introduction

The term assisted reproductive technology (ART) refers to all interventions that include the in vitro handling of both human oocytes and sperm or of embryos for the purpose of reproduction. This includes, but is not limited to in vitro fertilization IVF and embryo transfer (IVF-ET) and intracytoplasmic sperm injection (ICSI) (Zegers-Hochschild et al., 2017).

The first child was born following IVF in 1978 and since then there has been a steady increase in these treatments worldwide. In Israel, ART is funded by the Ministry of Health for the first two children, with no limit on the number of treatment cycles for women up to 45 years-of-age, and for oocyte donation up to age 54. Among the 38 members of the European ESHRE in 2013 the rate of IVF cycles per million women aged 15–45 ranged from 1207 in Moldova to 14,453 in the Czech Republic (Calhaz-Jorge et al., 2016). By comparison, the rate in Israel was higher by far, at 20,500 (Ministry of Health Israel Portal, 2017). Currently, 4.2% of all live births in Israel are conceived with ART.

Despite the wide use of ART treatments, there is still concern regarding its safety and effects on the children's physical health and emotional well-being. Two main types of concerns have been raised regarding the theoretical reasons for increased

A. Farhi · S. Glasser (✉) · L. Lerner-Geva
Women and Children's Health Research Unit, Gertner Institute for Epidemiology and Health Policy Research (Ltd.), Sheba Medical Center, Tel Hashomer 52621, Israel
e-mail: Saraleeg@gertner.health.gov.il

A. Farhi
e-mail: Dollyf@gertner.health.gov.il

L. Lerner-Geva
e-mail: Liatl@gertner.health.gov.il

L. Lerner-Geva
Sackler Faculty of Medicine, School of Public Health, Tel Aviv University, Tel Aviv, Israel

O. Taubman – Ben-Ari (ed.), *Pathways and Barriers to Parenthood*,
https://doi.org/10.1007/978-3-030-24864-2_6

risk for adverse short- and long-term outcomes: (a) those related to the technology itself, such as bypassing natural selection, use of medications for ovarian stimulation, exposure to biochemical agents in the culture medium, physical damage to the oocyte or sperm (in ICSI for which a single sperm is injected into the ovum), and damage during freezing or thawing processes; and (b) those related to the patients undergoing ART, including the cause and duration of infertility, maternal and paternal age, and chromosomal anomalies in the gametes used.

Short-term or adverse pregnancy and birth outcomes that have been found related to ART include higher rates of spontaneous abortions, pregnancy complications, such as gestational diabetes and preeclampsia, multiple births, prematurity, low birthweight and intrauterine growth retardation (i.e., small-for-gestational-age) (Qin et al., 2017), and congenital malformations (Hansen, Kurinczuk, Milne, de Klerk, & Bower, 2013). Longer-term concerns have been raised regarding childhood cancer (Hargreave, Jensen, Toender, Andersen, & Kjaer, 2013), autism spectrum disorders, attention deficit-hyperactivity disorder and developmental delay (Hart & Norman, 2013).

The following sections will focus on current findings regarding three of these potential adverse outcomes for children born following ART treatments:

1. The risk for congenital malformations
2. The risk for childhood cancer
3. Long-term growth, health and neurodevelopmental outcomes.

6.2 Congenital Malformations in ART Children

- Since the onset of ART treatments, concerns have been raised regarding the increased risk of congenital malformations (CM) (Sutcliffe, 2002). Over the years, studies have been conducted to clarify this concern, however the findings have been conflicting. As noted by Schieve, Ramussen, and Reefhuis (2005): "The inconsistency in results…is not surprising…studies are often plagued by one or more methodologic limitations." These include:
- Sample size—Both the exposure (ART) and the outcome (CM) are relatively rare, thus extremely large study samples are necessary in order determine conclusive findings.
- Definitions—Research studies have variously defined CM, with some including only major CM (fatal, causing severe impairment, or requiring surgery), or all CM as defined by the ICD-10.
- Timing of diagnosis–Many studies have reported only CM diagnosed at birth, while others consider diagnosis by a given age, which may not have been apparent at birth.

Despite these problems, a recent meta-analysis has concluded that accumulating data increasingly points to a positive association. Reviewing 57 studies involving nearly 120,000 infants conceived following ART, Qin et al. (2017) reported a relative risk of 1.33 (95% CI 1.24–1.43) for CM when compared to those who were spontaneously conceived (SC). Considering subgroups, the risk for those born following ICSI was greater than that for those born following IVF. This confirms findings of other meta-analyses investigating this issue (Hansen, Bower, Milne, de Klerk, & Kurinczuk, 2005; Rimm, Katayama, Diaz, & Katayama, 2004; Wen et al., 2012).

The largest Israeli study on this topic was a retrospective cohort study including 9,042 livebirths following ART and 213,288 SC livebirths during the period 1997–2004 (Farhi et al., 2013). The findings indicated an increased adjusted risk for all CM identified at birth in the ART group compared with SC [2.4% vs. 1.9%; ORadj. = 1.45; 95% CI 1.26–1.68] after adjusting for maternal age, ethnicity, education level, gender, and year of delivery. Increased risks were also observed in separate comparisons of IVF births versus SC [2.2% vs. 1.9%; ORadj. = 1.28; 95% CI 1.00–1.63], and ICSI births versus SC [2.46% vs. 1.9%; ORadj. = 1.56; 95% CI 1.31–1.84]. Although, the risk for CM was significantly higher in the non-Jewish population, this difference was probably related to the prevalence of consanguineous marriage, thus ethnicity was adjusted for in the multi-variable analysis. An interesting aspect of the Israeli research is that ART is covered by the National Health Insurance Law (as detailed above), thus the population undergoing ART is unselected and nationwide. Further, data on CM are collected routinely in a national birth registry, thereby reducing the possibility of ascertainment bias between the ART group and the reference group.

In addition to an increased risk for all congenital malformations, increased risks for organ-specific malformations have been reported, including circulatory system (Anthony et al., 2002; Katalinic, Rösch, & Ludwig, 2004; Klemetti et al., 2005; Koivurova et al., 2002; Olson et al., 2005; Reefhuis et al., 2009), cleft lip and cleft palate, digestive system (Reefhuis et al., 2009), hypospadias (Källén, Finnström, Nygren, & Otterblad Olausson, 2005; Reefhuis et al., 2009), and nervous system (Ericson, & Källén, 2001; Källén et al., 2005; Klemetti et al., 2005). In the Israeli study (Farhi et al., 2013), an increased risk was found for nervous, circulatory, digestive and genital systems in the ART-conceived singleton infants, similar to the findings of Koivurova et al. (2002). However, the study did not find an increased risk for chromosomal defects among ART-conceived infants, similar to reports of others (Davies et al., 2012; Källén et al., 2010a).

Regarding the underlying causes of the risk for CM, Olson et al. (2005) found a non-significant increased risk for malformations in pregnancies following insemination versus SC pregnancies, concluding that part of the increased risk for malformations is due to the infertility itself. Zhu, Basso, Obel, Bille, and Olsen (2006) attempted to untangle differences in risks associated with the technology and those associated with infertility per sê. A significant risk for malformations was evident among patients with infertility problems who conceived spontaneously and an even higher risk in the group that received infertility treatments, suggesting that infertility could be an independent risk factor in addition to the technology.

In summary, ART has been found to increase the risk for CM, with the risk somewhat higher in cases of ICSI than IVF. This risk may be due to characteristics of the parents and aspects of the infertility itself.

6.3 Cancer in ART Children

The potential for an increased risk for cancer among children born following ART has been the focus of attention, however most studies published to date included small sample sizes and short follow-up periods. Källén et al. (2010b) reported a significant hazard rate of 1.42 (95% CI 1.10–1.91), however Pinborg, Loft, Rasmussen, and Nyboe Andersen (2004) reported only borderline significance (OR 1.34 [95% CI 0.71–1.78]). In 2005, Raimondi, Pedotti, and Taioli (2005) conducted a meta-analysis of several studies, and reported a non-significant increased risk of childhood cancer associated with ART. In a 2013 meta-analysis, Hargreave et al. (2013) reported on a larger sample size and found childhood cancer significantly associated with maternal fertility treatments. An Israeli population-based cohort study reported a higher rate of neoplasms among children conceived after IVF or ovulation induction treatments (1.0/1000 person years), as compared to SC children (Wainstock et al., 2017). However, another Israeli study analyzing data from an historical cohort (Lerner-Geva et al., 2017) reported 21 cases of cancer in the ART group and 361 cases in the SC group (2.2 vs. 1.8 per 10,000 person-years, respectively), with the median age at diagnosis somewhat earlier for the ART group than for the SC group (4.6 $\pm$ 3.3 and 4.9 $\pm$ 4.8, respectively). Upon adjusting for maternal and infant characteristics, the relative risk for cancer in the ART group was elevated, but non-significantly 1.42 (95% CI 0.85–2.37). When singleton and multiple births were analyzed separately, a non-significant increased risk for cancer was also noted in the ART group. Williams et al. (2013) who conducted a historical cohort of over 100,000 subjects, also did not find a significant association between ART and childhood cancer.

Studies have reported a broad spectrum of specific cancers associated with ART.

Reigstad et al. (2016) found an increased risk for leukemia and Hodgkin's lymphoma among ART-conceived children. Akefeldt, Finnström, Gavhed, and Henter (2012) compared their historical cohort to the Brazilian population cancer rate, and reported a significantly increased risk for Langerhans cell histiocytosis among ART-conceived children. The meta-analysis of Hargreave et al. (2013) reported a significant risk for retinoblastoma (OR 1.62), similar to that found by Lerner-Geva et al. (2017). These findings are in contrast to a number of historical cohort studies that failed to find a significantly increased risk for this type of cancer (Källén et al., 2010b; Marees et al., 2009; Sundh et al., 2014; Williams et al., 2013). Interestingly, while Hargreave et al. (2013) noted an increased risk of hematological cancers, this was not noted in several other studies (Källén et al., 2010b; Lerner-Geva et al., 2017; Petridou et al., 2012; Sundh et al., 2014). The conflicting findings are likely due to differences in methodology and analysis.

Some factors that have been found to be associated with specific childhood cancers may be more prevalent among ART-conceived children (Kurinczuk & Bhattacharya, 2014), including very low birthweight, certain chromosomal abnormalities (e.g. Down syndrome, Trisomy 18, Turner syndrome and multiple births) (Heck et al., 2013; Stiller, 2004).

In summary, the results published thus far regarding the association of ART and childhood cancer are inconclusive. Two major problems in this type of research are: (a) the rarity of these multiple conditions makes it extremely difficult to accrue sufficient sample sizes; and (b) long-term follow-ups are necessary in light of the extended latency period of cancer.

6.4 Neurodevelopment of ART Children

A preponderance of the research on child outcomes of ART has been conducted on infancy and early childhood, thus studies following the children into middle childhood, i.e., into the early school years, are lacking and necessary to clarify longer-term neurodevelopmental outcomes. In addition to health, these include aspects such as cognitive, motor, and behavioral development. Below is a review of some of these issues that have received significant attention in recent literature.

Cognitive Development: The research considering ART with respect to cognitive development has produced mixed results. Some studies have reported that ART might actually have a positive effect on children's cognitive development. Comparing 423 children aged 8–17 conceived by IVF to national data, on the basis of parent interviews and test scores, Mains et al. (2010) reported that the IVF children had higher educational achievement. Specifically, they scored significantly above the national mean across all grades and subtests, and higher than their matched peers for grades 3–11. Leunens, Celestin-Westreich, Bonduelle, Liebaers, and Ponjaert-Kristoffersen (2006), studying 151 8-year-olds born following ICSI, found that compared to SC, they had higher IQ scores, although the effect was small and within the same range. Sacks et al. (2016) found that 4–5 year-olds who were born following IVF with preimplantation genetic diagnosis (PGD), an even more invasive procedure than IVF itself, had scores within the normal or above-normal ranges for all developmental outcomes. In a study of singleton ART children (IVF and ICSI), Punamäki et al. (2016) found no difference in parent reports of cognitive problems between that group and those in the SC group. However, interestingly, when analyzed by gender, the ART-conceived boys actually had fewer cognitive problems than did the SC boys, while the ART-conceived girls had more such problems than did the SC girls. This suggests that the role of gender-specific differences in ART should be considered.

On the other hand, some studies have indicated that conception by IVF or ICSI may be a risk factor for children's poor cognitive development. Sandin, Nygren, Iliadou, Hultman, and Reichenberg (2013) reported a non-significant increase of mental retardation in a Swedish population-based prospective cohort of 31,000 children born following IVF/ICSI compared to SC. Testing the IQ of 3–9 year old singletons born following ICSI, Knoester et al. (2008) found that cognitive development among this group was significantly lower than that of those born following SC, but there was no difference in the IQ categories (<85, etc.). Comparing IVF and ICSI children, Goldbeck, Gagsteiger, Mindermann, Strobele, and Izat (2009) did find slightly delayed cognitive development among the latter.

Despite these conflicting findings, there is a significant body of evidence indicating no negative impact of ART on children's cognitive functioning (Balayla et al., 2017). In a recent study, Schendelaar et al. (2016) found no difference in total IQ scores between children born following IVF compared to SC. Bay (2014) assessed the intelligence, attention and executive functions in 1,782 5-year-old singletons, and found no differences in test scores in children conceived following ART compared to SC. Similar findings were reported by Levy-Shiff et al. (1998) studying school-age children (mean age 9.7), as well as by Wagenaar et al. (2009a), who studied 9-18-year-olds, and by Halliday et al. (2014), who found no differences in educational achievement among IVF and SC who were 18–28 years old. These findings confirm those of a review of similar studies by Middelburg, Heineman, Bos, and Hadders-Algra (2008) who concluded that no increase in cognitive problems were documented in high quality studies of children born following IVF/ICSI.

Motor Development: Bay's (2014) large historical cohort study from the Danish registries indicated no significant difference in psychomotor development between ART and SC children. This confirms the findings of Leunens et al. (2006), who studied 300 8-year-old Dutch-speaking Belgian children born following ICSI and those of Knoester, Helmerhorst, van der Westerlaken, Walther, and Veen (2007), who found no difference in neuromotor development between children born following IVF and ICSI. Performance on the tests of visual-motor integration have also been found similar for children in ART and SC groups. Both Levy-Shiff et al. (1998) and Wagenaar et al. (2009b) found no differences between IVF and SC groups on these tests. In an international collaborative study of ART including five European countries, Ponjaert-Kristoffersen et al. (2005) found no differences in motor development between 5-year-old children conceived by IVF, ICSI or SC. Reviewing studies dealing with motor development of children conceived by ART, Zhan et al. (2013) found that in half of the studies motor development in the ART group was similar to those in the SC group, however some studies did find motor delay or poorer visual-motor competence among ART children. Here, too, it should be noted that studies variously dealt with IVF, ICSI and/or PGD groups.

Attention Deficit Hyperactivity Disorder: Beydoun, et al. (2010), in a study of 173 adults aged 18–26 born after IVF, found a marked increase in the risk of attention deficit disorder (27% compared to an expected 3–5%). In a large registry-based study in Sweden, Källén et al. (2011) found a weak but significant association between IVF and drug-treated ADHD, however the significance was not maintained when adjusting for length of involuntary infertility. Bay's (2014) Danish registry-based study found no significant association between ART and SC children in the rate of ADHD. Wagenaar et al.'s (2009b) findings confirmed this result in their sample of 8–18-year-olds, with no significant differences in either speed or accuracy of responses. It should be noted that their SC control group was comprised of children of subfertile parents, further highlighting the difficulty of comparing study findings.

Autistic Spectrum Disorder (ASD). Studies exploring the link between ART and autism or ASD, have reported inconsistent results. While Bay's (2014) Danish large registry-based study found no difference between ASD rates for ART and SC children, Maimburg and Vaeth's (2007) study, drawing from Danish registry records of 461 children aged 2–11 born after ART and matched controls, was the only study that reported a significant protective association of ART with diagnosis of infantile autism. They found a 59% decreased risk for developing infantile autism among children conceived after ART (odds ratio [OR] 0.41, 95% [0.19–0.89]) and a 63% decreased risk after adjusting for known risk factors (OR 0.37, 95% [0.14–0.98]). Finally, focusing on the few studies that report outcomes of children beyond early childhood, most have found ART to be neither a risk factor nor protective for autism or ASD. For example, in a Finnish study, Lehti et al. (2013) investigated over 4,000 children aged 2–16 born following ART, compared to over 16,000 children born of SC, and found no differences in rates of ASD overall, or in subtypes-child autism, Asperger's syndrome or other pervasive developmental disorder, and no associations were confirmed following adjustment for known risk factors. Sandin et al. (2013) also reported in a Swedish population-based cohort of 31,000 4–17-year-olds born of ART compared to 2.5 million SC, that there was no significant association with autistic disorder, even when analyzing by type of ART, type of embryo transfer (fresh or frozen), or sperm source. Similar findings were reported after adjustment for maternal age, birthweight, etc., in a Danish population-based study of Hvidtjørn et al. (2009) studying over 33,000 4–13-year-olds (median age 9 years) born after IVF/ICSI, compared to over 500,000 SC children. In a large population-based study in the U.S. Fountain et al. (2015) found that the rate of autism among ART children was not increased when only singletons were considered. Zachor and Ben Itzchak (2011) reported higher rates of ART among children diagnosed with ASD, compared to the general Israeli population (10.7% vs. 3.1%, respectively). It should be noted, however, that this study was cross-sectional and included children of a very broad age-range: 9 months to 18 years.

6.5 Summary and Conclusions

The majority of long-term outcome studies have observed no significant differences in health and developmental outcomes of assisted reproductive technology (ART) children, as compared to spontaneously-conceived children (SC). These findings are also confirmed by the multinational Evian Annual Reproduction Workshop Group (Fauser et al., 2014) that evaluated the impact of IVF/ICSI on the health of children born thereof, which concluded that despite variations in assessment scales, growth, development and cognitive function of children born after assisted reproductive technology are similar to those of spontaneously-conceived children.

However, while most have indeed not found significant associations, it is difficult to compile a cumulative body of data, due to several issues: study design, data source, differing follow-up periods; population-based vs. case-control study groups; specific comparison groups (IVF vs. ICSI; ART vs. SC, etc.); inclusion of twins; definitions of disorders (e.g., for autism/ASD the terms sometimes used interchangeably); confounders adjusted for; and ART-related independent variables, such as ET/FET/ovulation induction; infertility cause, source of sperm, duration of infertility, etc. It is hoped that the results of a comprehensive prospective long-term study will improve the quality of information given to those considering ART (Middelburg et al., 2008).

References

Akefeldt, S. O., Finnström, O., Gavhed, D. C. E., & Henter, J. I. (2012). Langerhans cell histiocytosis in children born 1982–2005 after in vitro fertilization. *Acta Paediatrica, 101*(11), 1151–1155.

Anthony, S., Buitendijk, S. E., Dorrepaal, C. A., Lindner, K., Braat, D. D., & den Ouden, A. L. (2002). Congenital malformations in 4224 children conceived after IVF. *Human Reproduction, 17*(8), 2089–2095.

Balayla, J., Sheehy, O., Fraser, W. D., Séguin, J. R., Trasler, J., Monnier, P., … Bérard, A. (2017). Neurodevelopmental outcomes after assisted reproductive technologies. *Obstetrics & Gynecology, 129*(2), 265–272.

Bay, B. (2014). Fertility treatment: Long-term growth and mental development of the children. *Danish Medical Journal, 61*(10), B4947.

Beydoun, H. A., Sicignano, N., Beydoun, M. A., Matson, D. O., Bocca, S., Stadtmauer, L., et al. (2010). A cross-sectional evaluation of the first cohort of young adults conceived by in vitro fertilization in the United States. *Fertility and Sterility, 94*(6), 2043–2049.

Calhaz-Jorge, C., de Geyter, C., Kupka, M. S., de Mouzon, J., Erb, K., Mocanu, E., … Goossens, V. (2016). Assisted reproductive technology in Europe, 2012: Results generated from European registers by ESHRE. *Human Reproduction, 31*(8), 1638–1652.

Davies, M. J., Moore, V. M., Willson, K. J., Van Essen, P., Priest, K., Scott, H., … Chan, A. (2012). Reproductive technologies and the risk of birth defects. *The New England Journal of Medicine, 366*(19), 1803–1813.

Ericson, A., & Källén, B. (2001). Congenital malformations in infants born after IVF: A population-based study. *Human Reproduction, 16*(3), 504–509.

Farhi, A., Reichman, B., Boyko, V., Mashiach, S., Hourvitz, A., Margalioth, E. J., … Lerner-Geva, L. (2013). Congenital malformations in infants conceived following assisted reproductive technology in comparison with spontaneously conceived infants. *The Journal of Maternal-Fetal & Neonatal Medicine, 26*(12), 1171–1179.

Fauser, B. C., Devroey, P., Diedrich, K., Balaban, B., Bonduelle, M., Delemarre-van de Waal, H. A., … Wells, D. (2014). Health outcomes of children born after IVF/ICSI: A review of current expert opinion and literature. *Reproductive Biomedicine Online, 28*(2), 162–182.

Fountain, C., Zhang, Y., Kissin, D. M., Schieve, L. A., Jamieson, D. J., Rice, C., et al. (2015). Association between assisted reproductive technology conception and autism in California, 1997–2007. *American Journal of Public Health, 105*(5), 963–971.

Goldbeck, L., Gagsteiger, F., Mindermann, I., Strobele, S., & Izat, Y. (2009). Cognitive development of singletons conceived by intracytoplasmic sperm injection or in vitro fertilization at age 5 and 10 years. *Journal of Pediatric Psychology, 34*(7), 774–781.

Halliday, J., Wilson, C., Hammarberg, K., Doyle, L.W., Bruinsma, F., McLachlan, R., … Amor, D. (2014). Comparing indicators of health and development of singleton young adults conceived with and without assisted reproductive technology. *Fertility and Sterility, 101*(4), 1055–1063.

Hansen, M., Bower, C., Milne, E., de Klerk, N., & Kurinczuk, J. J. (2005). Assisted reproductive technologies and the risk of birth defects - A systematic review. *Human Reproduction, 20*(2), 328–338.

Hansen, M., Kurinczuk, J. J., Milne, E., de Klerk, N., & Bower, C. (2013). Assisted reproductive technology and birth defects: A systematic review and meta-analysis. *Human Reproduction Update, 19*(4), 330–353.

Hargreave, M., Jensen, A., Toender, A., Andersen, K. K., & Kjaer, S. K. (2013). Fertility treatment and childhood cancer risk: A systematic meta-analysis. *Fertility and Sterility, 100*(1), 150–161.

Hart, R., & Norman, R. J. (2013). The longer-term health outcomes for children born as a result of IVF treatment. Part II–mental health and development outcomes. *Human Reproduction Update, 19*(3), 244–250.

Heck, J. E., Meyers, T. J., Lombardi, C. A., Park, A. S., Cockburn, M. G., Reynolds, P., et al. (2013). Case-control study of birth characteristics and the risk of hepatoblastoma. *Cancer Epidemiology, 37*(4), 390–395.

Hvidtjørn, D., Schieve, L., Schendel, D., Jacobsson, B., Svaerke, C., & Thorsen, P. (2009). Cerebral palsy, autism spectrum disorders, and developmental delay in children born after assisted conception: A systematic review and meta-analysis. *Archives of Pediatrics and Adolescent Medicine, 163*(1), 72–83.

Källén, B., Finnström, O., Lindam, A., Nilsson, E., Nygren, K. G., & Olausson Otterblad, P. (2010a). Congenital malformations in infants born after in vitro fertilization in Sweden. *Birth Defects Research, Part A: Clinical and Molecular Teratology, 88*(3), 137–143.

Källén, B., Finnström, O., Lindam, A., Nilsson, E., Nygren, K. G., & Otterblad Olausson, P. (2010b). Cancer risk in children and young adults conceived by in vitro fertilization. *Pediatrics, 126*(2), 270–276.

Källén, B., Finnström, O. O., Lindam, A. P., Nilsson, E. M., Nygren, K. G., & Otterblad Olausson, P. M. (2011). Is there an increased risk for drug treated attention deficit/hyperactivity disorder in children born after in vitro fertilization? *European Journal of Paediatric Neurology, 15*(3), 247–253.

Källén, B., Finnström, O., Nygren, K. G., & Otterblad Olausson, P. (2005). In vitro fertilization (IVF) in Sweden: Risk for congenital malformations after different IVF methods. *Birth Defects Research, Part A: Clinical and Molecular Teratology, 73*(3), 162–169.

Katalinic, A., Rösch, C., & Ludwig, M. (2004). Pregnancy course and outcome after intracytoplasmic sperm injection: A controlled, prospective cohort study. *Fertility and Sterility, 81*(6), 1604–1616.

Klemetti, R., Gissler, M., Sevon, T., Koivurova, S., Ritvanen, A., & Hemminki, E. (2005). Children born after assisted fertilization have an increased rate of major congenital anomalies. *Fertility and Sterility, 84*(5), 1300–1307.

Knoester, M., Helmerhorst, F. M., van der Westerlaken, L. A., Walther, F. J., & Veen, S. (2007). Matched follow-up study of 5 8-year-old ICSI singletons: Child behaviour, parenting stress and child (health-related) quality of life. *Human Reproduction, 22*(12), 3098–3107.

Knoester, M., Helmerhorst, F. M., Vandenbroucke, J. P., van der Westerlaken, L. A., Walther, F. J., & Veen, S. (2008). Cognitive development of singletons born after intracytoplasmic sperm injection compared with in vitro fertilization and natural conception. *Fertility and Sterility, 90*(2), 289–296.

Koivurova, S., Hartikainen, A. L., Gissler, M., Hemminki, E., Sovio, U., & Järvelin, M. R. (2002). Neonatal outcome and congenital malformations in children born after in-vitro fertilization. *Human Reproduction, 17*(5), 1391–1398.

Kurinczuk, J. J., & Bhattacharya, S. (2014). Rare chromosomal, genetic, and epigenetic-related risks associated with infertility treatment. *Seminars in Fetal and Neonatal Medicine, 19*(4), 250–253.

Lehti, V., Brown, A. S., Gissler, M., Rihko, M., Suominen, A., & Sourander, A. (2013). Autism spectrum disorders in IVF children: A national case-control study in Finland. *Human Reproduction, 28*(3), 812–818.

Lerner-Geva, L., Boyko, V., Ehrlich, S., Mashiach, S., Hourvitz, A., Haas, J., … Farhi, A. (2017). Possible risk for cancer among children born following assisted reproductive technology in Israel. *Pediatric Blood & Cancer, 64*(4), e26292.

Leunens, L., Celestin-Westreich, S., Bonduelle, M., Liebaers, I., & Ponjaert-Kristoffersen, I. (2006). Cognitive and motor development of 8-year-old children born after ICSI compared to spontaneously conceived children. *Human Reproduction, 21*(11), 2922–2929.

Levy-Shiff, R., Vakil, E., Dimitrovsky, L., Abramovitz, M., Shahar, N., Har-Even, D., … Fish B. (1998). Medical, cognitive, emotional, and behavioral outcomes in school-age children conceived by in-vitro fertilization. *Journal of Clinical Child Psychology, 27*(3), 320–329.

Maimburg, R. D., & Vaeth, M. (2007). Do children born after assisted conception have less risk of developing infantile autism? *Human Reproduction, 22*(7), 1841–1843.

Mains, L., Zimmerman, M., Blaine, J., Stegmann, B., Sparks, A., Ansley, T., et al. (2010). Achievement test performance in children conceived by IVF. *Human Reproduction, 25*(10), 2605–2611.

Marees, T., Dommering, C. J., Imhof, S. M., Kors, W. A., Ringens, P. J., van Leeuwen, F. E., et al. (2009). Incidence of retinoblastoma in Dutch children conceived by IVF: An expanded study. *Human Reproduction, 24*(12), 3220–3224.

Middelburg, K. J., Heineman, M. J., Bos, A. F., & Hadders-Algra, M. (2008). Neuromotor, cognitive, language and behavioural outcome in children born following IVF or ICSI-a systematic review. *Human Reproduction Update, 14*(3), 219–231.

Ministry of Health Israel Portal. (2017). *In-vitro fertilization (IVF) treatments 2013*. https://www.health.gov.il/English/News_and_Events/Spokespersons_Messages/Pages/14072015_1.aspx. Updated 2015. Accessed October, 28, 2017.

Olson, C. K., Keppler-Noreuil, K. M., Romitti, P. A., Budelier, W. T., Ryan, G., Sparks, A. E. T., et al. (2005). In vitro fertilization is associated with an increase in major birth defects. *Fertility and Sterility, 84*(5), 1308–1315.

Petridou, E. T., Sergentanis, T. N., Panagopoulou, P., Moschovi, M., Polychronopoulou, S., Baka, M., … Kieler, H. (2012). In vitro fertilization and risk of childhood leukemia in Greece and Sweden. *Pediatric Blood & Cancer, 58*(6), 930–936.

Pinborg, A., Loft, A., Rasmussen, S., & Nyboe Andersen, A. (2004). Hospital care utilization of IVF/ICSI twins followed until 2–7 years of age: A controlled Danish national cohort study. *Human Reproduction, 19*(11), 2529–2536.

Ponjaert-Kristoffersen, I., Bonduelle, M., Barnes, J., Nekkebroeck, J., Loft, A., Wennerholm, U. B., … Sutcliffe, A. G. (2005). International collaborative study of intracytoplasmic sperm injection-conceived, in vitro fertilization-conceived, and naturally conceived 5-year-old child outcomes: Cognitive and motor assessments. *Pediatrics, 115*(3), e283–289.

Punamäki, R. L., Tiitinen, A., Lindblom, J., Unkila-Kallio, L., Flykt, M., Vänskä, M., … Tulppala, M. (2016). Mental health and developmental outcomes for children born after ART: A comparative prospective study on child gender and treatment type. *Human Reproduction, 31*(1), 100–107.

Qin, J., Sheng, X., Wu, D., Gao, S., You, Y., Yang, T., et al. (2017). Adverse obstetric outcomes associated with in vitro fertilization in singleton pregnancies. *Reproductive Sciences, 24*(4), 595–608.

Raimondi, S., Pedotti, P., & Taioli, E. (2005). Meta-analysis of cancer incidence in children born after assisted reproductive technologies. *British Journal of Cancer, 93*(9), 1053–1056.

Reefhuis, J., Honein, M. A., Schieve, L. A., Correa, A., Hobbs, C. A., & Rasmussen, S. A. (2009). Assisted reproductive technology and major structural birth defects in the United States. *Human Reproduction, 24*(2), 360–366.

Reigstad, M. M., Larsen, I. K., Myklebust, T. A., Robsahm, T. E., Oldereid, N. B., Brinton, L. A., et al. (2016). Risk of cancer in children conceived by assisted reproductive technology. *Pediatrics, 137*(3), e20152061-2061.

Rimm, A. A., Katayama, A. C., Diaz, M., & Katayama, K. P. (2004). A meta-analysis of controlled studies comparing major malformation rates in IVF and ICSI infants with naturally conceived children. *Journal of Assisted Reproduction and Genetics, 21*(12), 437–443.

Sacks, G. C., Altarescu, G., Guedalia, J., Varshaver, I., Gilboa, T., Levy-Lahad, E., et al. (2016). Developmental neuropsychological assessment of 4- to 5-year-old children born following Preimplantation Genetic Diagnosis (PGD): A pilot study. *Child Neuropsychology, 22*(4), 458–471.

Sandin, S., Nygren, K. G., Iliadou, A., Hultman, C. M., & Reichenberg, A. (2013). Autism and mental retardation among offspring born after in vitro fertilization. *JAMA, 310*(1), 75–84.

Schendelaar, P., La Bastide-Van Gemert, S., Heineman, M., Middelburg, K. J., Seggers, J., Van den Heuvel, E. R., et al. (2016). Subfertility factors rather than assisted conception factors affect cognitive and behavioural development of 4-year-old singletons. *Reproductive BioMedicine Online, 33*(6), 752–762.

Schieve, L. A., Ramussen, S. A., & Reefhuis, J. (2005). Risk of birth defects among children conceived with assisted reproductive technology: Providing an epidemiologic context to the data. *Fertility and Sterility, 84*(5), 1320–1324.

Stiller, C. A. (2004). Epidemiology and genetics of childhood cancer. *Oncogene, 23*(38), 6429–6444.

Sundh, K. J., Henningsen, A. A., Källen, K., Bergh, C., Romundstad, L. B., Gissler, M., … Wennerholm, U. B. (2014). Cancer in children and young adults born after assisted reproductive technology: A Nordic cohort study from the committee of Nordic ART and safety (CoNARTaS). *Human Reproduction, 29*(9), 2050–2057.

Sutcliffe, A. G. (2002). *IVF children, the first generation: Assisted reproduction and child development*. London, UK: The Parthenon Publishing Group.

Wagenaar, K., van Weissenbruch, M. M., Knol, D. L., Cohen-Kettenis, P. T., Delemarre-van de Waal, H. A., & Huisman, J. (2009a). Behavior and socioemotional functioning in 9-18-year-old children born after in vitro fertilization. *Fertility and Sterility, 92*(6), 1907–1914.

Wagenaar, K., van Weissenbruch, M. M., Knol, D. L., Cohen-Kettenis, P. T., Delemarre-van de Waal, H. A., & Huisman, J. (2009b). Information processing, attention and visual-motor function of adolescents born after in vitro fertilization compared with spontaneous conception. *Human Reproduction, 24*(4), 913–921.

Wainstock, T., Walfisch, A., Shoham-Vardi, I., Segal, I., Harlev, A., Sergienko, R., … Sheiner, E. (2017). Fertility treatments and pediatric neoplasms of the offspring: results of a population-based cohort with a median follow-up of 10 years. *American Journal of Obstetrics and Gynecology, 216*(3), 314.e1–314.e14.

Wen, J., Jiang, J., Ding, C., Dai, J., Liu, Y., Xia, Y., … Hu, Z. (2012). Birth defects in children conceived by in vitro fertilization and intracytoplasmic sperm injection: A meta-analysis. *Fertility and Sterility, 97*(6), 1331–1337.e4.

Williams, C. L., Bunch, K. J., Stiller, C. A., Murphy, M. F. G., Botting, B. J., Wallace, W. H., … Sutcliffe, A. G. (2013). Cancer risk among children born after assisted conception. *The New England Journal of Medicine, 369*(19), 1819–1827.

Zachor, D. A., & Ben Itzchak, E. (2011). Assisted reproductive technology and risk for autism spectrum disorder. *Research in Developmental Disabilities, 32*(6), 2950–2956.

Zegers-Hochschild, F., Adamson, G. D., Dyer, S., Racowsky, C., de Mouzon, J., Sokol, R., … van der Poel, S. (2017). The International Glossary on Infertility and Fertility Care, 2017. *Fertility and Sterility, 108*(3), 393–406.

Zhan, Q. T., Pan, P. P., Xu, X. R., Lou, H. Y., Lou, Y. Y., & Jin, F. (2013). An overview of studies on psychological well-being in children born following assisted reproductive technologies. *Journal of Zhejiang University Science B, 14*(1), 947–960.

Zhu, J. L., Basso, O., Obel, C., Bille, C., & Olsen, J. (2006). Infertility, infertility treatment, and congenital malformations: Danish national birth cohort. *BMJ, 333*(7570), 679.

Chapter 7
Psychological and Ethical Issues in Third Party Assisted Conception and Surrogate Motherhood

Olga van den Akker

7.1 Introduction

The transition to parenthood is one of the most important milestones in an individual's life which for some can be associated with a huge amount of distress and discomfort. The experience of traumatic events pre-pregnancy (when an individual realizes s/he cannot conceive; when a pregnancy is not yet desired; when a conception fails), or during pregnancy (such as miscarriages, foetal abnormalities or death) and post-delivery (such as neonatal death, delivery trauma, post-natal depression or psychosis) can be life changing (van den Akker, 2012). These life changing experiences, many of which are described in the chapters within this book, can also be experienced during AC treatment which in itself is known to be psychologically taxing for many individuals experiencing it (Domar, 2015). AC using third party input such as mitochondrial, gamete, embryo donation and surrogacy add another layer of complexity.

7.2 Third Party Assisted Conception

Third party AC requires the assistance of a donor or surrogate and a team of professionals to bring about a pregnancy. It refers to a number of AC treatments and processes which includes another person's (the third party's) mitochondria, gametes or embryo and or a contracted surrogate mother to carry a genetic or gestational pregnancy to term for another person (van den Akker, 2012, 2017). This chapter is concerned with gamete donation and surrogate motherhood, although some of the issues addressed also apply to the more recent practices of mitochondrial donation,

O. van den Akker (✉)
Middlesex University, The Burroughs, Hendon, London NW4 4BT, UK
e-mail: o.vandenakker@mdx.ac.uk

O. Taubman – Ben-Ari (ed.), *Pathways and Barriers to Parenthood*,
https://doi.org/10.1007/978-3-030-24864-2_7

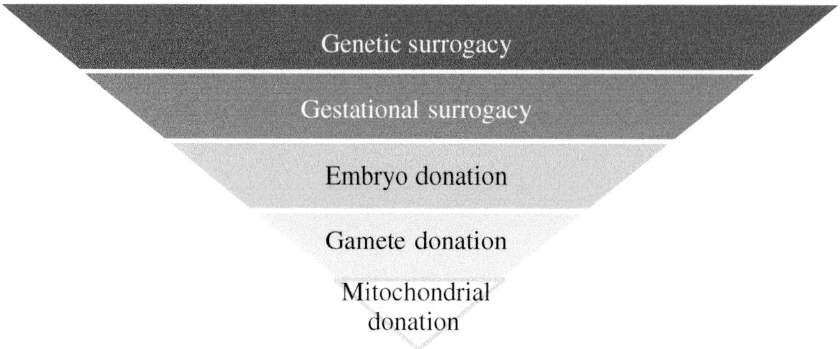

Fig. 7.1 The amount of third party genetic and gestational input provided and lost via third party AC, ranging from a pregnancy and oocytes belonging to the surrogate to at the other end of the scale, the addition of only third party mitochondria

(where the mother' faulty mitochondrial DNA is removed from her egg and replaced with healthy mitochondria from a donor egg). The amount of third party input necessary in building a family for recipients varies and is shown in Fig. 7.1. It also potentially relates to the loss of third party input or potential family members in those providing the third party input (Purewal & van den Akker, 2007).

7.3 Demand

Across the world in 2010, an estimated 48.5 million couples worldwide were unable to have a child after five years of trying (Mascarenhas, Flaxman, Boema, Vanderpoel, & Stevens, 2012) with many of them stigmatised in their communities (see for example, Bos et al., Chap. 4 in this volume). The demand for AC stems from the continuing desire for babies, preferably with a genetic or gestational link (van den Akker, 2007), and is also due to increasing numbers of individuals seeking AC against biological and social odds, such as women and men who are older, single or in same sex relationships (Carone, Baiocco, & Lingiardi, 2017). AC family units, like adoptive families, require parents able to disclose the use of third parties in their conceptions to ensure their children have accurate genetic and gestational information. In single and same sex parenting third party AC involvement is generally more obvious, but in heterosexual couples this is not always the case.

7.4 Open Versus Hidden Practices

Not all countries laws or their religions endorse third party AC practices. For example, Jewish religious authorities are generally 'pronatalist and gladly accommodate AC technologies' (Birenbaum-Carmeli, 2016, p. 16) whereas the Catholic Church although also pro-natal, does not condone third party conceptions (Chliaoutakis, Koukouli, & Papadakaki, 2002). In countries where third party AC is accepted it was (Barton, Walker, & Wiesner, 1945) and still is generally used for the benefit of the new parents with the genetic origins of the child never disclosed (Royal College of Obstetricians & Gynaecologists, 1987). Where third party AC is not accepted, people travel abroad and also often maintain secrecy about the child's origins. Since few countries monitor the numbers or origins of surrogate arrangements and gamete/embryo donations, and no records exist, the concern for the wishes of the parent(s) is adequately addressed but the welfare of the child's right to accurate genetic or gestational information is entirely ignored (Shidlow, 2011). In 2012, an Israeli public health committee recommended that since gay men and single women should be allowed to use a surrogate to have children, they also recommended non-anonymous sperm donation (Pritchard, 2012) as obviously single and same sex parents will have needed gametes and surrogates respectively. This marked a shift in line with other countries' consideration for the welfare of the child—albeit a relatively slow shift. Most countries continue to fail to consider the wider implications of third party AC on the donor or surrogate or on the person conceived.

7.5 Disclosure

Disclosure of information about third party assisted conception was recognised decades earlier by a number of other governments and sperm banks as more advantageous for the parties involved—including for the offspring (Blyth & Frith, 2015; Scheib, 2003), although some did not legislate for these changes until the turn of the century. Such changes in practice enabled donor-conceived individuals to understand their biogenetic (genetic/biological) information (Strathern, 2005), a part of their identity reported to be incomplete (Frith, Crawshaw, van den Akker & Blyth, 2017; van den Akker, Crawshaw, Blyth, & Frith, 2015), and also provided the opportunity for donors' to learn about the outcomes of their donation (Blyth & Frith, 2015; Raes, Ravelingien, & Pennings, 2013).

Access to accurate genetic information is increasingly important for health information (Harper, Kennett, & Reisel, 2016) and is a basic human right. The UK Government was the first to legislate for donors details and the outcomes of donations to be registered by the Human Fertilisation and Embryology Authority in 1991 (HFEA, state regulator) (Blyth & Frith, 2015), giving donor-conceived individuals the right to request non-identifying donor information from the HFEA from age 18 and in 2004, all prospective donors were required to agree to disclosure of their identity

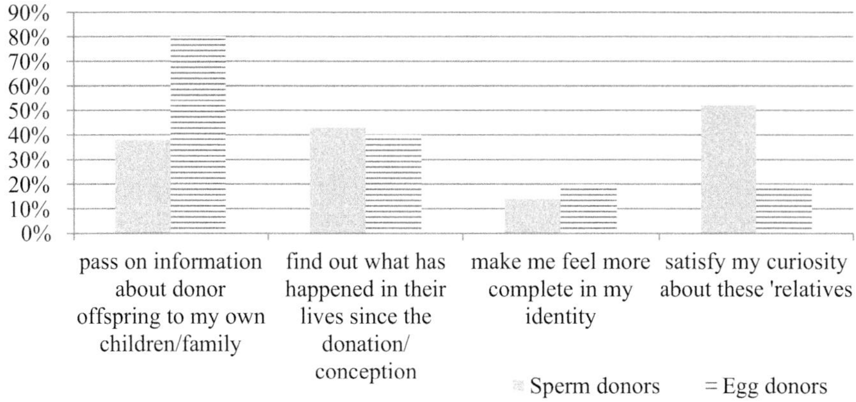

Fig. 7.2 Reasons for searching for genetic relatives. Adapted from Blyth et al. (2017)

(HFEA (Disclosure of Donor Information) Regulations 2004/1511). In a study of 21 sperm and 5 egg donors who registered on a voluntary DNA register for donors and donor conceived adult offspring, disclosure of information was welcomed by donors for very personal reasons (Blyth, Crawshaw, Frith, & van den Akker, 2017) as shown in Fig. 7.2. Family and identity also featured as reasons for disclosure for donor conceived adult offspring (van den Akker et al., 2015).

7.6 Fragmented Parenthood

Unlike gamete or embryo donation, in surrogate motherhood, the traditional motherhood/parenthood functions are more fragmented with the surrogate contributing to the prenatal, and the recipient parent(s) contributing to the postnatal epigenetic environments. Both epigenetic contributions can have life-long health effects upon the surrogate child (EpiHealth, 2016). The surrogate mother becomes pregnant (through AC as a gestational surrogate, or through insemination as a genetic surrogate) and carries, and then delivers a baby for another, usually infertile woman, or for a single man or heterosexual or gay couple who cannot achieve a pregnancy (the recipient or commissioning couple). The baby is usually handed over to the commissioning recipient(s) immediately or soon after birth (Sharma, 2006), who then raise it as their own. In gestational surrogacy, using in vitro fertilisation (IVF) treatment the embryo is entirely genetically unrelated to the surrogate mother, and may be (partly or fully) related to the commissioning couple or donors, and is transferred into the surrogates' uterus (American College of Obstetricians and Gynecologists, ACOG, 2008). The process requires medical intervention, and the resultant child could not exist without the explicit selection of gametes, the IVF process, the embryo transfer (ET) and the surrogate. In this case, the commissioning couple may be entirely genetically linked to the embryo or the embryo may come from donated gametes (ACOG, 2008), but the new intended couple were not involved in its gestation. The surrogate on the other hand, finds herself involved in a medical and technological conception, far removed from natural conception. The fragmentation of functions removes the historical reliability of motherhood; *mater semper est* (motherhood is always certain) is now no longer certain (van den Akker, 2017). Similar to the donor insemination trajectory, acceptability of surrogate motherhood is not universal.

7.7 Legal Parenthood

In most countries, parenthood is legally attributed to biological/birth motherhood because it was always certain, making the surrogate the legal mother. In gamete or embryo (and mitochondrial) donation, the 'route' to giving birth (origins of gametes/embryos from a third party) has no legal position. Consequently, in mitochondrial/gamete/embryo donation legal parenthood is bestowed upon the person giving birth, even if neither, only one or part of one of the new parents donated their own genetic material. The resultant children may never find out their true genetic origins unless they are accurately informed. In surrogacy, the surrogate birth mother is usually the legal mother of the child. The new commissioning parent(s) may or may not have contributed some or all of their genes to the resultant child. These parents, in for example the UK, need to apply for parental responsibility of the child, even if it is entirely genetically related to them. Legal parenthood is therefore not based upon genetic but birth parenthood as shown in Fig. 7.3a, b. The implications for the offspring are many fold since birth records tend not to show the true genetic or gestational origins. Importantly, depending upon differing national laws, the genetic and or gestational difference brought about via third party reproduction continues to be hidden, marginalized or denied (van den Akker, 2001, 2007). Parents create a new reality or script (Strathern, 2002) which has left many thousands of now grown up third party offspring with inaccurate family histories (Frith, Blyth, Crawshaw, & van den Akker, 2018).

Governments have a difficult task legislating for or against third party AC treatments as they need to consider current laws across many different departments (child welfare, human rights, birth registrations, legal parenthood, immigration, education and so on) and across different countries—each with their own complex national laws. In the USA the reproductive industry has been referred to as the 'wild west' of AC because of its 'relatively lax and sparse regulation' of third-party and AC transactions, as no federal legislation effectively regulates the rights and responsibilities of the parties involved including clinicians, intended parents, donors, surrogates, and donor-conceived children (Markens, 2016). In the UK on the other hand, many aspects of surrogacy have remained relatively unaltered over the course of several decades following the Brazier Committee in 1998 (Brazier, Campbell, & Golombok, 1998). The HFEA Act (2008) finally suggested changes to the ways legal parenthood can be ascribed in third party reproduction, taking into account changes to

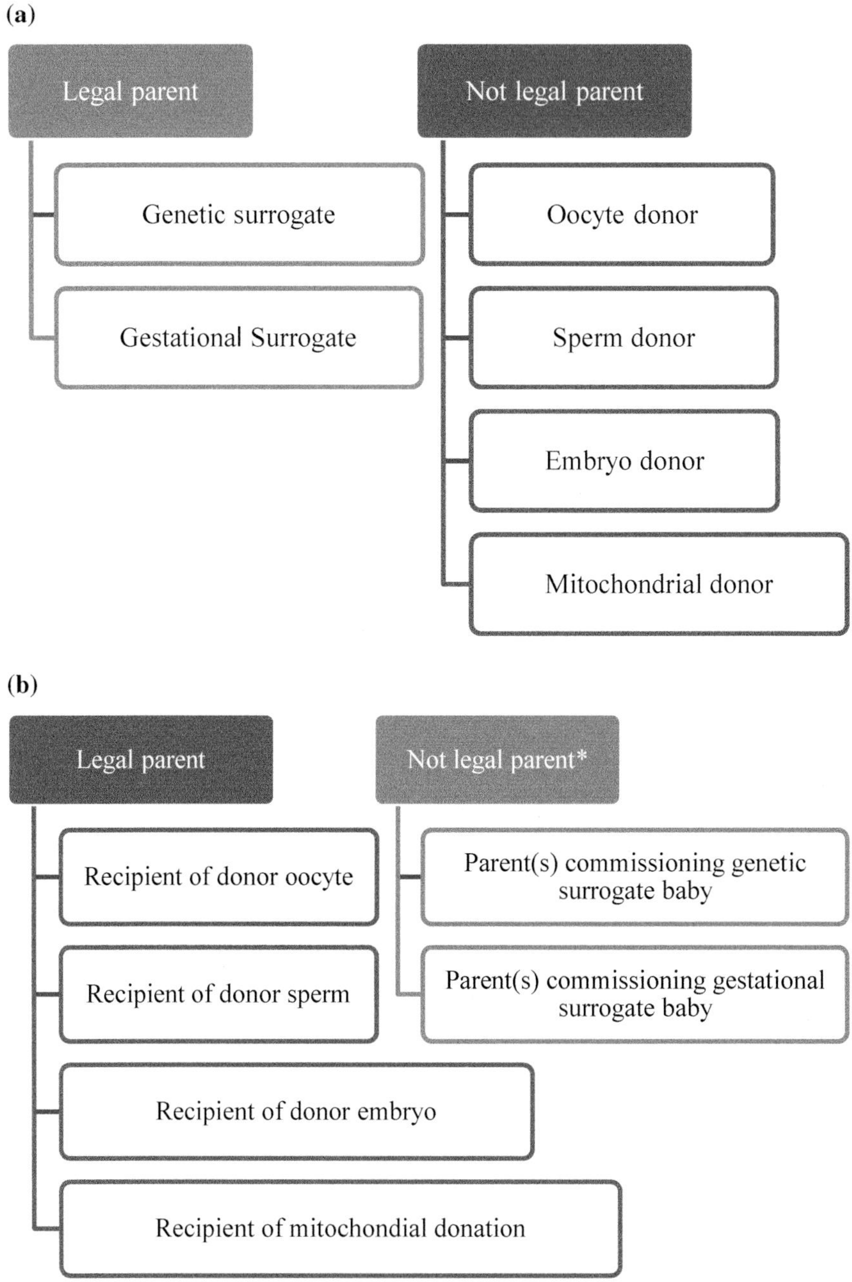

Fig. 7.3 **a** Legal and contributing parentage of third party conceived children in the UK, **b** legal recipient parentage of third party conceived children in the UK. *Until an application for parental responsibility is made

legal parentage for couples in civil partnerships and same sex relationships. Many countries still do not recognise any form of same sex relationships or for single men or women to wish to build a family, making cross border AC even more difficult to legislate for.

7.8 Commercialisation, Commodification and Inequalities

Third party AC is expensive and time consuming, involving a range of medical interventions to obtain the gametes, create embryos ex-utero and implant these into the mother requesting these or into a surrogate mother. In most countries, these expensive and time consuming treatment processes are (with few exceptions such as Israel) not freely available to all who need it. Third party AC and surrogacy are therefore generally only available to those who can afford these, which has led to substantial inequalities in access to these services world-wide. Such inequalities compound the marginalisation and stigmatisation of individuals who cannot have children (Inhorn & Serour, 2011; van den Akker, 2017). In countries offering commercially available third party reproduction the resultant children are therefore socially the children from relatively affluent parents. Genetically or gestationally they are the children of less affluent or extremely poor parents. The inequalities in access pose breaches in human rights and liberties. It also paves the way for the commodification of commissioning children, based upon the perceived quality of the donors and surrogates. Commercialisation and commodification open up opportunities for market forces delivering babies according to demand, a demand led by purchase preferences. It is unethical to treat human beings as resources to satisfy another person's interests (Orlov & Orlov, 2007) in the same way as it is unethical to partake in people trafficking, sexual exploitation or organ trafficking (Wilkinson, 2003). Some of these practices are known to exist under the pretence of surrogacy (van den Akker, 2017). Finally, commodification via eugenics or genetic selection of the perfect offspring (Pande, 2016) is also unethical.

7.9 International Commercialization

As surrogacy, gamete and embryo donation are not permitted in some countries, cross border opportunities offer an alternative route to obtaining a new born baby through surrogacy or to selecting gametes and embryos for own use (Ruiz-Robledillo & Moya-Albiol, 2016). It is always a commercial arrangement. Permissive laws, excellent English speaking clinics and cheaper services make cross border options attractive to Western individuals (Kumar, Inder, & Sharma, 2013). Commercial cross border surrogates such as those available in India, Thailand and Cambodia have been popular in the last decade, although new laws now prohibit Western couples' access to these surrogates. The Indian Surrogacy Bill 2016 for example proposed a ban on gay, foreign and unmarried couples and single people from using Indian surrogates. This proposed law, assumes Indian surrogates are not in control. It also discriminates against gay and single people (BBC, 2016). To date, it is estimated that more than 25,000 babies have been born through surrogacy arrangements in India many commissioned by Western commissioning couples (Shetty, 2012). The complexity of bringing home babies commissioned in another country (Crawshaw, Blyth, & van den Akker, 2012) add further fuel to the ethical and moral rights and wrongs of inequalities between the developed and developing nations. It potentially allows for the masking of the trafficking and buying of babies and the using and exploitation of poor women by those with substantially more wealth. Participating in arrangements which have been likened to baby 'factories' or 'farms' where poor (or abducted) women live to produce babies (Kroløkke & Pant, 2012; Kumar et al., 2013; Riggs & Due, 2010; van den Akker, 2017) cannot be condoned. Future generations resulting from such origins may wonder about the human costs of their conception.

7.10 Epigenetic Influences

Individuals conceived via surrogacy particularly if donor gametes are used, may also have been conceived under financially determined conditions, or via malpractice on behalf of unscrupulous brokers, donors, surrogates or clinics. Recently, a donor who was registered as 'handsome and healthy, with several degrees and a genius-level IQ' was in fact exposed as a convicted criminal and college dropout with schizophrenia. The 36 children born from his sperm were therefore at a genetic risk for schizophrenia (Stapleton, 2016 CNN news). The importance of genetics is increasingly relevant to third party reproduction. However, the importance of epigenetic influences—factors relating to the developing embryo's developmental flexibility to its environment including the quantity and quality of nutrient availability and the embryo/foetus's compensatory responses interacting with the delivery of the needs for the foetus (EpiHealth, 2016)—are not yet sufficiently considered in third party AC research, policy and practice.

Research into the outcome of genetic and gestational surrogate pregnancies considers the importance of pregnancy and live birth rates. Little attention is paid to the effects of the clinical 'in vitro' route to the pregnancy (Gardner & Lane, 2004) or the psychological state and physiological competence of the surrogate mother during the pregnancy which will contribute to determining the growth and wellbeing of the foetus. Surrogates are known not to attach to the foetus and their health behaviours, including drug, alcohol, dietary, smoking and exercise behaviours during the pregnancy will influence the foetus's epigenetic health and future wellbeing.

Although it is reassuring to know that malformations in gestational surrogate babies are comparable to those reported in the general population (Parkinson, Tran, Tan, Nelson, & Serafini, 1999) infertile couples using IVF or ICSI are at a greater risk of a number of adverse outcomes (Yeung et al., 2016). Premature deliveries (Koudstaal et al., 2000), pregnancy complications and low birthweight babies

(Schieve et al., 2002) have been reported. It is not yet known if factors related to the IVF techniques or prenatal factors are responsible for these adverse outcomes, since adverse outcomes are reportedly lower after surrogate pregnancies (Schieve et al., 2002). On the other hand, there is an association between oocyte donation and low birthweight, pregnancy complications and caesarean sections (Savasi et al., 2016). Since gestational surrogates undergo embryo transfer with 'donated' oocytes (from the commissioning mother or a donor) these pregnancies are likely to be at the same risks as oocyte recipients and their babies in IVF treated cycles. Finally, psychologically, not bonding with the foetus in pregnancy may benefit a surrogate and make the relinquishment easier (van den Akker, 2003, 2007), but the foetus is influenced by her (the surrogate's) behaviours and mental state. Some surrogates' behaviours may therefore have consequences for the developing foetus (Egliston, McMahon, & Austin, 2007; Ombelet, De Sutter, Van der Elst, & Martens, 2005) and these effects are under investigated in general (Purewal, Chapman, & van den Akker, 2017) and in surrogacy in particular.

7.11 Welfare Issues

Surrogate motherhood may disadvantage the child or surrogate mother (Agnafors, 2014), and ethical and legal complications have been reported in surrogate motherhood arrangements (Brinsden, 2003). There are also numerous reports indicating surrogates experience of surrogacy tends to be positive rather than negative and separation from the child is generally problem free. Neither do surrogate mothers show major psychological problems following the surrogacy arrangement (Jadva, Murray, Lycett, MacCallum, & Golombok, 2003; MacCallum, Lycett, Murray, Jadva, & Golombok, 2003; Ruiz-Robledillo & Moya-Albiol, 2016; Söderström-Anttila et al., 2016; van den Akker, 2003). Surrogate mothers are even reported to be empowered by the process (DasGupta & Dasgupta, 2014). Altruistic surrogates in particular, are happy with their choice and felt empowered by their surrogate experiences (Blyth, 1994; van den Akker, 2005). They reject some of the commodification arguments and assert their right to decide what to do with their own body (Bromfield, 2016). In Western contexts the main reasons that lead women to become altruistic surrogate mothers are not primarily financial, but a relatively altruistic desire to help others (Imrie & Jadva, 2014; Markens, 2012; van den Akker, 2003), although they do receive payment which they acknowledge as important.

Gestational surrogate children's psychological adjustment does not differ from naturally conceived children and the lack of the genetic/gestational link between the commissioning parent(s) and their child(ren) does not impact negatively upon parent–child relationships (Bos & van Balen, 2010; Golombok et al., 2006, 2011; Ruiz-Robledillo & Moya-Albiol, 2016; Shelton et al., 2009). There is some evidence that adjustment problems have been reported in surrogate children compared to children born through gamete donation (Golombok, Blake, Casel, Roman, & Jadva, 2012). Importantly, the surrogate's own children do not experience negative consequences after their mother's surrogate pregnancy and relinquishment of the baby in altruistic surrogacy (Jadva & Imrie, 2014). It is probable that support for all involved in third party AC is likely to be necessary in the foreseeable future, particularly where non-disclosure has been practiced (Crawshaw, Frith, van den Akker, & Blyth, 2016).

7.12 Summary

The competing interests and interactions between legal, organizational, health, personal, social, psychological and cultural issues in transitioning to non-biological and non-genetic parenthood are under explored. Third party assisted reproductive healthcare and surrogate motherhood services result in the creation of families with part or full genetic and gestational difference from the parent(s) seeking the services. Genetic and gestational differences in these families are often hidden. At the other end of the spectrum, biological and genetic (half) siblings and grandparents with partial or full genetic and gestational similarity are in too many cases denied knowledge of and nearly always, denied contact with the third party offspring. The psychological adaptation required to changes in public opinions, technology and legislation in third party reproduction and surrogate motherhood impacts at individual, societal and global levels. The evidence that some donors, surrogates, recipients and offspring demonstrate conflict or dissonance about their involvement in third party conception indicates a need to address these concerns in future research, policy and practice.

References

Agnafors, M. (2014). The harm argument against surrogacy revisited: Two versions not to forget. *Medicine, Health Care and Philosophy, 17*(3), 357–363.

American College of Obstetricians and Gynecologists. (2008). Surrogate motherhood. ACOG committee opinion No. 397. *Obstetrics and Gynaecology, 111,* 465–470.

Barton, M., Walker, K., & Wiesner, B. (1945). Artificial insemination. *British Medical Journal, 1,* 40–43.

BBC. (2016, August 25). India unveils plans to ban surrogacy. *BBC News*. Retrieved from http://www.bbc.com/news/world-asia-india-37182197.

Birenbaum-Carmeli, D. (2016). Thirty-five years of assisted reproductive technologies in Israel. *Reproductive Biomedicine and Society Online, 2,* 16–23.

Blyth, E. (1994). "I wanted to be interesting. I wanted to be able to say 'I've done something interesting with my life'": Interviews with surrogate mothers in Britain. *Journal of Reproductive and Infant Psychology, 12*(3), 189–198.

Blyth, E., Crawshaw, M., Frith, L., & van den Akker, O. B. A. (2017). Gamete donors' reasons for, and expectations and experiences of, registration with a voluntary donor linking register. *Human Fertility, 20*(4), 268–278.

Blyth, E., & Frith, L. (2015). Access to genetic and biographical history in donor conception: An analysis of recent trends and future possibilities. In K. Horsey (Ed.), *Revisiting the regulation of human fertilisation and embryology* (pp. 136–152). London: Routledge.

Bos, H., & van Balen, F. (2010). Children of the new reproductive technologies: Social and genetic parenthood. *Patient Education and Counselling, 81*(3), 429–435.

Brazier, M., Campbell, A., & Golombok, S. (1998). *Surrogacy review for health ministers of current arrangements for payments and regulation*. Report of the review team. Cm 4068. London: Department of Health.

Brinsden, P. R. (2003). Gestational surrogacy. *Human Reproduction Update, 9*(5), 483–491.

Bromfield, N. F. (2016). "Surrogacy has been one of the most rewarding experiences in my life": A content analysis of blogs by US commercial gestational surrogates. *IJFAB: International Journal of Feminist Approaches to Bioethics, 9*(1), 192–217.

Carone, N., Baiocco, R., & Lingiardi, V. (2017). Single fathers by choice using surrogacy: Why men decide to have a child as a single parent. *Human Reproduction, 32*(9), 1871–1879.

Chliaoutakis, J., Koukouli, S., & Papadakaki, M. (2002). Using attitudinal indicators to explain the public's intention to have recourse to gamete donation and surrogacy. *Human Reproduction, 17*(11), 2995–3002.

Crawshaw, M., Blyth, E., & van den Akker, O. B. A. (2012). The changing profile of surrogacy in the UK—Implications for policy and practice. *Journal of Social Welfare and Family Law, 34*(3), 267–277.

Crawshaw, M., Frith, L., van den Akker, O. B. A., & Blyth, E. (2016). Voluntary DNA-based information exchange and contact services following donor conception: An analysis of service users' needs. *New Genetics and Society, 35*(4), 372–392.

DasGupta, S., & Dasgupta, S. D. (Eds.). (2014). *Globalization and transnational surrogacy in India: Outsourcing life*. Maryland: Lexington Books.

Domar, A. (2015). Creating a collaborative model of mental health counselling for the future. *Fertility and Sterility, 104*(2), 277–280.

Egliston, K., McMahon, C., & Austin, M. (2007). Stress in pregnancy and infant HPA axis function: Conceptual and methodological issues relating to the use of salivary cortisol as an outcome measure. *Psychoneuroendocrinology, 32*(1), 1–13.

EpiHealth. (2016). http://www.epihealthnet.org/. Accessed 12/05/2016.

Frith, L., Crawshaw, M., van den Akker, O. B. A., & Blyth, E. (2017). Searching for 'relations' using a DNA linking register: Constructions of identity, relatedness and kinship by adults conceived following sperm donation. *BioSocieties*, 1–20.

Frith, L., Blyth, E., Crawshaw, M., & van den Akker, O. B. A. (2018). Secrets and disclosure in donor conception. *Sociology of Health and Illness, 40*(1), 188–203.

Gardner, D. K., & Lane, M. (2004). Ex vivo early embryo development and effects on gene expression and imprinting. *Reproduction, Fertility, and Development, 17*(3), 361–370.

Golombok, S., Blake, L., Casel, P., Roman, G., & Jadva, V. (2012). Children born through reproductive donation: A longitudinal study of psychological adjustment. *Journal of Child Psychology and Psychiatry, 54*(6), 653–660.

Golombok, S., Murray, C., Jadva, V., Lycett, E., MacCallum, F., & Rust, J. (2006). Non-genetic and non-gestational parenthood: Consequences for parent–child relationships and the psychological well-being of mothers, fathers and children at age 3. *Human Reproduction, 21*(7), 1918–1924.

Golombok, S., Readings, J., Blake, L., Casey, P., Marks, A., & Jadva, V. (2011). Families created through surrogacy: Mother–child relationships and children's psychological adjustment at age 7. *Developmental Psychology, 47*(6), 1579–1588.

Harper, J., Kennett, D., & Reisel, D. (2016). The end of donor anonymity: How genetic testing is likely to drive anonymous gamete donation out of business. *Human Reproduction, 31*(6), 1135–1140.

HFEA. (2004). *Disclosure of Donor Information Regulations 2004/1511*. http://www.legislation.gov.uk/uksi/2004/1511/pdfs/uksi_20041511_en.pdf. Accessed 23/11/2018.

HFEA Act. (2008). SCHEDULE 6 Amendments relating to parenthood in cases involving assisted reproduction. https://www.legislation.gov.uk/ukpga/2008/22/schedule/6. Accessed 23/11/2018.

Imrie, S., & Jadva, V. (2014). The long-term experiences of surrogates: Relationships and contact with surrogacy families in genetic and gestational surrogacy arrangements. *Reproductive Biomedicine Online, 29*(4), 424–435.
Inhorn, M., & Serour, G. (2011). Islam, medicine, and Arab-Muslim refugee health in America after 9/11. *The Lancet, 378*(9794), 935–943.
Jadva, V., & Imrie, S. (2014). Children of surrogate mothers: Psychological well-being, family relationships and experiences of surrogacy. *Human Reproduction, 29*(1), 90–96.
Jadva, V., Murray, C., Lycett, E., MacCallum, F., & Golombok, S. (2003). Surrogacy: The experiences of surrogate mothers. *Human Reproduction, 18*(10), 2196–2204.
Koudstaal, J., Braat, D. D. M., Bruinse, H. W., Naaktgeboren, N., Vermeiden, J. P. W., & Visser, G. H. A. (2000). Obstetric outcome of singleton pregnancies after IVF: A matched control study in four Dutch university hospitals. *Human Reproduction, 15*(8), 1819–1825.
Kroløkke, C. H., & Pant, S. (2012). "I only need her uterus": Neo-liberal discourses on transnational surrogacy. *NORA-Nordic Journal of Feminist and Gender Research, 20*(4), 233–248.
Kumar, P., Inder, D., & Sharma, N. (2013). Surrogacy and women's right to health in India: Issues and perspective. *Indian Journal of Public Health, 57*(2), 65–70.
MacCallum, F., Lycett, E., Murray, C., Jadva, V., & Golombok, S. (2003). Surrogacy: The experience of commissioning couples. *Human Reproduction, 18*(6), 1334–1342.
Markens, S. (2012). The global reproductive health market: US media framings and public discourses about transnational surrogacy. *Social Science and Medicine, 74*(11), 1745–1753.
Markens, S. (2016). Third-party reproductive practices: Legislative inertia and the need for nuanced empirical data. *Journal of Law and the Biosciences, 3*(3), 666–672.
Mascarenhas, M., Flaxman, S., Boema, T., Vanderpoel, S., & Stevens, G. (2012). National, regional, and global trends in infertility prevalence since 1990: A systematic analysis of 277 Health Surveys. *PLOS,* Dec 8th.
Ombelet, W., De Sutter, P., Van der Elst, J., & Martens, G. (2005). Multiple gestation and infertility treatment: Registration, reflection and reaction—The Belgian project. *Human Reproduction Update, 11*(1), 3–14.
Orlov, S., & Orlov, D. (2007). Commercial surrogacy: Commodification or choice? *University of Toronto Medical Journal, 84*(3), 177–179.
Pande, A. (2016). Global reproductive inequalities, neo-eugenics and commercial surrogacy in India. *Current Sociology, 64*(2), 244–258.
Parkinson, J., Tran, C., Tan, T., Nelson, J., & Serafini, P. (1999). Perinatal outcome after in-vitro fertilization surrogacy. *Human Reproduction, 14*(3), 671–676.
Pritchard, S. (2012). Israel gives gay men the right to conceive children via a surrogate. *BioNews,* 659.
Purewal, S., Chapman, S., & van den Akker, O. B. A. (2017). A systematic review and meta-analysis of lifestyle and body mass index predictors of successful assisted reproductive technologies. *Journal of Psychosomatic Obstetrics and Gynecology, 27,* 1–17.
Purewal, S., & van den Akker, O. B. A. (2007). The socio-cultural and biological meaning of parenthood. *Journal of Psychosomatic Obstetrics and Gynaecology, 28*(3), 79–86.
Raes, I., Ravelingien, A., & Pennings, G. (2013). The right of the donor to information about children conceived from his or her gametes. *Human Reproduction, 28*(3), 560–565.
Riggs, D. W., & Due, C. (2010). Gay men, race privilege and surrogacy in India. *Outskirts, 22.*
Royal College of Obstetricians and Gynaecologists. (1987). *Donor insemination.* London: RCOG.
Ruiz-Robledillo, N., & Moya-Albiol, L. (2016). Gestational surrogacy: Psychosocial aspects. *Psychosocial Intervention, 25*(3), 187–193.
Savasi, V. M., Mandai, L., Laoreti, A., & Cetin, I. (2016). Maternal and fetal outcomes in oocyte donation pregnancies. *Human Reproduction, 22*(5), 620–633.
Scheib, J. E. (2003). Choosing identity-release sperm donors: The parents' perspective 13–18 years later. *Human Reproduction, 18*(5), 1115–1127.

Schieve, L. A., Meikle, S. F., Ferre, C. C., Peterson, H. B., Jeng, G., & Wilcox, L. S. (2002). Low and very low birth weight infants conceived with use of assisted reproductive technology. *New England Journal of Medicine, 346*, 731–737.
Sharma, B. (2006). Forensic considerations of surrogacy—An overview. *Journal of Clinical Forensic Medicine, 13*(2), 80–85.
Shelton, K. H., Boivin, J., Hay, D., van den Bree, M. B., Rice, F. J., Harold, G. T., et al. (2009). Examining differences in psychological adjustment problems among children conceived by assisted reproductive technologies. *International Journal of Behavioral Development, 33*(5), 385–392.
Shetty, P. (2012). India's unregulated surrogacy industry. *The Lancet, 380*(9854), 1633–1634.
Shidlow, R. (2011). Of family and finance. Israeli citizens without rights and HFEA remuneration. *BioNews, 637*.
Söderström-Anttila, V., Wennerholm, U. B., Loft, A., Pinborg, A., Aittomäki, K., Romundstad, L. B., et al. (2016). Surrogacy: Outcomes for surrogate mothers, children and the resulting families—A systematic review. *Human Reproduction Update, 22*(2), 260–276.
Stapleton, A. C. (2016, April 20). Sperm donor lied about criminal and mental health history, lawsuit alleges. *CNN updated* 1407 GMT (2207 HKT). http://edition.cnn.com/2016/04/19/health/sperm-donor-criminal-mental-health-history/. Accessed February 2017.
Strathern, M. (2002). Still giving nature a helping hand? Surrogacy: A debate about technology and society. *Journal of Molecular Biology, 319*(4), 985–993.
Strathern, M. (2005). *Kinship, law and the unexpected: Relatives are always a surprise*. Cambridge: Cambridge University Press.
van den Akker, O. B. A. (2001). The acceptable face of parenthood: The relative status of biological and cultural interpretations of offspring in infertility treatment. *Psychology, Evolution and Gender, 3*(2), 137–153.
van den Akker, O. B. A. (2003). Genetic and gestational surrogate mothers' experience of surrogacy. *Journal of Reproductive and Infant Psychology, 21*(2), 145–161.
van den Akker, O. B. A. (2005). A longitudinal pre pregnancy to post delivery comparison of genetic and gestational surrogate and intended mothers: Confidence and gynecology. *Journal of Psychosomatic Obstetrics and Gynecology, 26*(4), 277–284.
van den Akker, O. B. A. (2007). Psychosocial aspects of surrogate motherhood. *Human Reproduction Update, 13*(1), 53–62.
van den Akker, O. B. A. (2012). *Reproductive health psychology*. London, UK: Wiley.
van den Akker, O. B. A. (2017). *Surrogate motherhood families*. London, UK: Palgrave MacMillan.
van den Akker, O. B. A., Crawshaw, M. A., Blyth, E. D., & Frith, L. J. (2015). Expectations and experiences of gamete donors and donor-conceived adults searching for genetic relatives using DNA linking through a voluntary register. *Human Reproduction, 30*(1), 111–121.
Wilkinson, S. (2003). The exploitation argument against commercial surrogacy. *Bioethics, 17*(2), 169–187.
Yeung, E. H., Sundaram, R., Bell, E. M., Drushell, C., Kus, C., Xie, Y., et al. (2016). Infertility treatment and children's longitudinal growth between birth and 3 years of age. *Human Reproduction, 31*(7), 1621–1628.

Chapter 8
Resilience to Prenatal Stress

Michael Ungar, Kristin Hadfield, Nicole Bush, Amélie Quesnel-Vallée and Igor Pekelny

8.1 Introduction

There is epidemiological evidence that women are particularly vulnerable to structural disadvantage, violence, and the burden of psychological and physical health concerns during pregnancy and during the period immediately afterwards (Burns, Farr, & Howards, 2015; Ward, Kanu, & Robb, 2017). These same biological, psychological and sociological challenges that women face pre- and postnatally can also influence the developmental trajectories of their children. Fetal in utero experiences are known to have long lasting effects on postnatal child development and health. While many children born to mothers that experience severe stress during pregnancy have more negative developmental outcomes, a surprisingly large number of children nevertheless thrive. Much of the focus to date in this field of study has, however, been on negative outcomes related to stress exposure in contexts of adversity and how these become biologically embedded in the foetus. Fortunately, there is

M. Ungar (✉)
Canada Research Chair in Child, Family and Community Resilience, Resilience Research Centre, Dalhousie University, Halifax, Canada
e-mail: Michael.ungar@dal.ca

K. Hadfield
Positive Psychology, Queen Mary University of London, London, UK
e-mail: k.hadfield@qmul.ac.uk

N. Bush
Center for Health and Community, University of California, San Francisco, California, USA
e-mail: Nicole.Bush@ucsf.edu

A. Quesnel-Vallée
Canada Research Chair in Policies and Health Inequalities, McGill University, Montreal, Canada
e-mail: amelie.quesnelvallee@mcgill.ca

I. Pekelny
Resilience Research Centre, Dalhousie University, Halifax, Canada
e-mail: igor.pekelny@dal.ca

O. Taubman – Ben-Ari (ed.), *Pathways and Barriers to Parenthood*,
https://doi.org/10.1007/978-3-030-24864-2_8

growing interest in the promotive and protective factors related to resilience that buffer or moderate the effects of exposure to a mother's stressed environment. In this chapter, we review the impact of mothers' stress exposure on mother and foetus, and subsequently on the child's epigenetics, gene expression, and emotional and behavioural development. We then review potential protective factors and processes related to resilience. Throughout, we will use a social ecological perspective of resilience that defines resilience as the result of multisystemic interactions that facilitate access to the resources required for optimal development (Ungar, 2011, 2012). By studying both mothers' contexts of adversity and the social ecologies of resilience, we will be able to recommend interventions that promote the protective factors and processes which are most likely to decrease the threats to both the capacity of mothers to prevent their children's risk exposure and the conditions that support positive development when risks are present.

8.2 A Multisystemic Understanding of Risk and Resilience

Given that threats to women during and after pregnancy arise from psychological, social and economic sources, it follows that promotive and protective processes should also be ecologically complex. Indeed, as other chapters in this volume show (see Ayers & Sawyer, Chap. 12; Scharf et al., Chap. 13 in this volume), there are many potentially traumatizing experiences that women are exposed to during pregnancy, birth, and during the postnatal period (Dikmen-Yildiz, Ayers, & Phillips, 2017). Most of these stressors are the result of suboptimal environments and could therefore be ameliorated through interventions and better social policies. In this respect, the resilience of mothers and their newborns is a function of the resilience of the multiple systems with which they interact (e.g., a women's relationship with an intimate partner; government policies related to health care; Sawyer, Ayers, Young, Bradley, & Smith, 2012). This description of resilience during pregnancy, childbirth and immediately afterwards is an example of the emerging science of resilience which describes positive development in stressful environments as a cluster of multisystemic processes in which co-occurring and nested systems respond to developmental risks by creating new regimes of behaviour (Masten, 2014). These adaptive regimes increase the viability of the focal system (in the present case, the mother and the newborn child).

Ungar (2011) has suggested that resilience needs to be understood in relation to people's interactions with both their social and physical ecologies and the opportunities individuals experience to navigate and negotiate for needed resources that are culturally and contextually relevant. This same systemic thinking is evident in work by researchers studying resilient environmental systems, community resilience, and other types of resilience in response to economic challenges (positive or negative), disasters and catastrophic events (Abramson, Park, Stehling-Ariza, & Redlener, 2010). Rather than focusing on dysfunction and problems exclusively, the concept of resilience broadens the focus of research to the protective and promotive factors that mediate the impact of social, economic, institutional and structural factors contributing to vulnerability (Southwick, Douglas-Palumberi, & Pietrzak, 2014). Given the many challenges that put women (and their children) at risk during and after pregnancy, it is reasonable to assume that the conditions that will protect women and bolster their capacity to cope well under stress will also largely depend on their experience of their social and physical ecologies. This ecological understanding of resilience shifts the focus from individual coping to the capacity of social and physical ecologies to create the conditions for resilience to occur.

Social ecological resilience may be especially relevant when considering biological processes that make it possible for external stressors to "get under the skin" and influence patterns of gene expression and neurological functioning. An ecological understanding of resilience challenges a discourse of resilience that emphasizes motivation to change, adaptation to one's attribution style, or individual changes to behaviour as the most important mechanisms for individual success when exposure to stress is abnormally high (see Ungar, 2015). These personal efforts to do well are unlikely to be sufficient to mitigate long-term exposure to risk if a women's environment continues to present threats to her and her child's optimal biopsychosocial development (Sternthal et al., 2009). A multisystemic understanding of resilience suggests that environments potentiate positive development in contexts of adversity when resources are sufficient to trigger healthy biological, psychological and social reactions to stress. Individual resilience is always dependent to some extent upon the quality of external resources (Masten, 2014). Indeed, the term resilience has been misused as a way of blaming victims of oppression and violence for the persistence of their problems (i.e., if someone does not thrive, it must be her fault). Women and children's positive adaptation during and after pregnancy, however, are far more likely to result from social bonding, better communication between caregivers, the quality of the mother and child's neighbourhood, a mother's educational opportunities, as well as individual traits including stress- and adaptation-related physiology, when these are triggered by supportive environments (Stein et al., 2000; Ungar, 2015; Walsh, 2016).

Recently, resilience research has become more sophisticated and the modelling more complex. Research on differential susceptibility to stressors (such as parental neglect) and the protective factors that decrease that susceptibility (e.g., a kinship network) at biological, psychological and family levels (Bush & Boyce, 2014) suggests that phenotypical protective factors like sensitivity to one's environment may enhance one's capacity to succeed in a low risk environment but increase one's risk of failure when risk exposure is high. Genotypical features are similarly variable (Belsky & Pluess, 2009; Pluess, 2015). Meanwhile, there is emerging evidence for the differential impact of the environment on populations under stress (Ungar, 2017). In higher risk contexts, some protective factors such as out-of-home placement for children when there is intimate partner violence (IPV) may be highly beneficial, while a similar placement can be neutral or even potentially harmful when risk exposure is low (Rutter, 2013). Both theories of differential susceptibility and differential impact suggest the need for greater specificity with regard to which biological and social factors at what dosage are protective against which stressors at different points during pregnancy and afterwards throughout a child's life.

With this complexity in mind, we will explore in detail the stressors that affect women and children pre- and postnatally, as well as the potential protective factors and processes that are the most likely candidates to positively influence development when the environment is suboptimal.

8.3 Threats to Women's Health During Pregnancy

Pregnancy is a highly stressful time, during which women must cope with a number of physical and social changes resulting from their pregnancies while also dealing with the stressors that existed before their pregnancies. Globally, at least 25% of mothers can be expected to cope with heightened levels of overall life stress during the pre-natal period (Lynn, Alderdice, Crealey, & McElnay, 2011) while 60% of women report experiencing at least one significant stressful life event (a legal matter, relationships, finances, physical injury, and family illness or death) immediately before or during their pregnancy (Burns et al., 2015; Ward et al., 2017; Whitehead, Brogan, Blackmore-Prince, & Hill, 2003). Pregnant women most commonly report financial strain (compounded by a lack of employment, transportation, and affordable housing options), violence exposure, and feelings of intense isolation and loneliness as stressors (Bloom, Bullock, & Parsons, 2012; Bloom, Glass, Curry, Hernandez, & Houck, 2013). They also may experience stress from their romantic relationships and experiences with racial or ethnic discrimination. Many pregnant women experience more than one of these stressors at the same time (Braveman et al., 2010; Burns et al., 2015). Pfost, Stevens and Lum (1990) have argued that the experience of pregnancy itself should also be considered a stressful event. Below, we outline rates of exposure to stressors during pregnancy, as well as how exposure may change during pregnancy.

8.3.1 *Financial Strain*

Financial strain has been identified as the most common stressor during pregnancy in a number of studies (e.g., Bloom et al., 2012). Pregnancy may lead to changes in women's lives which affect their socioeconomic status. Their food intake is increased requiring greater expenditure (Laraia, Siega-Riz, Gundersen, & Dole, 2006), they experience discrimination at work as a result of their pregnancies (Masser, Grass, & Nesic, 2007; Williams & Segal, 2004), and they have increased medical expenses. Extant data from the United States indicates that childbearing women have lower incomes than women of childbearing age overall, with 50% of pregnant women being low-income (30% in poverty, 20% near-poor, Braveman et al., 2010). Most low-income women in the US experience at least one additional major hardship during their pregnancy, including food insecurity, the inability to pay bills, and homelessness. Poorer women are also more likely to move during pregnancy (Fell, Dodds, & King, 2004), and to do so for negative reasons or because of homelessness than women with a higher socioeconomic status (Tunstall, Pickett, & Johnsen, 2010). In this way, financial strain during poverty may lead to residential mobility, itself a stressor.

8.3.2 Intimate Partner Violence (IPV)

Studies comparing women's experiences of IPV before getting pregnant, during pregnancy, and after pregnancy suggest that the intimate partner violence to which many women are exposed does not stop during pregnancy (Kendall-Tackett, 2007; Sternthal et al., 2009) and, indeed, pregnancy onset may be associated with increases in psychological aggression and sexual violence victimization (Martin et al., 2004). A small proportion of women's first experiences of IPV occur during pregnancy (Daoud et al., 2012). Thus, for many women, IPV continues, worsens, or begins during their pregnancies. Differences in methodology, measurement, and rates of reporting make determining rates of IPV during pregnancy challenging (Devries et al., 2010). Devries and colleagues' (2010) analysis of trends across 19 countries found that prevalence of IPV victimization during pregnancy ranges from 2 to 14%, with rates in most countries ranging between 4 and 9%. Prevalence tended to be higher in African and Latin American countries than in the European and Asian countries surveyed. Studies carried out in individual countries also suggest IPV during pregnancy is commonplace (e.g., García-Moreno, Jansen, Ellsberg, Heise, & Watts, 2005). IPV during pregnancy is most prevalent among women who are marginalized by their race and socioeconomic status (Aizer, 2011; Daoud et al., 2012; Gazmararian et al., 1996; Taillieu & Brownridge, 2010), compounding the impact of those stressors.

8.3.3 Romantic Relationships

The quality of the romantic relationship is particularly critical for maternal well-being during pregnancy (Hagen, 1999). However, pregnancy is a challenging time for both men and women for a range of reasons, not the least of which is the decrease in romantic relationship satisfaction across the trimesters (Figueiredo & Conde, 2015). For example, nearly half of pregnant women meet criteria for "sexual distress", reporting that pregnancy reduces women's sexual desire, whereas it does not do the same for men (Sagiv-Reiss, Birnbaum, & Safir, 2012; Vannier & Rosen, 2017). This mismatch in sexual desire and distress during pregnancy may be stressful to the women and negatively affect functioning within couples.

8.3.4 Racial or Ethnic Discrimination

Racism is a distinct form of stress that predicts psychological and physiological distress over and above other stressors (Klonoff, Landrine, & Ullman, 1999). As during other periods of their lives, many racial or ethnic minority women report individual and institutional discrimination during their pregnancies. In a representative sample from Oregon, for instance, about one in five (19%) pregnant women accessing prenatal care, labour, or delivery reported recent experiences of discrimination (Marco, Thorburn, & Zhao, 2008). These women may experience discrimination in many areas, including their prenatal care. Minority women accessing prenatal care are more likely than non-minority women to report harsh, rude, or impersonal treatment from healthcare workers, long wait times for short prenatal visits, and inadequate information (Novick, 2009). Discrimination may be particularly deleterious for more marginalized women: for instance, minority and immigrant women in New Zealand were more likely to feel angry or upset in response to ethnic discrimination than white women born in New Zealand (Thayer & Kuzawa, 2015).

8.4 Effects of Stress on Mother and Infant Health

A growing body of research suggests that women's prenatal stress exposure can affect the development and health of their infants directly (i.e., neurobiological development) and indirectly (i.e., adverse birth outcomes for the mother, perinatal depression, conflict in their relationship with their partner) (Coussons-Read, 2013; Stanton, Lobel, Sears, & Del Luca, 2002; Yali & Lobel, 1999). Higher levels of maternal perceived stress have been shown to predict higher cortisol (Pruessner, Hellhammer, & Kirschbaum, 1999), poor eating, drinking and sleeping practices (Cohen & Williamson, 1988), and worse general health behaviours during pregnancy (Guardino & Schetter, 2014), which can affect fetal development. Prenatal exposure to stress is linked to low infant birth weight, impairment of serotonin systems, caesarean section delivery, and gestational age (Bussières et al., 2015; Gavin, Hill, Hawkins, & Maas, 2011). Heightened prenatal stress also increases an infant's risk for morbidity and mortality over the life course (Witt, Litzelman, Cheng, Wakeel, & Barker, 2014).

This stress exposure appears to worsen mothers' mental health which in turn affects the health of their children. Pregnant women are at greater risk than women in general to suffer from generalized anxiety, social phobia, and various disorders (major depressive disorders, eating disorders, panic disorder and obsessive-compulsive disorder). Pregnant women with psychiatric symptoms are also more likely than those without psychiatric symptoms to report physical symptoms (Andersson et al., ndersson 2003), and give birth preterm (Grote et al., 2010; Männistö et al., 2016). However, pregnancy 'per se' has not been associated with an increase in psychiatric disorders (Vesga-López et al., 2008). Instead, stress exposure is accentuated during pregnancy, predisposing women with vulnerabilities (psychological, social, economic) and their children to problems during pregnancy and after a child's birth.

Building upon this deeper understanding of women's experiences of stress during pregnancy, the concept of "fetal programming of health and disease risk" (c.f., Barker, 1998, 2007; Wadhwa, Buss, Entringer, & Swanson, 2009) suggests that fetal development, followed from genotype to phenotype, involves the embryo/foetus seeking, receiving, and responding to the intrauterine environment created by the mother's body (but shaped by her social and physical ecology) throughout gestation, particularly during sensitive periods of development. This embryonic or fetal responsiveness results in structural and functional changes in cells, tissues, organ systems, and individual set points for achieving homeostasis (balance across these systems). This developmental plasticity can result in changes, which, independently or through interactions with subsequent environments and biological milieus, confer immediate consequences for fetal development and birth outcomes (Cruceanu, Matiosin, & Binder, 2017; Girchenko et al., 2017). A mother's stress is one such environment, as are her biological changes resulting from stress.

Not surprisingly, such fetal programming can have important long-term consequences for health and disease susceptibility across the life course (Entringer et al., 2012; Gluckman & Hanson, 2004; Glynn & Sandman, 2011; Wadhwa et al., 2009). Just as we know that stress exposure is common among women during pregnancy globally, so too is there epidemiologic evidence for disease susceptibility across the life cycle when there is excessive prenatal stress (e.g., Kleinhaus et al., 2013; Nolvi et al., 2016; Ramchandani, Richter, Norris, & Stein, 2010). Importantly, exposure to prenatal stress may not directly cause offspring disease, but may, instead, alter the offspring's susceptibility for a broad range of developmental and health outcomes in later life by shaping an individual's phenotypic responsivity to social and physical environmental exposures related to disease risk, or protection from that risk.

While not unique to women during pregnancy, studies suggest that stressful major life events, as well as chronic adversity, can affect myriad biologic processes, but the candidate system most examined as a transducer of maternal stress effects is the hypothalamic-pituitary-adrenal (HPA) axis and its expression of the glucocorticoid, cortisol. With regard to women who are pregnant, substantial animal and human research demonstrates that stress 'signals', predominantly in the form of maternal glucocorticoids, are transmitted from the mother to the foetus throughout gestation via the placenta (Moisiadis & Matthews, 2014; Wadhwa, Dunkel-Schetter, Chicz-DeMet, Porto, & Sandman, 1996). The placenta is integral to fetal development, providing nutrient transfer, immune protection, and endocrine regulation of developmental processes that continue postnatally (Gilbert, 2013; Maltepe, Bakardjiev, & Fisher, 2010) and can thus have functional consequences for fetal and infant development (Monk, Spicer, & Champagne, 2012; Cox, Leavey, Nosi, Wong, & Kingdom, 2015; Pappas et al., 2015).

Indeed, human studies find that high levels of stress hormones, such as placental corticotropin-releasing hormone (pCRH) and maternal cortisol, predict impaired fetal maturation (Sandman et al., 2003; Wadhwa et al., 2004), premature birth (Ruiz et al., 2015), infant mental and motor development, infant temperament (Davis et al.,

2005), child IQ (LeWinn et al., 2009), and depression (Howland, Sandman, Glynn, Crippen, & Davis, 2016). Differential activation and expression of genes within the placenta has also been associated with adverse birth outcomes (e.g., preterm birth, pre-eclampsia, and intrauterine growth restriction, Lee et al., 2010; McCarthy et al., 2007; Monk et al., 2012). In addition to association with numerous changes in placental hormones, psychosocial stress in pregnancy has been associated with variation in maternal inflammation, and more recently with increased gene expression within stress pathways in mitochondria, the energy-creating powerhouses of our cells (Lambertini, Chen, & Nomura, 2015; Monk et al., 2012). Epigenetic mechanisms that impact on fetal development are also an emerging area of research (Moisiadis & Matthews, 2014; Monk et al., 2012). It is important to note though, that despite the potential importance of prenatal psychosocial stressors on offspring development, the cumulative impact of multiple stressors on biological mechanisms has not been well investigated (Dunkel-Schetter, 2011) as most studies focus on one type of stress exposure and one or two biological processes. For example, cumulative lifetime adversity—particularly trauma—may lead to persistent physiological changes in women (Bush & Boyce, 2014; Shalev et al., 2013) that have implications for the developing child. Recently, attention has been drawn to "intergenerational transmission" of stress effects (Entringer, Buss, & Wadhwa, 2015; Heim & Binder, 2012; Meaney, 2001), such as a mother's own childhood adversity (adverse childhood experiences, or ACES) affecting her own biology (Anda et al., 2006; Hillis et al., 2004), reproductive health, fetal development, and risk for fetal death (Hillis et al., 2004). Comprehensive understanding of these processes will require more sophisticated models that incorporate the complex, often co-occurring, challenges, as well as the protective factors that mitigate those experiences and resulting biological impacts.

Although the full picture of the precise mechanisms for such inter- and transgenerational effects are not yet well understood, there is a considerable evidence base for the association between prenatal stress and subsequent offspring behavioral, emotional, and biological regulation (Bush et al., 2017; Buss et al., 2012; DiPietro, 2004; Dunkel-Schetter, 2011; Entringer et al., 2015; Moisiadis & Matthews, 2014; Monk et al., 2012; Sandman, Davis, Buss, & Glynn, 2011). Evidence from a smaller, but growing, body of research reveals prenatal stress effects on offspring brain structure and function as well (e.g., Buss, Davis, Muftuler, Head, & Sandman, 2010; Buss et al., 2012). Animal research has also demonstrated mechanistic links between prenatal stress and altered immune function in offspring (Coe, Kramer, Kirschbaum, Netter, & Fuchs, 2002; Pincus-Knackstedt et al., 2006; Wright, 2005), which suggests additional biological pathways between maternal exposure to adversity and later offspring health outcomes, such as asthma, infections, and PTSD. There is less research on the role of stress-related variation in epigenetics and placental gene expression in prediction of later childhood health outcomes, though work in this domain is also growing (Boyce & Kobor, 2015).

8.5 Protective Factors During the Pre- and Postnatal Periods

While there are many reasons for concern regarding the amount of stress exposure for women during pregnancy, and the precariousness state that stress leaves children in, there is also an emerging understanding of the many biological, psychological, social and environmental factors and processes which are likely to either prevent exposure to stressors or moderate the effect of those stressors once exposure has occurred.

8.5.1 Biological Protective Factors

As the study of resilience gains traction, examination of biological factors related to adversity has broadened to explore the neurobiology of resilience (for a review, see Masten, 2016). Collectively, this emerging body of evidence has provided important insights into the roles of specific hormones, neurotransmitters, neuropeptides, and genetic factors in the neurobiology of resilience (Pfau & Russo, 2015). This work has been largely focused on animal research, and although evidence in humans is expanding, there is relatively little work specifically examining neurobiological resilience during pregnancy, in relation to effects on offspring. However, research from several key domains suggests this is an important area for greater investment.

Individual differences in sensitivity. Researchers from a "developmental psychopathology" perspective have emphasized that many individual factors thought to confer "risk" for problems actually can lead to vulnerability in the context of negative environments but may also promote particularly favourable outcomes in positive environments—a concept articulated by both differential susceptibility and biological sensitivity to context theories (see Bush & Boyce, 2016, for a review). Both theories posit that such factors confer 'sensitivity' to a range of environmental exposures across individual, family, community, and larger socio-political contexts. Sensitivity can result from varying levels of individual differences, including variations in temperament (e.g., irritability or positive affect), stress physiology (e.g., HPA-axis or autonomic nervous system reactivity), and genetics—at both the candidate gene level (e.g., the serotonin transporter), and more recently at the polygenic level. These sensitivity factors for enhancing risk or resilience have been applied specifically to the prenatal period (Pluess & Belsky, 2011). For example, in a large Dutch cohort study, genetic variation in 5-HTTLPR (a repeat polymorphic region of the gene that codes for the serotonin transporter gene) predicted sensitivity to the adverse effects of prenatal stress on offspring negative emotionality, with infants who were homozygous for the long allele being protected from the effects (Pluess et al., 2011). For women with the GG genotype of the oxytocin receptor gene (OXTR), higher levels of DNA methylation at the OXTR CpG during pregnancy predicted greater risk of postpartum depression, whereas A-allele carriers did not show this greater risk (Bell et al., 2015).

A child's sex may also be an important individual difference that impacts resilience to prenatal adversity. In particular, females appear to demonstrate less risk for maladaptive developmental outcomes associated with maternal adversity during gestation (Moisiadis & Matthews, 2014; Oberlander et al., 2008; Radtke et al., 2011), and it is well known that male and female foetuses respond differently to similar intrauterine environments (Banszegi, Altbacker, & Bilko, 2009; Ryan & Vandenbergh, 2002).

While our understanding of these nuanced interactions between genes and environments is growing rapidly, this work—particularly in terms of examining factors that promote resilience—is only just beginning. Characterizing individual differences that confer sensitivity to the environment may shed light on key biological systems that distinguish, or underlie, differences between more maladaptive versus more resilient pathways of development.

8.5.2 Variation in Perceptions of Stress May Protect

Although stress is a central concept in research on developmental processes and prenatal programming, there is no single measure used to assess it. Cognitions, including styles of attribution (Kalisch, Müller, & Tüsher, 2015), appear to influence whether a particular stressor will affect functioning. Events some people perceive as stressful may not be perceived as such by other individuals. Dunkel-Schetter (2011) suggests that the perception of adversity, followed by experiences of distress resulting from that adversity, are more likely to affect maternal biology and subsequent fetal development than the experience of adversity alone. Recent work has revealed that maternal experiences of stressful life events during pregnancy positively predicted infant autonomic nervous system reactivity, but only for women who reported average or higher-than-average levels of perceived stress, whereas babies born to women experiencing major negative events, but not reporting that they felt stressed, were buffered from those effects (Bush et al., 2017).

Women experiencing chronic adversity, such as limited access to financial resources or frequent exposure to neighborhood violence, may have habituated to such events and therefore may not perceive or report exposures to negative life events as particularly distressing. Habituation to stressful exposures is an important element of adaptation to the environment and helps our bodies achieve and maintain homeostasis, although it can lead to "allostatic load" and later health problems (Juster et al., 2016; McEwen, 2012). Minimizing acknowledgement of stress may be adaptive for high-risk populations or those in a particular cultural context (Kuo, 2014), although recent evidence for racial differences in measures of self-reported psychosocial states during pregnancy suggests minority women may report the highest levels of stress (Grobman et al., 2015). This pattern appears to refute the notion of habituation to above normal allostatic load.

8.5.3 Protective Interpersonal Factors and Processes

Partners, family members, friends, and community members can increase mothers' stress, but may also act as important sources of support. Social support can aid with coping and reduce the psychological impact of the stressful experiences many women encounter during their pregnancies. Social resources such as the size of a mother's social support network, her degree of social integration, and the availability of needed support all act as buffers against stressors which increase the risk of preterm birth (Kramer, Séguin, Lydon, & Goulet, 2000). When pregnant women are satisfied with their social support, they are at less risk for a diagnosis of depression (Coburn, Gonzales, Luecken, & Crnic, 2016) and experience reductions in depression symptoms during pregnancy (Ritter, Hobfoll, Lavin, Cameron, & Hulsizer, 2000). However, studies indicate that prenatal social stress can negatively impact maternal mental health, even while social support can simultaneously attenuate these negative effects (e.g., Coburn et al., 2016). In this way, social influences can be experienced as both risk and protective factors.

While relationships bring the potential for both positive and negative outcomes, the lack of an intimate relationship altogether is associated with leading to worse pre- and postnatal outcomes. Indeed, the literature on maternal romantic relationships has suggested an association between marital status and adverse postnatal outcomes, such as low birth weight and preterm births (Luo, Wilkins, & Kramer, 2004; Peacock, Bland, & Anderson, 1995; Raatikainen, Heiskanen, & Heinonen, 2005; Zeitlin, Saurel-Cubizolles, & Ancel, 2002). Zain, Low, and Othman (2015) reported that unmarried women, when compared to a married sample, had a higher prevalence of depressive symptoms (67.0% vs. 15%) and poor psychological well-being (68.5% vs. 25.4%) during the prenatal stage, and displayed significant differences in low birth weight (28.5% vs. 12.2%) and preterm births (31.0% vs. 19.7%). Research by Lurie, Zalmanovitch, Golan, and Sadan (2010) also reported unmarried women to be more likely to smoke during prenatal and postnatal periods (35.2% vs. 15.2%).

A healthy relationship with an intimate partner can be protective during pregnancy (Røsand, Slinning, Eberhard-Gran, Røysamb, & Tambs, 2011). However, the quality of the romantic relationship is critical. Social support from a partner can act as a buffer against the impacts of stress during pregnancy, with a good partner relationship having a protective effect on mothers' distress. This intimate relationship can be an important social resource, buffering against stressors which increase the risk of preterm birth (Kramer et al., 2000). Dissatisfaction with the partner relationship, though, is a significant predictor of mother's prenatal emotional distress (Røsand et al., 2011) and, consequently, of adverse child outcomes (Ramchandani et al., 2010). When pregnant mothers rate their relationships as being more negative, they report more depression and anxiety symptoms (Field et al., 2008). Experiences of IPV can result in fetal insults, thereby leading to a greater risk of perinatal death, pretermness, and low birth weight (Coker, Sanderson, & Dong, 2004; Huth-Bocks, Levendosky, & Bogat, 2002; Saltzman, 1990). The newborns of pregnant women who require hospitalization as a result of abuse by their partners are 163 g smaller than newborns of mothers who were not hospitalized for IPV (Aizer, 2011).

Women's support from their family and friends is also critical to their well-being. In general, family support reduces psychological distress during pregnancy (Sanguanklin et al., 2014). This support is most critical when women are feeling most anxious: those with pregnancy-related anxiety particularly appreciate and rely on their family, friends, and neighbours as sources of knowledge and support (Rosario, Premji, Nyanza, Bouchal, & Este, 2017). When women have family problems and unstable family relationships, however, this increases their likelihood of receiving inadequate prenatal care (Heaman et al., 2014) and is associated with heightened levels of depression during pregnancy (Bolton, Hughes, Turton, & Sedgwick, 1998). Low-income and minority women may also be less likely to have available sources of social support, given the demands on the time and resources of their family and friends (Dauner, Wilmot, & Schultz, 2015; Garrett-Peters & Burton, 2016). These women are thus disadvantaged in two ways, both of which affect health outcomes: they are likely to have more stressors and they have fewer consistent sources of social support available to them.

As expected, then, throughout pregnancy woman show a pattern of gradually rising oxytocin levels. Oxytocin has been shown to increase the salience of certain social stimuli, particularly for women (Theodoridou, Penton-Voak, & Rowe, 2013). Recent writing suggests that during pregnancy, increased oxytocin may enhance maternal awareness of potential harm to her developing foetus, which parallel the "protective pathogen avoidance" behaviors women exhibit during the first trimester that prevents them from consuming foods that present significant risk to the developing foetus (Bakermans-Kranenburg & van IJzendoorn, 2017). Experiences of positive social support and emotional connection are, however, associated with a range of positive psychobiogiological indices, such as higher levels of circulating oxytocin, decreased inflammation, and better physiological regulation in times of stress (see for reviews: Hostinar & Gunnar, 2015; Ozbay et al., 2007; Pilcher & Bryant, 2016; Taylor, 2011). Women who have strong social support, either through partners, family, or community, may thus demonstrate healthier physiologies that support fetal development and their own postnatal well-being, thereby promoting resilient outcomes in offspring exposed to prenatal maternal stress.

8.5.4 Education, Employment and Income as Protective Factors

A mothers' level of education may act as an overarching mechanism structuring stressful exposures and their buffers. Education is very strongly associated with early life social conditions emerging from the socioeconomic status of one's parents and conditions many other social determinants later in life, first for the mother, and afterwards for her child. Parents' and offspring's levels of educational attainment are very highly correlated across the world, even in countries with more equitable educational systems, such as Canada (Statistics Canada, 2016). This association extends to offspring' adult health (Quesnel-Vallée & Taylor, 2012), and even across three generations (Modin & Fritzell, 2009). Furthermore, the relationship between education and health is mostly indirect, mediated by other factors that act as more proximal stressors or buffers. Those other factors include employability, income, psychosocial resources, and health behaviours.

Both employment and income act as buffers to stress, facilitating access to a variety of psychosocial resources (Pearlin, 1999). The beneficial effects of education on one's health are largely mediated by income (Ross & Wu, 1995). Individuals with poor education are more likely to occupy jobs of lower quality, which often offer lower benefits and do not pay well (Kalleberg, Reskin, & Hudson, 2000). Conversely, findings show that education does provide long-term advantages since individuals with more education earn more than their less educated counterparts (Day & Newburger, 2002). Even when controlling for income, however, better-educated people have been found to suffer less from economic hardship, in part because of an improved ability to cope with stress (Ross & Wu, 1995).

It follows, then, that a mother's education and income are protective factors for the health of her infant and a proxy for her risk of experiencing socioeconomic inequalities. Low socioeconomic status is associated with increased depressive symptoms in late pregnancy (Goyal, Gay, & Lee, 2010), with poorer women having a greater likelihood of meeting diagnostic criteria for major and minor depression during pregnancy than middle class women (20–25% vs. 9–13%; Grote et al., 2010). Poorer mothers indicate feeling stereotyped and discriminated against by healthcare workers, which deters their engagement with prenatal care (Novick, 2009).

Unemployment during pregnancy may be associated with increased stress and, therefore, with adverse affects on infant health. Indeed, given the difficulties of being unemployed during pregnancy, pregnant women report that interventions which increase their employability would be most effective at reducing their stress (Bloom et al., 2012). Cyclical unemployment has been associated with decreased gestational age and increased likelihood of lower birth weight for infants (Kaplan, Collins, & Tylavsky, 2017). A recent review of related research indicates that higher education of the mother can reduce the risk of low birth weight by as much as 33% (Silvestrin et al., 2013). Additionally, Weitzman (2017) suggests that education increases women's healthcare visits before giving birth and increases the odds that labour will take place in a formal healthcare centre.

Socioeconomic factors also confer protection related to health behaviors. In general, the better educated a woman is, the more likely she is to adopt healthier lifestyle habits, including being less likely to smoke, drink, or overeat (Ross & Wu, 1995), all significant health-related concerns during pregnancy. Better educated women are also more likely to seek routine medical care, not only because of their knowledge of the importance of these behaviours and the higher value attributed to health in general (Link & Phelan, 1995), but also because they have the financial resources, insurance and social networks required to do so. As expected, in developing countries, a community's education level positively correlates with increased use of prenatal care, child health prevention, and adequate nutrition (Kravdal, 2004).

8.5.5 *Protection Conferred by Social Justice*

At a broader level, more equitable societies with stronger anti-discrimination laws should, reasonably, be a protective factor for pregnant women and their children. We arrive at this conclusion from a review of studies of social marginalization. Research on racial discrimination, for example, has highlighted its adverse effects on birth outcomes. An integrative review found a significant association between racial discrimination and adverse birth outcomes (preterm birth, low birth weight, or small for gestational age) in the majority of examined studies (Alhusen, Bower, Epstein, & Sharps, 2016). Further, independent of ethnicity and socioeconomic status, women who experienced discrimination during their pregnancies had worse self-rated health, higher evening cortisol, and their newborns had higher cortisol reactivity than those who did not experience discrimination (Thayer & Kuzawa, 2015).

8.6 Strategies to Improve the Resilience of Mothers and Their Children

The above summary of risk and protective factors influencing mothers and their children pre- and postnatal suggests many possible ways to intervene. Critically, no single strategy in isolation is likely to be sufficient to ensure a child's positive development. Risk factors cluster. Likewise, promotive and protective factors are cumulative (Cicchetti, 2013). A systemic understanding of the interactions between these factors can inform a deeper understanding of which factors are most likely to have the greatest impact on the well-being of mothers and children. Changes to a mother's social and physical ecology are expected to moderate the impact of environmental stressors, preventing their deleterious effect on a mother's genes and behaviour. While the list of possible interventions would fill volumes, we present here a few of the best researched: psychosocial interventions and supportive policies for education, childcare, nutrition and income.

8.6.1 *Psychosocial Interventions*

In a systematic review of the English-language literature on coping behaviours and coping styles in pregnancy (45 studies involving 16,060 participants published between 1990 and 2012), authors found some evidence that avoidant coping behaviours or styles and poor coping skills in general are associated with postpartum depression, preterm birth and infant development (Guardino & Schetter, 2014). Studies in both the U.S. and Finland have found that greater levels of maternal positive affect, and/or increases in affect over pregnancy, were positively associated with length of gestation and reduced risk of preterm delivery (Pesonen et al., 2016; Voellmin, Entringer, Moog, Wadhwa, & Buss, 2013). This effect was not accounted for by the lower stress levels associated with higher positive affect (Voellmin et al., 2013).

These findings point to the possibility of providing resources to reduce the experience of stress or improve adaptive coping for pregnant women exposed to adverse events in order to minimize their impact on the foetus. For example, prenatal mindfulness interventions have been shown to reduce pregnancy-related anxiety, perceived stress, and depression in pregnant women (Guardino, Schetter, Bower, Lu, & Smalley, 2014; see Hall, Beattie, Lau, East, & Biro, 2016 for review of some programs across U.S., Australia, and New Zealand), reduce the harmful impacts of poor sleep on perinatal well-being (Felder et al., 2017), and improve parent-child interactions during infancy (Setterberg, Nissen, Jonas, & Niemi, 2017). Moreover, mindfulness and meditation therapies have been shown to affect a range of biological outcomes associated with chronic disease and mood (see McEwen, 2016) which are likely to relate to physiology during pregnancy and offspring development. Group-based centering interventions during pregnancy can reduce perinatal depression and improve infant outcomes, likely through improved social support (Chae, Chae, Kandula, & Winter, 2017; Felder et al., 2017; Fiset, Hoffman, & Ehrenthal, 2016).

8.6.2 Supportive Policies

Animal research has demonstrated how enriched environments before and during pregnancy predict better maternal and offspring functioning postnatally. For example, enriching maternal environments after early stress, reduces anxious behaviour and improves brain development in rat offspring, as well as improving maternal stress physiology after birth (see Taouk & Schulkin, 2016 for a review). Intuitively, providing enriched environments to humans—through neighbourhood resources, income supplementation, social interaction and support, and equity-promoting policies—should result in better outcomes for stress-affected pregnancies, though empirical evidence is still lacking.

One of the most efficient ways to reduce health inequalities for women and children is to invest in universal education for all (Commission on Social Determinants of Health, 2008). In Canada, research shows that such social investments in education have succeeded in improving the socioeconomic position of most Canadians who undergo compulsory education (Oreopoulos, 2005). While investments in young women's education could alleviate multiple stressors before they become pregnant, Low, Low, Baumler, and Huynh (2005) have proposed an "Education Starts at Birth" policy scheme, which would involve combining comprehensive childcare, parental education, and childhood education initiatives into a single policy goal to improve educational outcomes for women who lack educational opportunities before they became mothers. Such initiatives are expected to reduce health disparities within one generation by transferring the benefits of the mother's education to her child.

Similarly, the World Health Organization's Commission on the Social Determinants of Health (2008) recommended "equity from the start," which includes universal child care, education, and early childhood programs, regardless of ability to pay. Policies such as these are designed to stop the cycle of intergenerational disadvantage and strengthen early childhood development programs, making them universally accessible. Doing so would help to ensure that all children begin school on an equal footing, regardless of their social background. Ultimately, though, the most efficient policies for women and children will ensure a coherent strategy that engages the multiple systems required for child health. An example of such a concerted effort is the "Every Child Matters" agenda in Britain, which promotes children's health, safety, academic achievement, civic involvement and responsibility, and economic well-being (Winchester, 2008).

Just as access to education can reduce a mother's stress exposure, so too can programs that improve nutrition, especially in contexts of extreme stress such as war and poverty. In addition to reducing experiences of stress, interventions targeting diet/nutrition or exercise can improve biomarkers of brain function, HPA-axis activation, inflammation, and cellular aging in adults (McEwen, 2016). Such interventions should help to counteract stress-related impacts to maternal physiology during pregnancy, though this is not often tested. Recently, a nutritional supplementation intervention that included high levels of antioxidants provided immediately after birth was shown to reduce risk of postpartum depression (Dowlati et al., 2017). Improved nutrition is possible at a relatively small cost. Programs such as OLO (*oeuf, lait, orange* [egg, milk, orange]), which provides one egg, one pint of milk, and one orange a day to pregnant women in need, are a relatively inexpensive way to improve perinatal outcomes among low income populations (Haeck & Lefebvre, 2016).

In sum, as the WHO Commission on Social Determinants of Health (2008) concluded, investments prioritizing equity in mothers' access to healthy food, housing security, and education offer tremendous intergenerational benefits. More generally, it also argued for a need to provide adequate employment, education, training, housing, and childcare opportunities for low-income families to mitigate the effects of their social circumstances on their health and that of their offspring. Meanwhile, considering that work on these structural determinants takes a long time to show effects, more immediate interventions could include encouraging clinicians to look beyond women's personal risk factors for disease during pregnancy, broadening their scope to social factors, such as income and violence exposure, which may be affecting their patients' health and the long-term health of their children (Bloch et al., 2008). As with individual protective factors, these population-wide processes are even more important to the resilience of mothers and children with multiple vulnerabilities.

8.7 A Framework for Resilience

Though the factors and processes associated with resilience have been presented as nested, recent advances in research suggest that there is no hierarchy between systems when it comes to predicting positive development under stress. Each system has the potential to influence other systems while also being influenced itself. These reciprocal relationships illustrate the mutual dependency of systems to produce resilience of both mothers and children. For example, much of the trauma mothers experience during pregnancy and childbirth can be avoided if pre-natal and post-natal care is changed in our hospitals and clinics, giving women the information they need to anticipate the stress they could experience and address the potential for violence in their relationships. An ecological understanding of resilience provides a multisystemic framework for both the study of women's stress exposure and the multiple levels at which protective processes improve outcomes. Therefore, resilience is both the capacity of women to prepare themselves for the experience of birth and the design of our medical systems to minimize the chances of exposure to atypical stress.

It is because sources of resilience occur at so many different levels that resilience is a relatively common experience for women and their children even when they experience structural disadvantage. In one Turkish study, for example, almost two-thirds of women who had traumatic births avoided negative outcomes (Dikmen-Yildiz et al., 2017). Likewise, a study of UK women showed that a traumatic birth actually produced an overall experience of post-traumatic growth depending on the meaning a woman attaches to her experience and the cultural norms which influence her individual perceptions (Sawyer et al., 2012; see also Ayers & Sawyer, Chap. 12; Taubman – Ben-Ari, Chap. 16 in this volume). Building on this body of research, there are a number of systemic interventions that are likely to enhance the resilience of women and newborns.

Minimize exposure to violence. A woman in an emotionally or physically abusive relationship is at much greater risk for psychological problems after her child's birth. If she is experiencing violence (and intimate partner violence, when it does occur, usually increases during pregnancy), then interventions by health care provider to assess for violence and legal assistance to deal with dangerous situations can improve biological and psychological outcomes.

Build a network of social supports. It is important that women build a set of relationships that will meet their needs if the prenatal or postnatal periods become unduly complicated. Women tend to report very specific "hotspots" when it comes to trauma causing experiences. These can be attributed to their experience of health care and health care providers, their child's challenges (especially if the child is born premature), and to problems with the mother's interpersonal relationships. Mothers who set clear expectations of others and ask for help when it's needed appear to cope better with a traumatic pregnancy and birth.

Improve health care. The experience of neonatal units and other aspects of a mother's time in hospital can cause heightened levels of stress (Ayers & Pickering,

2001). These stressors inhibit both the mother's capacity to provide care for her child and the neurological development of children. Well-designed primary and tertiary health care and social service systems, including the physical wards used to house mothers and children, may help to improve the resilience of mothers and newborns even when children are born prematurely.

Prevent problems before they occur. Much of trauma can be avoided if health-care professionals assessed women for vulnerability (and strengths) during the early phases of pregnancy. In partnership with institutional change, knowing if women are at risk for anxiety, depression or relationship violence can inform early interventions known to be effective. Postnatal, too, women need their healthcare professionals to screen for PTSD and if it does appear, to provide access to psychological counselling as quickly as possible. These interventions will not only decrease symptoms, they can also help women draw meaning from their experience of traumatic events and improve their resistance to future stress.

All of these interventions reflect a multisystemic understanding of resilience which focuses attention on the capacity of systems and their reciprocal influence. A resilience-promoting environment during prenatal and postnatal periods can ensure mothers, children and fathers have the resources they need to survive this complex life transition even when it is atypically stressful.

8.8 Conclusion

While the risks women face during pregnancy are many, and the impact of stress exposure long lasting for both mothers and children, there are many resilience-promoting factors that can buffer the impact of stress and improve developmental outcomes. Our summary of this vast literature suggests the need to think about the problem of stress on mothers multi-systemically, considering the impact of stress at multiple levels from the genetic, to the neurological, psychological, social, and economic. Solutions need to be equally complex. Future research is needed, however, to better understand how all these systems can work together to the advantage of mothers and the subsequent development of the broader community. Good interventions and social policies targeting resilience are those which reflect a multi-systemic approach to well-being that is a catalyst for changes to vulnerability across generations.

References

Abramson, D. M., Park, Y. S., Stehling-Ariza, T., & Redlener, I. (2010). Children as bellwethers of recovery: Dysfunctional systems and the effects of parents, households, and neighborhoods on serious emotional disturbance in children after Hurricane Katrina. *Disaster Medicine and Public Health Preparedness, 4*(Supp. 1), S17–S27.

Aizer, A. (2011). Poverty, violence and health: The impact of domestic violence during pregnancy on newborn health. *The Journal of Human Resources, 46*(3), 518–538.

Alhusen, J. L., Bower, K. M., Epstein, E., & Sharps, P. (2016). Racial discrimination and adverse birth outcomes: An integrative review. *Journal of Midwifery and Women's Health, 61*(6), 707–720.
Anda, R. F., Felitti, V. J., Bremner, J. D., Walker, J. D., Whitfield, C., Perry, B. D., … Giles, W. H. (2006). The enduring effects of abuse and related adverse experiences in childhood: A convergence of evidence from neurobiology and epidemiology. *European Archives of Psychiatry and Clinical Neuroscience, 256*(3), 174–186.
Andersson, L., Sundström-Poromaa, I., Bixo, M., Wulff, M., Bondestam, K., & Åstrom, M. (2003). Point prevalence of psychiatric disorders during the second trimester of pregnancy: A population-based study. *American Journal of Obstetrics and Gynecology, 189*(1), 148–154.
Ayers, S., & Pickering, A. D. (2001). Do women get posttraumatic stress disorder as a result of childbirth? *A prospective study of incidence. Birth, 28*(2), 111–118.
Bakermans-Kranenburg, M. J., & van IJzendoorn, M. H. (2017). Protective parenting: Neurobiological and behavioral dimensions. *Current Opinion in Psychology, 15*((Suppl C)), 45–49.
Banszegi, O., Altbacker, V., & Bilko, A. (2009). Intrauterine position influences anatomy and behavior in domestic rabbits. *Physiology and Behavior, 98*(3), 258–262.
Barker, D. J. (1998). In utero programming of chronic disease. *Clinical Science, 95*(2), 115–128.
Barker, D. J. (2007). The origins of the developmental origins theory. *Journal of Internal Medicine, 261*(5), 412–417.
Bell, A. F., Carter, C. S., Steer, C. D., Golding, J., Davis, J. M., Steffen, A. D., et al. (2015). Interaction between oxytocin receptor DNA methylation and genotype is associated with risk of postpartum depression in women without depression in pregnancy. *Frontiers in Genetics, 6,* 243.
Belsky, J., & Pluess, M. (2009). Beyond diathesis stress: Differential susceptibility to environmental influences. *Psychological Bulletin, 135*(6), 885–908.
Bloch, G., Etches, V., Gardner, C., Pellizzari, R., Rachlis, M., Scott, F., et al. (2008). Why poverty makes us sick: Physician backgrounder. *Ontario Medical Review, 75,* 32–37.
Bloom, T. L., Bullock, L., & Parsons, L. (2012). Rural pregnant women's stressors and priorities for stress reduction. *Issues in Mental Health Nursing, 33*(12), 813–819.
Bloom, T., Glass, N., Curry, M. A., Hernandez, R., & Houck, G. (2013). Maternal stress exposures, reactions, and priorities for stress reduction among low-income urban women. *Journal of Midwifery and Women's Health, 58*(2), 167–174.
Bolton, H. L., Hughes, P. M., Turton, P., & Sedgwick, P. (1998). Incidence and demographic correlates of depressive symptoms during pregnancy in an inner London population. *Journal of Psychosomatic Obstetrics and Gynaecology, 19*(4), 202–209.
Boyce, W. T., & Kobor, M. S. (2015). Development and the epigenome: The 'synapse' of gene–environment interplay. *Developmental Science Review, 18*(1), 1–23.
Braveman, P., Marchi, K., Egerter, S., Kim, S., Meltzer, M., Stancil, T., et al. (2010). Poverty, near-poverty, and hardship around the time of pregnancy. *Maternal and Child Health Journal, 14*(1), 20–35.
Burns, E. R., Farr, S. L., & Howards, P. P. (2015). Stressful life events experienced by women in the year before their infants' births–United States, 2000–2010. *Morbidity and Mortality Weekly Report, 64,* 247–251.
Bush, N. R., & Boyce, W. T. (2014). The contributions of early experience to biological development and sensitivity to context. In M. Lewis & K. D. Rudolph (Eds.), *Handbook of developmental psychopathology* (3rd ed., pp. 287–309). New York: Springer.
Bush, N. R., & Boyce, W. T. (2016). Differential sensitivity to context: Implications for developmental psychopathology. In D. Cicchetti (Ed.), *developmental psychopathology*. Hoboken, NJ: Wiley.
Bush, N. R., Jones-Mason, K., Coccia, M., Caron, Z., Alkon, A., Thomas, M., … Epel, E. (2017). Effects of pre- and postnatal maternal stress on infant temperament and autonomic nervous system reactivity and regulation in a diverse, low-income population. *Development and Psychopathology, 29*(5), 1553–1571.

Buss, C., Davis, E. P., Muftuler, L. T., Head, K., & Sandman, C. A. (2010). High pregnancy anxiety during mid-gestation is associated with decreased gray matter density in 6–9-year-old children. *Psychoneuroendocrinology, 35*(1), 141–153.

Buss, C., Davis, E. P., Shahbaba, B., Pruessner, J. C., Head, K., & Sandman, C. A. (2012). Maternal cortisol over the course of pregnancy and subsequent child amygdala and hippocampus volumes and affective problems. *PNAS, 109*(20), E1312–E1319.

Bussières, E.-L., Tarabulsy, G. M., Pearson, J., Tessier, R., Jean-Claude Forest, J.-C., & Giguère, Y. (2015). Maternal prenatal stress and infant birth weight and gestational age: A meta-analysis of prospective studies. *Developmental Review, 36,* 179–199.

Chae, S. Y., Chae, M. H., Kandula, S., & Winter, R. O. (2017). Promoting improved social support and quality of life with the Centering Pregnancy® group model of prenatal care. *Archives of Women's Mental Health, 20*(1), 209–220.

Cicchetti, D. (2013). Annual research review: Resilient functioning in maltreated children—past, present, and future perspectives. *Journal of Child Psychology and Psychiatry, 54*(4), 402–422.

Coburn, S. S., Gonzales, N. A., Luecken, L. J., & Crnic, K. A. (2016). Multiple domains of stress predict postpartum depressive symptoms in low-income Mexican American women: The moderating effect of social support. *Archives of Women's Mental Health, 19*(6), 1009–1018.

Coe, C. L., Kramer, M., Kirschbaum, C., Netter, P., & Fuchs, E. (2002). Prenatal stress diminishes the cytokine response of leukocytes to endotoxin stimulation in juvenile rhesus monkeys. *The Journal of Clinical Endocrinology and Metabolism, 87*(2), 675–681.

Cohen, S., & Williamson, G. (1988). Perceived stress in a probability sample of the United States. In S. Spacapam & S. Oskamp (Eds.), *The social psychology of health: Claremont symposium on applied social psychology* (pp. 31–67). Newbury Park, CA: Sage.

Coker, A. L., Sanderson, M., & Dong, B. (2004). Partner violence during pregnancy and risk of adverse pregnancy outcomes. *Paediatric and Perinatal Epidemiology, 18*(4), 260–269.

Commission on Social Determinants of Health. (2008). Closing the gap in a generation: Health equity through action on the social determinants of health. Retrieved from: http://apps.who.int/iris/bitstream/10665/43943/1/9789241563703_eng.pdf.

Coussons-Read, M. E. (2013). Effects of prenatal stress on pregnancy and human development: Mechanisms and pathways. *Obstetric Medicine, 6*(2), 52–57.

Cox, B., Leavey, K., Nosi, U., Wong, F., & Kingdom, J. (2015). Placental transcriptome in development and pathology: Expression, function, and methods of analysis. *American Journal of Obstetrics and Gynecology, 213*(4 Suppl), S138–S151.

Cruceanu, C., Matosin, N., & Binder, E. B. (2017). Interactions of early-life stress with the genome and epigenome: From prenatal stress to psychiatric disorders. *Current Opinion in Behavioral Sciences, 14,* 167–171.

Daoud, N., Urquia, M. L., O'Campo, P., Heaman, M., Janssen, P. A., Smylie, J., et al. (2012). Prevalence of abuse and violence before, during, and after pregnancy in a national sample of Canadian women. *American Journal of Public Health, 102*(10), 1893–1901.

Dauner, N. K., Wilmot, N. A., & Schultz, J. F. (2015). Investigating the temporal relationship between individual-level social capital and health in fragile families. *BMC Public Health, 15,* 1130.

Davis, E. P., Glynn, L. M., Schetter, C. D., Hobel, C., Chicz-Demet, A., & Sandman, C. A. (2005). Corticotropin releasing hormone during pregnancy is associated with infant temperament. *Developmental Neuroscience, 27*(5), 299–305.

Day, J. C., & Newburger, E. C. (2002). *The big payoff: Educational attainment and synthetic estimates of work-life earnings (Current Population Report P23–210).* Washington, DC: U.S. Census Bureau.

Devries, K. M., Kishor, S., Johnson, H., Stöckl, H., Bacchus, L. J., Garcia-Moreno, C., et al. (2010). Intimate partner violence during pregnancy: Analysis of prevalence data from 19 countries. *Reproductive Health Matters, 18*(36), 158–170.

Dikmen-Yildiz, P., Ayers, S., & Phillips, L. (2017). Longitudinal trajectories of post-traumatic stress disorder (PTSD) after birth and associated risk factors. *Journal of Affective Disorders, 229,* 377–385.

DiPietro, J. A. (2004). The role of prenatal maternal stress in child development. *Current Directions in Psychological Science, 13*(2), 71–74.

Dowlati, Y., Ravindrana, A. V., Segald, Z. V., Stewartb, D. E., Steinerb, M., & Meyera, J. H. (2017). Selective dietary supplementation in early postpartum is associated with high resilience against depressed mood. *PNAS, 114*(13), 3509–3514.

Dunkel-Schetter, C. (2011). Psychological science on pregnancy: Stress processes, biopsychosocial models, and emerging research issues. *Annual Review of Psychology, 62,* 531–558.

Entringer, S., Buss, C., Swanson, J. M., Cooper, D. M., Wing, D. A., Waffarn, F., & Wadhwa, P. D. (2012). Fetal programming of body composition, obesity, and metabolic function: The role of intrauterine stress and stress biology. *Journal of Nutrition and Metabolism*, 632548.

Entringer, S., Buss, C., & Wadhwa, P. D. (2015). Prenatal stress, development, health and disease risk: A psychobiological perspective—2015 Curt Richter Award Paper. *Psychoneuroendocrinology, 62,* 366–375.

Felder, J. N., Epel, E., Lewis, J. B., Cunningham, S. D., Tobin, J. N., Rising, S. S., et al. (2017). Depressive symptoms and gestational length among pregnant adolescents: Cluster randomized control trial of Centering Pregnancy® plus group prenatal care. *Journal of Consulting and Clinical Psychology, 85*(6), 574–584.

Fell, D. B., Dodds, L., & King, W. D. (2004). Residential mobility during pregnancy. *Paediatric and Perinatal Epidemiology, 18*(6), 408–414.

Field, T., Figueiredo, B., Hernandez-Reif, M., Diego, M., Deeds, O., & Ascencio, A. (2008). Massage therapy reduces pain in pregnant women, alleviates prenatal depression in both parents and improves their relationships. *Journal of Bodywork and Movement Therapies, 12*(2), 146–150.

Figueiredo, B., & Conde, A. (2015). First- and second-time parents' couple relationship: From pregnancy to second year postpartum. *Family Science, 6*(1), 346–355.

Fiset, K. L., Hoffman, M. K., & Ehrenthal, D. B. (2016). Centering prenatal care: Can a care model impact preterm birth rates? *Obstetrics and Gynecology, 127,* 17S.

García-Moreno, C., Jansen, H. A. F. M., Ellsberg, M., Heise, L., & Watts, C. (2005). *WHO multi-country study on women's health and domestic violence against women: Initial results on prevalence, health outcomes and women's responses*. Geneva: World Health Organization.

Garrett-Peters, R., & Burton, L. M. (2016). Tenuous ties: The nature and costs of kin support among low-income rural Black mothers. *Women, Gender, and Families of Color, 4*(1), 4–35.

Gavin, A. R., Hill, K. G., Hawkins, D., & Maas, C. (2011). The role of maternal early-life and later-life risk factors on offspring low birth weight: Findings from a three-generational study. *Journal of Adolescent Health, 49*(2), 166–171.

Gazmararian, J. A., Lazorick, S., Spitz, A. M., Ballard, T. J., Saltzman, L. E., & Marks, J. S. (1996). Prevalence of violence against pregnant women. *JAMA, 275*(24), 1915–1920.

Gilbert, S. (2013). *Developmental biology* (10th ed.). Sunderland (MA): Sinauer Associates.

Girchenko, P., Lahti, J., Czamara, D., Knight, A. K., Jones, M. J., Suarez, A., … Reynolds, R. M. (2017). Associations between maternal risk factors of adverse pregnancy and birth outcomes and the offspring epigenetic clock of gestational age at birth. *Clinical Epigenetics, 9*(1), 49.

Gluckman, P. D., & Hanson, M. A. (2004). Living with the past: Evolution, development, and patterns of disease. *Science, 305*(5691), 1733–1736.

Glynn, L. M., & Sandman, C. A. (2011). Prenatal origins of neurological development: A critical period for fetus and mother. *Current Directions in Psychological Science, 20*(6), 384–389.

Goyal, D., Gay, C., & Lee, K. A. (2010). How much does low socioeconomic status increase the risk of prenatal and postpartum depressive symptoms in first-time mothers? *Women's Health Issues, 20*(2), 96–104.

Grobman, W. A., Bailit, J. L., Rice, M. M., Wapner, R. J., Reddy, U. M., Varner, M. W., … VanDorsten, J. P. (2015). Racial and ethnic disparities in maternal morbidity and obstetric care. *Obstetrics Gynecology, 125*(6), 1460–1467.

Grote, V., Vik, T., von Kries, R., Luque, V., Socha, J., Verduci, E., … Koletzko, B. (2010). Maternal postnatal depression and child growth: A European cohort study. *BMC Pediatrics, 12*, 10–14.

Guardino, C. M., & Schetter, C. D. (2014). Coping during pregnancy: A systematic review and recommendations. *Health Psychology Review, 8*(1), 70–94.

Guardino, C. M., Schetter, C. D., Bower, J. E., Lu, M. C., & Smalley, S. L. (2014). Randomised controlled pilot trial of mindfulness training for stress reduction during pregnancy. *Psychology and Health, 29*(3), 334–349.

Haeck, C., & Lefebvre, P. (2016). A simple recipe: The effect of a prenatal nutrition program on child health at birth. *Labour Economics, 41*, 77–89.

Hagen, E. H. (1999). The functions of postpartum depression. *Evolution and Human Behavior, 20*, 325–359.

Hall, H. G., Beattie, J., Lau, R., East, C., & Biro, M. A. (2016). Mindfulness and perinatal mental health: A systematic review. *Women and Birth, 29*(1), 62–71.

Heaman, M. I., Moffatt, M., Elliott, L., Sword, W., Helewa, M. E., Morris, H., … Cook, C. (2014). Barriers, motivators and facilitators related to prenatal care utilization among inner-city women in Winnipeg, Canada: A case–control study. *BMC Pregnancy and Childbirth, 14*, 227.

Heim, C., & Binder, E. B. (2012). Current research trends in early life stress and depression: Review of human studies on sensitive periods, gene-environment interactions, and epigenetics. *Experimental Neurology, 233*(1), 102–111.

Hillis, S. D., Anda, R. F., Dube, S. R., Felitti, V. J., Marchbanks, P. A., & Marks, J. S. (2004). The association between adverse childhood experiences and adolescent pregnancy, long-term psychosocial consequences, and fetal death. *Pediatrics, 113*(2), 320–327.

Hostinar, C. E., & Gunnar, M. R. (2015). Social support can buffer against stress and shape brain activity. *AJOB Neuroscience, 6*(3), 34–42.

Howland, M. A., Sandman, C. A., Glynn, L. M., Crippen, C., & Davis, E. P. (2016). Fetal exposure to placental corticotropin-releasing hormone is associated with child self-reported internalizing symptoms. *Psychoneuroendocrinology, 67*, 10–17.

Huth-Bocks, A. C., Levendosky, A. A., & Bogat, G. A. (2002). The effects of domestic violence during pregnancy on maternal and infant health. *Violence and Victims, 17*(2), 169–185.

Juster, R.-P., Seeman, T., McEwen, B. S., Picard, M., Mahar, I., Mechawar, N., et al. (2016). Social inequalities and the road to allostatic load: From vulnerability to resilience. In D. Cicchetti (Ed.), *Developmental psychopathology*. Hoboken, NJ: Wiley.

Kalisch, R., Müller, M. B., & Tüsher, O. (2015). A conceptual framework for the neurobiological study of resilience. *Behavioral and Brain Science, 38*, 1–21.

Kalleberg, A. L., Reskin, B. F., & Hudson, K. (2000). Bad jobs in America: Standard and nonstandard employment relations and job quality in the United States. *American Sociological Review, 65*(2), 256–278.

Kaplan, E. K., Collins, C. A., & Tylavsky, F. A. (2017). Cyclical unemployment and infant health. *Economics and Human Biology, 27*, 281–288.

Kendall-Tackett, K. A. (2007). Violence against women and the perinatal period: The impact of lifetime violence and abuse on pregnancy, postpartum, and breast feeding. *Trauma Violence Abuse, 8*(3), 344–353.

Kleinhaus, K., Harlap, S., Perrin, M., Manor, O., Margalit-Calderon, R., Opler, M., … Malaspina, D. (2013). Prenatal stress and affective disorders in a population birth cohort. *Bipolar Disorders, 15*(1), 92–99.

Klonoff, E. A., Landrine, H., & Ullman, J. B. (1999). Racial discrimination and psychiatric symptoms among Blacks. *Cultural Diversity and Ethnic Minority Psychology, 5*(4), 329–339.

Kramer, M. S., Séguin, L., Lydon, J., & Goulet, L. (2000). Socio-economic disparities in pregnancy outcome: Why do the poor fare so poorly? *Paediatric and Perinatal Epidemiology, 14*(3), 194–210.

Kravdal, Ø. (2004). Child mortality in India: The community-level effect of education. *Population Studies, 58*(2), 177–192.

Kuo, B. C. H. (2014). Coping, acculturation, and psychological adaptation among migrants: A theoretical and empirical review and synthesis of the literature. *Health Psychology and Behavioral Medicine, 2*(1), 16–33.

Lambertini, L., Chen, J., & Nomura, Y. (2015). Mitochondrial gene expression profiles are associated with maternal psychosocial stress in pregnancy and infant temperament. *PLoS ONE, 10*(9), e0138929.

Laraia, B. A., Siega-Riz, A. M., Gundersen, C., & Dole, N. (2006). Psychosocial factors and socioeconomic indicators are associated with household food insecurity among pregnant women. *The Journal of Nutrition, 136*(1), 177–182.

Lee, M. H., Jeon, Y. J., Lee, S. M., Park, M. H., Jung, S. C., & Kim, Y. J. (2010). Placental gene expression is related to glucose metabolism and fetal cord blood levels of insulin and insulin-like growth factors in intrauterine growth restriction. *Early Human Development, 86*(1), 45–50.

LeWinn, K. Z., Stroud, L. R., Molnar, B. E., Ware, J. H., Koenen, K. C., & Buka, S. L. (2009). Elevated maternal cortisol levels during pregnancy are associated with reduced childhood IQ. *Interntaional Journal of Epidemiolology, 38*(6), 1700–1710.

Link, B. G., & Phelan, J. (1995). Social conditions as fundamental causes of disease. *Journal of Health and Social Behavior, 1*, 80–94.

Low, M. D., Low, B. J., Baumler, E. R., & Huynh, P. T. (2005). Can education policy be health policy? Implications of research on the social determinants of health. *Journal of Health Politics, Policy and Law, 30*(6), 1131–1162.

Luo, Z. C., Wilkins, R., & Kramer, M. S. (2004). Disparities in pregnancy outcomes according to marital and cohabitation status. *Obstetrics and Gynecology, 103*, 1300–1307.

Lurie, S., Zalmanovitch, A., Golan, A., & Sadan, O. (2010). The effect of marital status on pregnancy outcome in Israel: A retrospective case-control study. *The Journal of Obstetrics and Gynaecology Research, 36*(6), 1161–1164.

Lynn, F. A., Alderdice, F. A., Crealey, G. E., & McElnay, J. (2011). Associations between maternal characteristics and pregnancy-related stress among low-risk mothers: An observational cross-sectional study. *International Journal of Nursing Studies, 48*(5), 620–627.

Maltepe, E., Bakardjiev, A. I., & Fisher, S. J. (2010). The placenta: Transcriptional, epigenetic, and physiological integration during development. *The Journal of Clinical Investigation, 120*(4), 1016–1025.

Männistö, T., Mendola, P., Kiely, M., O'Loughlin, J., Werder, E., Chen, Z..., … Grantz, K. L. (2016). Maternal psychiatric disorders and risk of preterm birth. *Annals of Epidemiology, 26*(1), 14–20.

Marco, M. D., Thorburn, S., & Zhao, W. (2008). Perceived discrimination during prenatal care, labor, and delivery: An examination of data from the Oregon pregnancy risk assessment monitoring system, 1998–1999, 2000, and 2001. *American Journal of Public Health, 98*(10), 1818–1822.

Martin, S. L., Harris-Britt, A., Li, Y., Moracco, K. E., Kupper, L. L., Jacquelyn, C., et al. (2004). Changes in intimate partner violence during pregnancy. *Journal of Family Violence, 19*(4), 201–210.

Masser, B., Grass, K., & Nesic, M. (2007). We like you, but we don't want you: The impact of pregnancy in the workplace. *Sex Roles, 57*(9–10), 703–712.

Masten, A. S. (2014). Global perspectives on resilience in children and youth. *Child Development, 85*(1), 6–20.

Masten, A. S. (2016). Resilience in developing systems: The promise of integrated approaches. *European Journal of Developmental Psychology, 13*(3), 297–312.

McCarthy, C., Cotter, F. E., McElwaine, S., Twomey, A., Mooney, E. E., Ryan, F., et al. (2007). Altered gene expression patterns in intrauterine growth restriction: Potential role of hypoxia. *American Journal of Obstetrics and Gynecology, 196*(1), e71–e76.

McEwen, B. S. (2012). Brain on stress: How the social environment gets under the skin. *PNAS Proceedings of the National Academy of Sciences of the United States of America, 109*(Suppl 2), 17180–17185.

McEwen, B. S. (2016). In pursuit of resilience: Stress, epigenetics, and brain plasticity. *Annals of the New York Academy of Sciences, 1373*(1), 56–64.

Meaney, M. J. (2001). Maternal care, gene expression, and the transmission of individual differences in stress reactivity across generations. *Annual Review of Neuroscience, 24,* 1161–1192.

Modin, B., & Fritzell, J. (2009). The long arm of the family: Are parental and grandparental earnings related to young men's body mass index and cognitive ability? *International Journal of Epidemiology, 38*(3), 733–744.

Moisiadis, V. G., & Matthews, S. G. (2014). Glucocorticoids and fetal programming part 1: Outcomes. *National Reviews. Endocrinology, 10*(7), 391–402.

Monk, C., Spicer, J., & Champagne, F. A. (2012). Linking prenatal maternal adversity to developmental outcomes in infants: The role of epigenetic pathways. *Development and Psychopathology, 24*(4), 1361–1376.

Nolvi, S., Karlsson, L., Bridgett, D. J., Korja, R., Huizink, A. C., Kataja, E.-L., et al. (2016). Maternal prenatal stress and infant emotional reactivity six months postpartum. *Journal of Affective Disorders, 199,* 163–170.

Novick, G. (2009). Women's experience of prenatal care: An integrative review. *Journal of Midwifery and Women's Health, 54*(3), 226–237.

Oberlander, T. F., Weinberg, J., Papsdorf, M., Grunau, R., Misri, S., & Devlin, A. M. (2008). Prenatal exposure to maternal depression, neonatal methylation of human glucocorticoid receptor gene (NR3C1) and infant cortisol stress response. *Epigenetics, 3*(2), 97–106.

Oreopoulos, P. (2005). Stay in school: New lessons on the benefits of raising the legal school-leaving age. C.D. Howe Institute Commentary.

Ozbay, F., Johnson, D. C., Dimoulas, E., Morgan, C. A., Charney, D., & Southwick, S. (2007). Social support and resilience to stress: From neurobiology to clinical practice. *Psychiatry (Edgmont), 4*(5), 35–40.

Pappas, A., Chaiworapongsa, T., Romero, R., Korzeniewski, S. J., Cortez, J. C., Bhatti, G., … Tarca, A. L. (2015). Transcriptomics of maternal and fetal membranes can discriminate between gestational-age matched preterm neonates with and without cognitive impairment diagnosed at 18–24 months. *PloS One, 10*(3), e0118573.

Peacock, J. L., Bland, J. M., & Anderson, H. R. (1995). Preterm delivery: Effects of socioeconomic factors, psychological stress, smoking, alcohol, and caffeine. *BMJ, 311*(7004), 531–535.

Pearlin, L. I. (1999). The stress process revisited. In C. S. Aneshensel & J. C. Phelan (Eds.), *Handbook of the sociology of mental health. Handbooks of sociology and social research* (pp. 395–415). Boston, MA: Springer.

Pesonen, A.-K., Lahti, M., Kuusinen, T., Tuovinen, S., Villa, P., Hämäläinen, E., et al. (2016). Maternal prenatal positive affect, depressive and anxiety symptoms and birth outcomes: The PREDO study. *PLoS ONE, 11*(2), e0150058.

Pfau, M. L., & Russo, S. J. (2015). Peripheral and central mechanisms of stress resilience. *Neurobiology of Stress, 1*((Supplement C)), 66–79.

Pfost, K. S., Stevens, M. J., & Lum, C. U. (1990). The relationship of demographic variables, antepartum depression, and stress to postpartum depression. *Journal of Clinical Psychology, 46*(5), 588–592.

Pilcher, J. J., & Bryant, S. A. (2016). Implications of social support as a self-control resource. *Frontiers in Behavioral Neuroscience, 10,* 228.

Pincus-Knackstedt, M. K., Joachim, R. A., Blois, S. M., Douglas, A. J., Orsal, A. S., Klapp, B. F., Arck, P. C. (2006). Prenatal stress enhances susceptibility of murine adult offspring toward airway inflammation. *Journal of Immunology, 177*(12), 8484–8492.

Pluess, M. (2015). Individual differences in environmental sensitivity. *Child Development Perspectives, 9*(3), 138–143.

Pluess, M., & Belsky, J. (2011). Prenatal programming of postnatal plasticity? *Development and Psychopathology, 23*(1), 29–38.

Pluess, M., Velders, F. P., Belsky, J., van IJzendoorn, M. H., Bakermans-Kranenburg, M. J., Jaddoe, V. W. V., … Tiemeier, H. (2011). Serotonin transporter polymorphism moderates effects of prenatal maternal anxiety on infant negative emotionality. *Biological Psychiatry, 69*(6), 520–525.

Pruessner, J. C., Hellhammer, D. H., & Kirschbaum, C. (1999). Burnout, perceived stress, and cortisol responses to awakening. *Psychosomatic Medicine, 61*(2), 197–204.

Quesnel-Vallée, A., & Taylor, M. (2012). Socioeconomic pathways to depressive symptoms in adulthood: Evidence from the National Longitudinal Survey of Youth 1979. *Social Science and Medicine, 74*(5), 734–743.

Raatikainen, K., Heiskanen, N., & Heinonen, S. (2005). Marriage still protects pregnancy. *BJOG: An International Journal of Obstetrics and Gynaecology, 112*(10), 1411–1416.

Radtke, K. M., Ruf, M., Gunter, H. M., Dohrmann, K., Schauer, M., Meyer, A., et al. (2011). Transgenerational impact of intimate partner violence on methylation in the promoter of the glucocorticoid receptor. *Translational Psychiatry, 1*(7), e21.

Ramchandani, P. G., Richter, L. M., Norris, S. A., & Stein, A. (2010). Maternal prenatal stress and later child behavioral problems in an urban South African setting. *Journal of the American Academy of Child and Adolescent Psychiatry, 49*(3), 239–247.

Ritter, C., Hobfoll, S. E., Lavin, J., Cameron, R. P., & Hulsizer, M. R. (2000). Stress, psychosocial resources, and depressive symptomatology during pregnancy in low-income, inner-city women. *Health Psychology, 19*(6), 576–585.

Røsand, G.-M. B., Slinning, K., Eberhard-Gran, M., Røysamb, E., & Tambs, K. (2011). Partner relationship satisfaction and maternal emotional distress in early pregnancy. *BMC Public Health, 11*, 161.

Rosario, M. K., Premji, S. S., Nyanza, E. C., Bouchal, S. R., & Este, D. (2017). A qualitative study of pregnancy-related anxiety among women in Tanzania. *British Medical Journal Open, 7*(8), e016072.

Ross, C. E., & Wu, C.-L. (1995). The links between education and health. *American Sociological Review, 60*(5), 719–745.

Ruiz, R. J., Gennaro, S., O'Connor, C., Dwivedi, A., Gibeau, A., Keshinover, T., et al. (2015). CRH as a predictor of preterm birth in minority women. *Biological Research for Nursing, 18*(3), 316–321.

Rutter, M. (2013). Annual research review: Resilience—clinical implications. *Journal of Child Psychology and Psychiatry, 54*(4), 474–487.

Ryan, B. C., & Vandenbergh, J. G. (2002). Intrauterine position effects. *Neuroscience and Biobehavioral Reviews, 26*(6), 665–678.

Sagiv-Reiss, D. M., Birnbaum, G. E., & Safir, M. P. (2012). Changes in sexual experiences and relationship quality during pregnancy. *Archives of Sexual Behavior, 41*(5), 1241–1251.

Saltzman, L. E. (1990). Battering during pregnancy: A role for physicians. *Medical Association of Atlanta, 64*(3), 45–48.

Sandman, C. A., Davis, E. P., Buss, C., & Glynn, L. M. (2011). Prenatal programming of human neurological function. *International Journal of Peptides, 2011*, 837596.

Sandman, C. A., Glynn, L., Wadhwa, P. D., Chicz-DeMet, A., Porto, M., & Garite, T. (2003). Maternal hypothalamic-pituitary-adrenal disregulation during the third trimester influences human fetal responses. *Developmental Neuroscience, 25*(1), 41–49.

Sanguanklin, N., Mcfarlin, B., Finnegan, L., Park, C., Giurgescu, C., White-Traut, R., et al. (2014). Job strain and psychological distress among employed pregnant Thai women: Role of social support and coping strategies. *Archives of Women's Mental Health, 17*(4), 317–326.

Sawyer, A., Ayers, S., Young, D., Bradley, R., & Smith, H. (2012). Posttraumatic growth after childbirth: A prospective study. *Psychology and Health, 27*(3), 362–377.

Setterberg, S. E., Nissen, E., Jonas, W., & Niemi, M. (2017). Perinatal stress, anxiety, and depression: Effects of a MBCP intervention on mother-infant interaction. *European Psychiatry, 41*(Suppl), S30–S31.

Shalev, C., Entringer, S., Wadhwa, P. D., Wolkowitz, O. M., Puterman, E., Lin, J., et al. (2013). Stress and telomere biology: A lifespan perspective. *Psychoneuroendocrinology, 38*(9), 1835–1842.

Silvestrin, S., da Silva, C. H., Hirakata, V. N., Goldani, A. A. S., Silveira, P. P., & Goldani, M. Z. (2013). Maternal education level and low birth weight: A meta-analysis. *Jornal de Pediatria (Versão em Português), 89*(4), 339–345.

Southwick, S. M., Douglas-Palumberi, H., & Pietrzak, R. H. (2014). Resilience. In M. J. Friedman, T. M. Keane, & P. A. Resnick (Eds.), *Handbook of PTSD: Science and practice* (2nd ed., pp. 590–606). New York: Guilford.

Stanton, A. L., Lobel, M., Sears, S., & Del Luca, R. S. (2002). Psychosocial aspects of selected issues in women's reproductive health: Current status and future direction. *Journal of Consulting and Clinical Psychology, 70*(3), 751–770.

Statistics Canada. (2016). *Education Indicators in Canada: An International Perspective 2016*. Available online at http://www.statcan.gc.ca/pub/81-604-x/2016001/toc-tdm-eng.htm.

Stein, D., Williamson, D. E., Birmaher, B., Brent, D. A., Kaufman, J., Dahl, R. E., … Ryan, N. D. (2000). Parent-child bonding and family functioning in depressed children and children at high-risk and low-risk for future depression. *Journal of the American Academy of Child and Adolescent Psychiatry, 39*(11), 1387–1395.

Sternthal, M. J., Enlow, M. B., Cohen, S., Canner, M. J., Staudenmayer, J., Tsang, K., et al. (2009). Maternal interpersonal trauma and cord blood IgE levels in an inner-city cohort: A life-course perspective. *Journal of Allergy and Clinical Immunology, 124*(5), 954–960.

Taillieu, T. L., & Brownridge, D. A. (2010). Violence against pregnant women: Prevalence, patterns, risk factors, theories, and directions for future research. *Aggression and Violent Behavior, 15*(1), 14–35.

Taouk, L., & Schulkin, J. (2016). Transgenerational transmission of pregestational and prenatal experience: Maternal adversity, enrichment, and underlying epigenetic and environmental mechanisms. *Journal of Developmental Origins of Health and Disease, 7*(6), 588–601.

Taylor, S. E. (2011). Social support: A review. In H. S. Friedman (Ed.), *The Oxford handbook of health psychology*. Oxford: Oxford University Press.

Thayer, Z. M., & Kuzawa, C. W. (2015). Ethnic discrimination predicts poor self-rated health and cortisol in pregnancy: Insights from New Zealand. *Social Science and Medicine, 128*, 36–42.

Theodoridou, A., Penton-Voak, I. S., & Rowe, A. C. (2013). A direct examination of the effect of intranasal administration of oxytocin on approach-avoidance motor responses to emotional stimuli. *PLoS ONE, 8*(2), e58113.

Tunstall, H., Pickett, K., & Johnsen, S. (2010). Residential mobility in the UK during pregnancy and infancy: Are pregnant women, new mothers and infants 'unhealthy migrants'? *Social Science and Medicine, 71*(4), 786–798.

Ungar, M. (2011). The social ecology of resilience: Addressing contextual and cultural ambiguity of a nascent construct. *American Journal of Orthopsychiatry, 81*(1), 1–17.

Ungar, M. (2012). Researching and theorizing resilience across cultures and contexts. *Preventive Medicine, 55*(5), 387–389.

Ungar, M. (2015). Practitioner review: Diagnosing childhood resilience—A systemic approach to the diagnosis of adaptation in adverse social and physical ecologies. *The Journal of Child Psychology and Psychiatry, 56*(1), 4–17.

Ungar, M. (2017). Which counts more? The differential impact of the environment or the differential susceptibility of the individual? *British Journal of Social Work, 47*(5), 1279–1289.

Vannier, S. A., & Rosen, N. O. (2017). Sexual distress and sexual problems during pregnancy: Associations with sexual and relationship satisfaction. *Journal of Sexual Medicine, 14*(3), 387–395.

Vesga-López, O., Blanco, C., Keyes, K., Olfson, M., Grant, B. F., & Hasin, D. S. (2008). Psychiatric disorders in pregnant and postpartum women in the United States. *Archives of General Psychiatry, 65*(7), 805–815.

Voellmin, A., Entringer, S., Moog, N., Wadhwa, P. D., & Buss, C. (2013). Maternal positive affect over the course of pregnancy is associated with the length of gestation and reduced risk of preterm delivery. *Journal of Psychosomatic Research, 75*(4), 336–340.

Wadhwa, P. D., Buss, C., Entringer, S., & Swanson, J. M. (2009). Developmental origins of health and disease: Brief history of the approach and current focus on epigenetic mechanisms. *Seminars in Reproductive Medicine, 27*(5), 358–368.

Wadhwa, P. D., Dunkel-Schetter, C., Chicz-DeMet, A., Porto, M., & Sandman, C. A. (1996). Prenatal psychosocial factors and the neuroendocrine axis in human pregnancy. *Psychosomatic Medicine, 50*(5), 432–446.

Wadhwa, P. D., Garite, T. J., Porto, M., Glynn, L., Chicz-DeMet, A., Dunkel-Schetter, C., et al. (2004). Placental corticotropin-releasing hormone (CRH), spontaneous preterm birth, and fetal growth restriction: A prospective investigation. *American Journal of Obstetrics and Gynecology, 191*(4), 1063–1069.

Walsh, F. (2016). Family resilience: A developmental systems framework. *European Journal of Developmental Psychology, 13*(3), 313–324.

Ward, T. S., Kanu, F. A., & Robb, S. W. (2017). Prevalence of stressful life events during pregnancy and its association with postpartum depressive symptoms. *Archives of Women's Mental Health, 20*(1), 161–171.

Weitzman, A. (2017). The effects of women's education on maternal health: Evidence from Peru. *Social Science and Medicine, 180,* 1–9.

Whitehead, N. S., Brogan, D. J., Blackmore-Prince, C., & Hill, H. A. (2003). Correlates of experiencing life events just before or during pregnancy. *Journal of Psychosomatic Obstetrics and Gynecology, 24*(2), 77–86.

Williams, J. C., & Segal, N. (2004). Beyond the maternal wall: Relief for family caregivers who are discriminated against on the job. *Harvard Women's Law Journal, 26,* 77–162.

Winchester, R. (2008). Changes for the better. *The Guardian.* Available online at https://www.theguardian.com/society/2008/oct/22/every-child-matters.

Witt, W. P., Litzelman, K., Cheng, E. R., Wakeel, F., & Barker, E. S. (2014). Measuring stress before and during pregnancy: A review of population-based studies of obstetric outcomes. *Maternal and Child Health Journal, 18*(1), 52–63.

Wright, R. J. (2005). Stress and atopic disorders. *The Journal of Allergy and Clinical Immunology, 116*(6), 1301–1306.

Yali, A. M., & Lobel, M. (1999). Coping and distress in pregnancy: An investigation of medically high risk women. *Journal of Psychosomatic Obstetrics and Gynecology, 20*(1), 39–52.

Zain, N. M., Low, W.-Y., & Othman, S. (2015). Impact of maternal marital status on birth outcomes among young Malaysian women: A prospective cohort study. *Asia-Pacific Journal of Public Health, 27*(3), 335–347.

Zeitlin, J. A., Saurel-Cubizolles, M. J., & Ancel, P. Y. (2002). Marital status, cohabitation, and risk of preterm birth in Europe: Where births outside marriage are common and uncommon. *Paediatric and Perinatal Epidemiology, 16*(2), 124–130.

Chapter 9
Parenting in Hetero-Gay Families: Motivations, Assumptions, Gender and Culture

Dorit Segal-Engelchin, Sarah Jen and Pauline I. Erera

9.1 Introduction

In recent decades, marriage has lost much of its power as the institutional anchor tying together the processes of family formation, childbearing, and child rearing (Amato, Booth, Johnson, & Rogers, 2007). The decoupling of marriage from family configuration has led to the establishment of new family arrangements, including post-divorce, step-, foster-, and those "living apart together"-families, where the family spans multiple households (Cherlin, 2010). These variations on the traditional, heteronormative, two-parent household vary in the degree to which they challenge or resist this normative ideal. Additionally, although both men and women choose to participate in alternative family arrangements, their relative gendered power imbalance and positions in society, tend to lead to differing motivations behind their respective choices to forego participation in traditional heteronormative marriage and parenting roles.

In this chapter, we explore Israeli men and women's motivations for forming hetero-gay families for the purpose of conceiving and raising children. These hetero-gay families consist of a heterosexual mother and a gay father who conceive and parent children together while residing in separate households. We focus our presen-

D. Segal-Engelchin (✉)
The Spitzer Department of Social Work, Ben-Gurion University of the Negev, POB 653, 84105 Beer-Sheva, Israel
e-mail: dorsegal@bgu.ac.il

S. Jen · P. I. Erera
School of Social Work, University of Washington, 4101-15th Ave. NE, Seattle, WA 98105-6299, USA
e-mail: srjen@uw.edu

P. I. Erera
e-mail: ererap@uw.edu

O. Taubman – Ben-Ari (ed.), *Pathways and Barriers to Parenthood*,
https://doi.org/10.1007/978-3-030-24864-2_9

tation and discussion of findings not only on the lived experiences of the heterosexual women and gay men who participated in this study, but also on issues of power and social justice within the economic and cultural context of their lives. We recognize the need to balance our critique of normative assumptions and discursive influences with the acknowledgement of individual agency, power, and resistance in the face of these influences.

Exploring the hetero-gay family configuration requires that we draw from literature on three separate dimensions of the family context: the situational circumstances and motivations of the heterosexual mother, the circumstances and motivations of the gay father, and the broader cultural context in which this configuration arises.

9.2 Single-by-Choice Heterosexual Mothers

In many industrialized countries, rates of non-marital motherhood have increased in recent decades (Burns & Scott, 1994) and in the specific context of Israel, rates of non-marital births have increased most among women aged 35–39 (Israel Central Bureau of Statistics, 2017). This shift has led to the emergence of a distinct subgroup of unmarried mothers, who have been referred to as single mothers by choice (Bock 2000; Jadva, Badger, Morrissette, & Golombok, 2009; Mannis, 1999). From a critical feminist perspective, it is crucial to distinguish single mothers by choice, who tend to be highly educated, employed, and financially secure, from those who are in lower socioeconomic positions and are discursively associated with single motherhood not by choice, but by their limited position of power (Bock, 2000). Additionally, there remains ambiguity around what this "choice" refers to. Is choice evident in women's intentional motherhood, their single relationship status, or both? The literature on single mothers by choice tends to theorize that these women choose motherhood *despite* their status as single parents, as a "second best choice" in the face of their inability to find an appropriate and desirable male partner (Ludtke, 1997). In exploring why male partners are unavailable, various reasons have been explored by qualitative studies, suggesting that these women often remain committed to a traditional view of their hypothetical marriage and hold specific beliefs about what this idealized institution will look like. Unwilling to settle for anything less than this valued ideal, they choose to conceive and raise children in alternative family arrangements when marriage to a heterosexual man is deemed unattainable (Bock, 1995; Siegel, 1995). Single mothers by choice may fear intimacy with men more so than their married counterparts (Segal-Engelchin, 2008). They also may have reservations about relationships with men, fearing that these may undermine their independence and autonomy (Bock, 1995).

These interpretations of the single mothers' motivations may over-emphasize a critical perspective of these women as unable to secure a male partner. In extending these interpretations to mothers who participate in hetero-gay families, alternative explanations might emphasize these women's agency in actively creating a close simulation of traditional child rearing circumstances despite being single or in consciously choosing not to marry and to create a new kind of household arrangement.

Indeed, findings from our previous study (Segal-Engelchin, Erera, & Cwikel, 2010), drawing on in-depth interviews with mothers who had established hetero-gay families, reveal that some of these mothers attribute their single status to their own free choice. These women make a clear distinction between couplehood and marriage, emphasizing their desire to establish a relationship with a male partner outside of marriage. This is demonstrated in the following quotes:

> I never wanted to get married. Not really. I had three opportunities and I ran away from them. I still don't know how to explain it, but it's true. I am still not sure that I want to get married, I want to be in a relationship, that I want, but I am not sure about marriage.

> Marriage was never, almost never an option for me. It is difficult for me to live with a romantic partner […] That's why I was looking for the ideal way to have a child […] I never had a fantasy of wearing a white dress. Almost 90% of the women have this fantasy. Well, I am not, not an ordinary person. My life is not, was never ordinary and conventional. I would certainly like to find a life partner, certainly. I don't want to grow old alone. Absolutely not. I assume that it will happen, when I will really want it to happen.

Several mothers, however, associated their single status with their difficulty in maintaining romantic relationships with men, believing that they will lose their personal freedom, independence and autonomy once they will marry. The following quote exemplifies this:

> There must be a reason why I didn't find a marital partner. Reasons that are related to me. It seems […] maybe I was unlucky, maybe I will meet him tomorrow, but one needs to be realistic, it didn't just happen. If I was looking for a partner and couldn't find one, then there is also something in me that led to it. No doubt […] I am also an independent person […] I do things on my own, I don't like being told what to do, and I don't like it when people make decisions for me, and this […] this is undoubtedly related to my inability to find a marital partner.

In wanting to secure their independence and autonomy in child-rearing, mothers in hetero-gay families may see an advantage to seeking out a non-heterosexual partner who is not as tightly bound by heteronormative expectations of parenting roles or who creates space for their desired individuality outside of a marriage (Gerson, 2009). These women may also benefit from changing perspectives of single parenting, whereby the resonance of the traditional, two-parent, heterosexual household is lessened, reducing the impact of stigmatized single motherhood, particularly when single motherhood is chosen by financially secure and highly educated women (Amato et al., 2007; Gibson-Davis, 2011). In the hetero-gay family, heterosexual women may see the potential for raising children in the context of single, but supported, motherhood with a gay man who does not offer the option of romantic or sexual partnership, but does offer a level of support and respite from child-rearing responsibilities. This arrangement may allow for the negotiation of parenting roles and responsibilities across multiple households among partners whose relationship is defined solely by what is best for the children, without the additional complications of maintaining a marital relationship and without challenging the mother's autonomy (Segal-Engelchin, Erera, & Cwikel, 2005).

9.3 Gay Fatherhood

Contemporaneous to changing views on heteronormative marriage and family structure, recent years have also seen a generational shift in parenthood among gay men in Westernized countries (Berkowitz, 2007; Mallon, 2004; Patterson & Tornello, 2010). Until recently, few pathways to parenthood have existed for gay men, producing two contrasting stereotypes: the single, childless, and uncommitted gay man, or the gay man who fathered children in a heterosexual marriage prior to coming out (Bergman, Rubio, Green, & Padron, 2010; Erera, 2002; Schacher, Auerbach, & Silverstein, 2005). However, an increase in options to attaining fatherhood have contributed to a baby boom among gay male communities (Johnson & O'Connor, 2002), and to the emergent category of "new gay fathers" (Bergman et al., 2010; Schacher et al., 2005), which challenges the lonely gay male stereotype as well as that of the heteronormative father. In breaking down these societal barriers, gay fathers create space for a new version of fatherhood less tied to traditional cultural expectations of fathers often characterized as absent, distant, uncaring, or lacking in paternal instincts.

Despite having new available options for parenting, recent statistics indicate that most gay men continue to be childless (Patterson & Tornello, 2010). According to the National Survey of Family Growth, conducted by the National Center for Health Statistics in 2002, only 16% of gay men in the United States have had a child compared to 35% of lesbian women (Gates, Badgett, Macomber, & Chambers, 2007). Currently, there are no reliable statistics or estimates of rates of fatherhood among gay men in Israel.

Low rates of fatherhood among gay men may be related to lower desires or intentions to parent (Patterson & Riskind, 2010), rather than their ability to find a pathway to fatherhood. Gates et al. (2007) found that among childless gay men, only 57% express a desire to have a child compared to 87% of childless heterosexual men, and 70% of childless bisexual men. However, it is notable that these statistics still indicate that more than half of gay men do wish to parent, suggesting that social institutions and contextual barriers may also play a role (Berkowitz, 2007; Goldberg, Downing, & Moyer, 2012; Golombok & Tasker, 2010; Mallon, 2004). Pervasive heteronormative discourses result in discrimination toward gay men who apply to adopt, foster, or have children through surrogacy (Goldberg, 2012; Goldberg et al., 2012; Golombok & Tasker, 2010), and gay couples in Israel have only been able to adopt children not biologically related to them since 2008.

Despite these obstacles, progress has been made in shifting the dual marginal status of gay fathers in which as men they are viewed as less natural caregivers than women, and as gay men they are viewed as unnatural parents altogether (Hicks, 2006). This shift is evidenced by the fact that gay men are pursuing fatherhood in unprecedented numbers through adoption, foster care, and surrogacy (Golombok & Tasker, 2010; Mallon, 2004; Peplau & Beals, 2004). In hetero-gay families, gay men have the capacity to father biological children, be active parents, and have a co-parent, regardless of their relationship status.

9.4 Cultural Context—Institutionalization of the Hetero-Gay Family

In Israel, traditional views of marriage maintain a significant cultural influence. Despite being an industrialized and urbanized country, Israeli society maintains traditional values and perceptions of the ideal family configuration, resulting in relatively high rates of marriage and fertility accompanying low rates of divorce, childlessness, and non-marital births (Fogiel-Bijaoui, 2006; Lavee & Katz, 2003; Lewin-Epstein, Stier, & Braun, 2008). Along these traditional families, there are also a host of diverse families in Israel, including the hetero-gay family which has been facilitated and institutionalized as an acceptable alternative, as evidenced by the establishment of the Alternative Parenting Center in 1994. This nongovernmental organization seeks to match single, heterosexual women with gay men who hope to parent together outside of marriage. The Center's offered services include creating opportunities to meet with potential parenting partners, providing professional guidance through legal processes, drafting of a parenting contract, and supporting the establishment of the family unit through and beyond the arrival of a newborn (Segal-Engelchin et al., 2005). To date, over 500 children have been born through the support of the Center (see http://www.alp.org.il for further information).

In the past decades, additional organizations and websites have been established to offer similar services (e.g. Gobaby.co.il and Babyli.co.il). Indeed, the hetero-gay family has gained increasing visibility and attention in the media and public discussion. However, very little empirical work exists that explores the emergence and maintenance of the hetero-gay family as a unique sociological phenomenon. Aside from our prior work (Erera & Segal-Engelchin, 2014), we know of only one additional study that examined the personal experiences of gay men who chose to conceive and co-parent with a woman (Oren, 2006). However, Oren's study was not limited to hetero-gay families, as it considered mothers who were either lesbian or heterosexual, and all the gay men were coupled. Furthermore, to our knowledge, no study to date, aside from our previous studies (Segal-Engelchin et al., 2010; Segal-Engelchin, Erera, & Cwikel, 2012), has investigated the motivations of heterosexual women for choosing the hetero-gay family context of parenting. To enrich our understanding of the factors associated with this unique family choice, this chapter aimed to examine whether there are gender differences in the reasons men and women provide for choosing the hetero-gay family context of parenting.

The findings, based on in-depth interviews with nine gay fathers and ten heterosexual mothers who had established hetero-gay families, focused on comparing and contrasting the motivations of gay fathers and heterosexual mothers for co-parenting in the hetero-gay family. In some occasions we included the participants' descriptions of the process of searching for and selecting a co-parent of the desirable attributes in a co-parent, to enhance our understanding of the reasoning behind particular motivations.

In our comparison, we identified differences and similarities that arose in three sequential steps in the process of establishing a hetero-gay family: (1) a man and woman coming together as co-parents, (2) defining the household unit, and (3) establishing a family routine. Similar to the life course (Elder, 1994), we do not conceptualize these as distinct linear stages, but rather as dimensions of a single process that blend together and may be renegotiated over time. In moving through these steps, we discuss various aspects of similarity and difference in the perspectives of the heterosexual mother and gay father. Laying their motivations side by side challenged us to interpret not only the glaring contrasts, but also the more subtle differences embedded within surface level similarities.

9.5 The Coming Together of a Man and Woman

Most men and women stated a strong desire to find a co-parent of the opposite sex. This desire was informed by a belief that having both a mother and father figure was important to support a child's best interest and founded on the normative assumption, or belief, that a child will miss out on not having both a father and a mother. This belief about the necessity of a biological father was described by one woman in contrast to absent fathers and conception through a sperm bank:

> The more I thought about going to the sperm bank … and asking and checking with women who did do it through the sperm bank, whose kids are a bit older, the more I decided that I wanted a father for my kid. Kids constantly search for a father figure, it doesn't matter how many brothers they have, or how many uncles or male friends they have, they look for a father and cling to anyone […]. Even if the mother is divorced and the father left for good, there are still photos, there's the father's family, there's something to hold on to … and when it's the sperm bank and there's nothing – there's just one big emptiness […]

This perspective is informed by heteronormative and widely held beliefs that having two parents in the household is necessary for a child's ideal development and that children will continually seek out a father figure. Another woman's statement illustrated the subtle influence of a normative belief in the man-woman co-parenting dyad. She began by stating that the sex of those two parents does not make a difference in the child's development, it is only the presence of two parents of any sex that presents the opportunity for "balance" in a child's life. After presenting this position, however, she reverts to her belief that having a father is truly better than two mothers, although she cannot say why.

> I felt it was really important for the kid to have another [parental] figure. Not necessarily a father figure, I don't believe in that stuff too much, but another figure. So that he [the child] doesn't base all his developing personality on one source and it was important to me that he have another parent. It was very clear to me. I know at least one lesbian couple who has a kid, and the fact that there are two moms is not a negative thing, that's what I think, because there are plenty of male figures and female figures around us. But I thought, not too deeply, that it's best for him to have a dad.

While this woman subtly denied and then adopted a normative belief in the need for a father and mother, another woman more directly resisted the perception that she was simply being influenced by normative values, stating:

> … a child needs a defined and tangible mom and dad. For me it has nothing to do with it being the norm, that's not it. It's balance. When there's only a mom, something about that is out of balance … and when a kid has two parents, he has two points of reference, he has more balance in his life. There's balance in the sense that things I may be less good at, the dad can do, and things the dad is less good at, I can do.

Overall, women showed more of a tendency to defend their positions against normative discursive influences, asserting that they were not simply following the norm, but were actively choosing what they felt was best for other reasons, a tendency that was largely absent from the interviews with gay fathers.

While several fathers also believed that both a father and mother were in the best interests of a child, their reasoning was also tied to biological factors and a belief in the need for the "essential mother," or as one participant put it: "*In my opinion, it's something biological that was created this way like […] That's, that's how human creatures were created, in this way. That there's a mother.*" One father described his fantasy of being able to father a biological child without a mother; however, later in life he came to acknowledge that in addition to being impossible, it was also not in the best for the child:

> At the time I had these thoughts, when I started to think of myself as a father, of how I meet some woman and let's say she dies and I'm left by myself. It really was a kind of fantasy that the mother is erased. But over the years I came to realize that this isn't the right and proper model. And also, two men to raise a child it didn't feel right to me. It didn't feel right, I don't know … I came to the conclusion that a kid needs a mom. I have this friend who says he and his [gay] partner want either to adopt or to have [a child] with a surrogate, and have the mother leave the picture … to me it's obvious that's really unhealthy for the kid. It's not in the kid's best interest.

Most of the fathers stressed that it is in the best interests of the child to have a mother, because mothers have unique qualities that fathers don't have, such as "mother's affection" and "a mother's worrying":

> I can't see a child growing up without a mother […] the moment [the baby] is born to this world, it needs its mom [smiles]. And that's something a man cannot provide. I can't take on the role of a mother […] even in the sense of the warmth of a mother, the worrying of a mother. […] I have no doubt that mothers offer affection that a father can't always offer, especially at the beginning, when the kid is only just growing […] I don't think any kid can grow up healthily without a mom, without a mother's touch, without being breastfed

The fathers' perceived inability to fulfill the mother's role, seems to reflect the traditional view, which posits that mothers are more "natural" caregivers than fathers, resulting in the expectation that mothers will be the principal caretakers of children. Interestingly, none of the mothers interviewed expressed a belief that fathers play a unique role in the child's life, nor did they mention any fatherly functions which they believed a mother cannot assume.

In addition to the essential mother discourse, there was another reason that gay men were highly motivated to form a biological family. Many men described an internal, personal sense of purpose in leaving a legacy behind or the responsibility of continuing their family line:

> I don't want to leave this world without leaving my seal on it [...] I didn't want my family's lineage to be discontinued with me. [...] It burned in my bones: no. I will not be the link that will break the family's dynasty. And that prompted me enormously.

The importance of a patrilineal legacy or lineage as opposed to matrilineal, was also evident in the fact that all children took on the last name of their fathers, which was a choice supported by and desired by virtually all mothers and fathers.

Men who did not cite biology or the essential mother as key motivations for parenting in a hetero-gay family, were more deeply involved in the parenting process and more consistently present in their children's lives. They took a more egalitarian or gender-neutral approach to the relative contributions of a mother and father, challenging heteronormative beliefs regarding gender roles and parenting. For example, one man stated that his motivations for choosing a co-parent follows: *There is no view here [for me and the co-parent] that the woman has one role and the man has another role. We are [equal] partners ... Each of us is providing based on our abilities, but the matter is equal.*

In this early stage of identifying a co-parent and choosing to co-parent with a woman, there emerged in the data an unexpected difference between fathers who wanted more involvement in their children's lives, more often single men, and those who wanted to take on a more distant or less frequent role, more often those who were partnered. This distinction was also apparent in the way fathers defined the boundaries of the household unit and establishing family roles.

9.6 Defining the Household Unit

A notable difference emerged when we compared the mother and father's conceptualized boundaries of the family unit. Both often defined the household as including the mother, father, and child as a family unit, but for men, particularly those with partners, setting boundaries between themselves and their co-parent took on heightened importance. In contrast, women described creating a family resonant with their own experiences in homes with two present parents:

> I wanted a family. The same kind of family I had [family of origin] ... mom, dad, a couple of kids and a dog, and a backyard as well ... anyway, kids without a father seemed to me like something they would feel is missing. That it's incomplete, not the kind of family ... in my mind I did see a family unit like the one I grew up in, maybe it's just because that's how it was when I was growing up that it seemed ideal to me. But when I saw that it wasn't going to happen, I looked for the closest alternative, maybe that's the best definition, it's the closest thing to what I really wanted.

Another woman viewed alternative configurations not only as a close simulation of the ideal family unit, but as a reimagined family that fit with her conception or expectation for her own life:

> When I was errr... 34 or 35, I saw an article on alternative parenting. There was a story at the time in the "Haaretz" newspaper and I said: 'wow that works for me! That's exactly what I

> want: there's parenting, there's family'. I really did see it as a family, while also not having the romantic commitment.

More involved fathers were also likely to view their co-parents as part of their family unit. These men had high expectations for their own involvement in their child's life and described celebrating holidays with their co-parent, talking with the co-parent daily on the phone, and visiting their children in the mother's home frequently. However, men who were partnered described the need for a conceptual and sometimes physical boundary between the co-parent relationship and their relationship with their significant other. One man described the change in the boundaries between himself and his co-parent after transitioning from being single to becoming coupled with a gay man:

> When [the kids] were with me on Saturday, then in the beginning, she came to stay over with me because she liked it, because she wanted couple-ness. After that, I set the boundaries a bit and suddenly [my gay partner] also came back [to live with me], so it wasn't convenient.

Some men, all of them coupled, thought of the boundary between their family life with their partner and their parenting life with their co-parent should be firm if not rigid. For example, one man emphasized that boundaries were crucial to having a healthy relationship with his co-parent:

> One needs to set boundaries [between the co-parents]! I state this phrase again because it's recorded: SET BOUNDARIES. Underline it with three lines. And sometimes it's difficult and sometimes I need to set boundaries. They're still not clear enough. Look, I'll give you an example […] she can say: 'WE'RE coming for the weekend'. Like she's coming with the kids. This is my Saturday with the kids. So 'WE'RE coming'?

This distinct boundary-setting process was perhaps deemed more important from the perspective of the father because of the real or perceived potential imbalance of attraction. While the fathers were assured of their own lack of attraction to women and did not see the opportunity for blending romance with their co-parenting relationship, they saw the mothers as prone to emotional attachment to significant males in their lives due to their heterosexuality:

> I think that in every relationship there's some kind of falling in love or, from the woman's side. There's also this phase that at some stage happens to everybody, to most of the girls [mothers in hetero-gay families], because they're usually straight. Some kind of […] falling in love a little. Like [the hetero-gay family], is destined for that … there's some kind of a situation here that's seemingly a bit unfair …, no, not unfair, as every person is responsible and makes their own choices. There's nobody to blame … that is, that she can fall in love with you … and I cannot fall in love with her.

Some men even stated that they would have preferred to co-parent with a lesbian as opposed to a heterosexual woman, specifically to avoid the possibility that heterosexual mothers might have or develop romantic expectations of the gay father, which might create conflict in their own romantic relationships with men. This view of straight women as vulnerable to falling in love with significant men in their lives reflects a stereotype of heterosexual women as prone to developing emotional intimacy in relationship with any man, evident in this man's statement:

> She [the co-parent] can confuse [a gay co-parent] more as an object [of intimacy …]. And there were cases like that! I have a friend who is trying to conceive a child with some woman and she has to have it through sex! Well, that's already [too much …] She is straight and he's gay. Of course if it's a homo and a lesbian [who co-parent] there is seemingly a separation [between parenting and intimacy] and … also emotionally there's a clearer [separation], which seems also more fair, but it's a minor issue.

Mothers did not interpret their own emotions in this way and many expressed the removal of a sexual or romantic relationship with the father of their children as a benefit: "*no competitiveness, no jealousy, no boy-girl stuff.*" For some women, the lack of sexual tension rendered the co-parenting relationship less volatile and more stable:

> In a relationship between a straight woman and a gay man it's an advantage not to have sexual tension. And it's really easy. It makes the whole thing devoid of emotional baggage, devoid of sexual baggage. I mean, we both know ahead of time that we can't fall in love, all that's left is for us to be friends.

Additionally, while men had varied views on whether it would be better to co-parent with a lesbian or heterosexual mother, women's motivation to co-parent with a gay man as a way to remove sexual or romantic tension appeared to be secondary to the perceived relative lack of heterosexual men who were ready and willing to parent. As one woman said:

> It's not hard to find a gay man who is ready to be a parent; there's a thousand of them! Show me one straight guy who is ready to be a parent! A straight guy who's ready to be a parent, ready for a relationship, who's normal … over the age of 35, doesn't exist. Simply hardly exists! The good ones are taken and some are also caught up in really bad marriages and come out all scarred and come off as the bad ones … we've met those kind of guys as well.

This perceived lack of "normal" straight men able to parent, supports the heterosexist power dynamic of women having to compete to secure a desirable male partner from a limited supply. The assumption that women in the hetero-gay families are a "failure" because they were not able to secure a heterosexual husband to parent, was expressed by both men and women in this study. The perception that co-parenting with a gay man is a "second best option," seems to reflect a social norm of the relative superiority and desirability of heterosexual partners, preferably husbands, over gay partners, and the relative superiority and desirability of heterosexual fathers over gay fathers.

9.7 Establishing a Family Routine

Beyond setting boundaries and defining the family unit early in the co-parenting relationship, men and women approached establishing a family routine with different expectations about their respective parenting involvement and level of autonomy. Most of the men and women in this study expected a home life setting in which the children spent the majority of the time at the mother's home and visited with their fathers throughout the week. The notable exceptions to this preferred arrangement were a few of the single men who expressed a desire to be highly involved in their children's lives. These fathers were not as motivated by protecting their own time, energy, and independence, and views intimate gay relationships as secondary to parenting.

Establishing congruent expectations was particularly important in the areas of finances and time. Expecting to undertake most of the child-rearing, women were more concerned than men about having control and independence in raising their children. However women also expected financial and emotional support contributed by a father as well as occasional respite from their caregiving duties:

> I had thought of doing it [parenting] by myself, through the sperm bank, because I'm a real individualist and I'm very independent. I hate it when people tell me what they think I should do and say – "do this, do that". But financially, I'm not all that independent, I mean I am independent, but my financial situation is not as great as to have a child on my own … financial security was important to me.

In contrast, men, and particularly those living with a partner, tended to be more protective over their time, seeking to maintain their relative autonomy of their lives prior to parenting, while also having the privileges of fatherhood through regular visits:

> I wanted [my kid] to be with the mom and the mom also wanted that the [child] will be with her. [I wanted] that I'll have privileges […] like that [the child] will be here [at my home], on a regular basis, that is, twice a week. We didn't want; I didn't want, and also [the co-parent] didn't want fifty, half-and-half [parental responsibilities].

In contrast, two men did in fact want equal parenting responsibilities with their copartner:

> It was important for me that the parenting agreement includes equality in everything. That we are equal parents. Not that there is one who is more valuable and another is less valuable. During my first meeting with [the co-parent] I told her: 'I want to hear from you that you're looking for a partner, not a sperm donor or a sponsor […] that they'd know who their father is […] I want to know that you're actually willing to have a fifty-fifty partnership.

Despite these declared expectations, however, in the case of these men, the children also lived with their mother the majority of the time, signaling that even when fathers stated they wanted to share responsibilities, this may not have always been carried out in practice.

From a financial perspective, men often recognized the need for two incomes to support raising children and some also described an awareness that women were at a disadvantage when it came to earning potential, or what one father termed "*the classical inequality*." While willing to provide financially, fathers were also concerned that they will not be the sole bread winners. This concern is reflected in the emphasis fathers placed on selecting a co-parent who was financially and emotionally independent:

> When I met her [the co-parent] she was financially secure, more secure than I was. She had a job, she had an income, she didn't need me to be a "wallet" ... she could have gone to the sperm bank, she didn't need my money. The financial thing was really important to me. I mean, I couldn't have gotten along with someone where I had to give two thirds. And I think that's legitimate.

> There are single women that didn't succeed establishing themselves financially. This drove me crazy! [...] Usually the woman earns less. But here there was no reason why women wouldn't launch a career [...] I mean, you both didn't marry and didn't launch a career?! Perhaps it's unfair to say so, but it incensed me a bit.

This fear of women becoming financially dependent, illustrates both the influence of a real gendered wage gap, but also the sexist perception that women will often become dependent on a man to support them and their children. In this instance, gay fathers at once are pushing back on the traditional notion of a bread-winner father, while also relying on stereotypical views of women.

9.8 Insights: Gendered Motivations for Pursuing a New Form of Family Structure

Throughout the emergent themes of this comparison, we see co-parents as both taking up traditional perspectives on family configurations informed by biology, the child's best interest, and their own gendered parenting roles, but also actively resisting normative values and creating new definitions of a family in their hetero-gay families.

It seems that the process of choosing to parent biological children reflects, at least to some extent, the emphasis of the Israeli society on pro-natal parenting. The motivations of the gay men in this study to parent within a hetero-gay family reflect heteronormative beliefs which privilege heterosexual men; heterosexual marriage; and the canons of the traditional heterosexual family, including the paradigm of the essential mother; biological parenting; and two parents of the opposite sex. Each one of these heteronormative norms were depicted as being 'in the best interest of the child', implying that all other forms of parenting and family life are harmful to children and somehow deviant (Riggs, 2006).

At the same time, as they uphold the important role of mothers, the fathers also place women in a domesticated role, upholding traditional divisions of labor in the family (Coltrane, 2004). These findings echo Burman's (1997) claim that, "What dominant groups prefer as the desirable way to rear children is portrayed as the natural way for everyone to rear children" (p. 134). Heteronormative values appear to influence the belief, largely held among participants, that the combination of a man and woman form the ideal parenting partnership (Biblarz & Stacey, 2010).

Women's interviews show more tension in accepting this "natural" father-mother parenting dyad, as they more actively put their own perspectives in conversation with societal norms. However, women varied in the degree to which they embrace these norms, even as they depict themselves as having their own minds rather than simply taking up societal beliefs. There remains a question regarding why women are more prone to distancing themselves from, or acknowledging the possible influence of these social norms on their parenting choices compared to gay men. It is possible that women, as marginal or oppressed in terms of their gender, are more attuned to developing a critical consciousness around how their own views are influenced by their cultural surroundings. They may also have more experience with having to justify their parenting choices as they feel the pressures and stigma associated with single motherhood. This tension between taking up and distancing oneself from social influences reflects a society in transition regarding the possible re-scripting of motherhood and woman's gendered roles in the family. There is at once a lingering influence of pro-natalist policy as well as the desire among mothers to push back on their normative role as the primary caregiver by maintaining their independence as self-sufficient women.

Women also showed varied levels of comfort with their choice to parent with a gay father. Some women described their new family configuration as a valid choice that reflected their own internalized sense of what an ideal family should look like. They seemed to opt for a more queer version of family out of choice rather than out of need. However, other women emphasized choosing a gay father due to the lack of available straight men to parent with, a dynamic that continues to depict single mothers as romantic failures, unable to succeed in marriage (Hertz, 2006; Ludtke, 1997) and pressed for time. In fact, the biological clock stands out as a unique pressure on women choosing to parent biological children. Our findings suggest that women may feel they have only a certain amount of time left to conceive children and their choice to parent with a gay father may reflect this subjective experience running out of time.

In defining the family unit and the mismatch in co-parent's sexual orientations, there is an additional tension that arises from the perceived imbalance of potential attraction among co-parents. Gay men were more likely to perceive their co-parents as emotionally invested in building a romantic relationship that may create problems in the man's relationship with his gay partner. This perception reinforces a sexist belief in the emotional vulnerability of women and their inability to differentiate between a parenting relationship and a romantic one. However, this concern appears to be more perceived than real, as the women themselves did not voice romantic attractions to their co-parents, but rather believed that the removal of a sexual or romantic dimension might strengthen the co-parenting arrangement. This separation between romance and parenting can be contrasted to that of the post-divorce family, in which the dissolution of the romantic bond threatens the ability of co-parents to amicably collaborate in raising their children. The relationship between a heterosexual mother and gay father is therefore a unique bond in which a mother, father, and child form a new family structure, surrounded and supported by extended family members and the father's gay partner.

While some men described their family unit as including their co-parent, others emphasized the need for boundaries between their two households and family units: the parenting unit consisting of the gay father, the mother and child, and the intimate unit of the gay-couple. Particularly, the presence of the father's gay partner seemed to trigger this concern, giving a certain amount of power to the normative heterosexual relationship in which the "naturally" developing bond between a man and woman might undermine the relationship between two men. This concern seems to be overemphasized by gay fathers who perceive mothers to be more of a romantic threat to their relationships than the women themselves do. Their concern may also reflect their own insecurities and internalized stigma around whether their romantic relationship with another man or the ability of two men to parent are valid, natural, or immune to threat (Armesto, 2002; Berkowitz, 2011; Mallon, 2004; Schacher et al., 2005). These varied concepts about the boundaries of the core family unit, illustrate one possible contribution of hetero-gay family exploration to the broader literature on family configuration. We see a need for further theorizing around this issue of family definition as these boundaries may become more skewed or create new possible family arrangements in other alternative family structures that extend beyond a single household or beyond biological ties, including post-divorce, step-, and adoptive or foster families.

In regard to establishing a family routine, securing congruent expectations around co-parents' contributions of time, energy, caregiving duties, autonomy, and finances were seen as important aspects of co-parent selection. The stereotypical financially and emotionally dependent woman remains a concern for gay men and plays a large role in the process of co-parent selection. Mothers also seem to reinforce this traditional perspective of financial imbalance, as they consistently name financial assistance as a reason to co-parent. For both men and women then, having a middle-to-high socioeconomic status appears to be a near prerequisite for entering into a hetero-gay family, as co-parents must prove a certain level of financial security to be selected as a co-parent and must also be able to contribute enough to financially maintain a two-household family. This renders the question whether hetero-gay families are potentially inaccessible options for individuals of lower economic status or who are not gainfully employed.

Also evident in the establishment of day-to-day routines is the prevalence of the traditional pattern in which childcare is primarily the responsibility of the mother, who houses the children on a regular basis and is afforded a limited amount of support from a father who visits or houses the children on a partial and limited basis. Single men and those most heavily invested in maintaining an equal share of the caregiving tasks remain in the minority, but also serve as models for a new standard of fatherhood engagement that pushes back on traditional gendered expectations to some degree.

Drawing on queer theory, this study examined "how the doings of family, sexuality, and gender are inextricably intertwined with one another" (Berkowitz & Ryan, 2011, p. 333). The hetero-gay family at once depicts a queer take on what constitutes a valid and "natural" family, but one that is also influenced by the lingering pressures of heterosexist, heteronormative, and traditional beliefs regarding the importance of biological connection, the mother and father as the ideal parenting team, and gendered expectations of parenting roles. We argue that examination of this unique family configuration has much to offer the broader literature on family arrangements beyond the hetero-gay family itself. It is crucial that we recognize and continually inform the value-based transitions occurring in Westernized societies by acknowledging that changing values is a long-term process that at times necessitates incremental shifts in the minds of individuals who participate in alternative family arrangements.

Our analysis recognizes research participants' capacity to actively and creatively resist normative structures and discourses by producing a new form of family structure that resist traditional binary distinctions between heterosexual and homosexual, men and women, and nature versus nurture (Berkowitz, 2011; Elia, 2003). By resisting or reimagining these distinctions, we, ourselves and our participants, collaborate to create space for new possibilities and interpretations of family and gendered roles in parenting.

This study also offers some insights about the gendered motivations for pursuing various family arrangements among same-sex couples and single mothers, including in vitro fertilization, surrogacy, adoption, and fostering.

References

Amato, P. R., Booth, A., Johnson, D. R., & Rogers, S. J. (2007). *Alone together: How marriage in America is changing*. Cambridge, MA: Harvard University Press.

Armesto, J. C. (2002). Developmental and contextual factors that influence gay fathers' parental competence: A review of the literature. *Psychology of Men and Masculinity, 3*(2), 67–78.

Bergman, K., Rubio, R. J., Green, R. J., & Padron, E. (2010). Gay men who become fathers via surrogacy: The transition to parenthood. *Journal of GLBT Family Studies, 6*(2), 111–141.

Berkowitz, D. (2007). A sociohistorical analysis of gay men's procreative consciousness. *Journal of GLBT Family Studies, 3*(2–3), 157–190.

Berkowitz, D. (2011). Maternal instincts, biological clocks, and soccer moms: Gay men's parenting and family narratives. *Symbolic Interaction, 34*(4), 514–535.

Berkowitz, D., & Ryan, M. (2011). Bathrooms, baseball, and bra-shopping: Lesbian and gay parents talk about engendering their children. *Sociological Perspectives, 54*(3), 329–350.

Biblarz, T. J., & Stacey, J. (2010). How does the gender of parents matter? *Journal of Marriage and Family, 72*(1), 3–22.

Bock, J. D. (1995). *Single mothers by choice: From here to maternity* (Unpublished doctoral dissertation). University of Southern California.

Bock, J. D. (2000). Doing the right thing? Single mothers by choice and the struggle for legitimacy. *Gender & Society, 14*(1), 62–86.

Burns, A., & Scott, C. (1994). *Mother-headed families and why they have increased*. Mahwah, NJ: Lawrence Erlbaum.

Burman, E. (1997). Developmental psychology and its discontents. In D. Fox & I. Prilleltensky (Eds.), *Critical psychology: An introduction*. London: Sage.

Cherlin, A. J. (2010). Demographic trends in the United States: A review of research in the 2000s. *Journal of Marriage and Family, 72*(3), 403–419.

Coltrane, S. (2004). Fathering: Paradoxes, contradictions, and dilemmas. In M. Coleman & L. H. Ganong (Eds.), *Handbook of contemporary families: Considering the past, contemplating the future* (pp. 224–241). Thousand Oaks, CA: Sage.

Elder, G. H. (1994). Time, human agency, and social change: Perspectives on the life course. *Social Psychology Quarterly, 57*(1), 4–15.

Elia, J. P. (2003). Queering relationships: Toward a paradigmatic shift. *Journal of Homosexuality, 45*(2–4), 61–86.

Erera, P. I. (2002). *Family diversity: Continuity and change in the contemporary family*. Thousand Oaks, CA: Sage.

Erera, P. I., & Segal-Engelchin, D. (2014). Gay men choosing to co-parent with heterosexual women. *Journal of GLBT Family Studies, 10*(5), 449–474.
Fogiel-Bijaoui, S. (2006). Family. In U. Ram & N. Berkowitz (Eds.), *Inequality* (pp. 265–273). Beer-Sheva, Israel: Ben Gurion University Press. (Hebrew).
Gates, G. J., Badgett, M. V. L., Macomber, J. E., & Chambers, K. (2007). *Adoption and foster care by gay and lesbian parents in the United States*. Washington, DC: The Urban Institute.
Gerson, K. (2009). Changing lives, resistant institutions: A new generation negotiates gender, work, and family change. *Sociological Forum, 24*(4), 735–753.
Gibson-Davis, C. M. (2011). Mothers but not wives: The increasing lag between nonmarital births and marriage. *Journal of Marriage and Family, 73*(1), 264–278.
Goldberg, A. E. (2012). *Gay dads: Transitions to adoptive fatherhood*. New York, NY: NYU Press.
Goldberg, A. E., Downing, J. B., & Moyer, A. M. (2012). Why parenthood, and why now? Gay men's motivations for pursuing parenthood. *Family Relations, 61*(1), 157–174.
Golombok, S., & Tasker, F. (2010). Gay fathers. In M. E. Lamb (Ed.), *The role of the father in child development* (pp. 319–340). New York: Wiley.
Hertz, R. (2006). *Single by chance, mothers by choice*. New York: Oxford University Press.
Hicks, S. (2006). Maternal men—Perverts and deviants? Making sense of gay men as foster carers and adopters. *Journal of GLBT Family Studies, 2*(1), 93–114.
Israel Central Bureau of Statistics. (2017). *Press release: International Women's Day 2017*. Jerusalem. Retrieved December 22, 2017, from http://www.cbs.gov.il. (Hebrew).
Jadva, V., Badger, S., Morrissette, M., & Golombok, S. (2009). Mom by choice, single by life's circumstance. Findings from a large-scale survey of the experiences of single mothers by choice. *Human Fertility, 12*(4), 175–184.
Johnson, S., & O'Connor, E. (2002). *The gay baby boom: The psychology of gay parenthood*. New York: New York University Press.
Lavee, Y., & Katz, R. (2003). The family in Israel: Between tradition and modernity. *Marriage and Family Review, 35*(1–2), 193–217.
Lewin-Epstein, N., Stier, H., & Braun, M. (2008). The division of household labor in Germany and Israel. *Journal of Marriage and Family, 68*(5), 1147–1164.
Ludtke, M. (1997). *On our own: Unmarried motherhood in America*. Berkeley: University of California Press.
Mallon, G. P. (2004). *Gay men choosing parenthood*. New York: Columbia University Press.
Mannis, V. S. (1999). Single mothers by choice. *Family Relations, 48*(2), 121–128.
Oren, A. (2006). *Involvement of a woman in the making of a homosexual family* (Unpublished master's thesis). University of Haifa, Israel.
Patterson, C. J., & Riskind, R. G. (2010). To be a parent: Issues in family formation among gay and lesbian adults. *Journal of GLBT Family Studies, 6*(3), 326–340.
Patterson, C. J., & Tornello, S. L. (2010). Gay fathers' pathways to parenthood: International perspectives. *Zeitschrift fur Familienforschung (Journal of Family Research), 5*, 103–116.
Peplau, L. A., & Beals, K. P. (2004). The family lives of lesbians and gay men. In A. L. Vangelisti (Ed.), *Handbook of family communication* (pp. 233–248). Mahwah, NJ: L. Erlbaum Associates.
Riggs, D. W. (2006). Developmentalism and the rhetoric of best interests of the child: Challenging heteronormative constructions of families and parenting in foster care. *Journal of GLBT Family Studies, 2*(2), 57–73.
Schacher, S. J., Auerbach, C. F., & Silverstein, L. B. (2005). Gay fathers expanding the possibilities for us all. *Journal of GLBT Family Studies, 1*(3), 31–52.
Segal-Engelchin, D. (2008). Fear of intimacy and hardiness among single mothers by choice: A comparison to divorced and married mothers. *Journal of Family Social Work, 11*(2), 95–116.
Segal-Engelchin, D., Erera, P., & Cwikel, J. (2005). The hetero-gay family: An emergent family configuration. *Journal of GLBT Family Studies, 1*(3), 85–104.
Segal-Engelchin, D., Erera, P., & Cwikel, J. (2010). The meaning of choosing a hetero-gay family configuration from the women's perspective. In O. Sarid, D. Segal-Engelchin, & J. Cwikel

(Eds.), *Mind-body mosaic: Women's health in Israel*. Beer-Sheva: Ben-Gurion University Press. (Hebrew).

Segal-Engelchin, D., Erera, P., & Cwikel, J. (2012). Having it all? Unmarried women choosing hetero-gay families. *AFFILIA: Journal of Women and Social Work, 27*(4), 391–405.

Siegel, J. M. (1995). Looking for Mr. Right? Older single women who become mothers. *Journal of Family Issues*, *16*(2), 194–211.

Chapter 10
Reproductive Autonomy: Sex Selection as a Defining Case Study

Gil Siegal

10.1 Introduction

The place and role of gender in our lives cannot be exaggerated. Not only does it have a powerful impact on our identity and the way we see ourselves, but it also determines how we are regarded by society and the opportunities available to us (Oakley, 2016). In a world moving from chance to choice, attempting to control for the sex of children could be seen as an essential component of parenthood and family planning.

At the outset, it must be noted that sex and gender are not synonymous. Sex is most often considered the sum of biological and physiological characteristics that distinguish males from females. In contrast, gender, defined primarily by society and individual behaviors, relates to the social construction and demonstration of masculinity or femininity (Archer & Lloyd, 2002). With developing medical and scientific tools now interacting directly with sex and gender, there is a need to consider a new issue: the implications of current medical practices in shaping and influencing gender discourse.

Scientifically, sex is defined by the presence of specific chromosomes in an individual's genetic makeup. Humans carrying two X chromosomes are classified as female, whereas those carrying an X and a Y chromosome are categorized as male. The biological distinction between men and women can thus be reduced to the difference in a single chromosome.

This chapter focuses on medical procedures that enable parents to determine the sex of their children at different stages of development, for example, by choosing an XX or XY pre-embryo for reimplantation in IVF. Gender assignment/reassignment

G. Siegal (✉)
University of Virginia School of Law, Charlottesville, VA, USA
e-mail: gs6x@virginia.edu; gil.siegal@ono.ac.il

The Israeli National Committee for Non-Medical Sex Selection, Jerusalem, Israel

Center for Health Law, Bioethics and Health Policy, Ono Academic College, Kiryat Ono, Israel

O. Taubman – Ben-Ari (ed.), *Pathways and Barriers to Parenthood*,
https://doi.org/10.1007/978-3-030-24864-2_10

procedures and hormonal therapy that allow an individual of one sex to exhibit biological (phenotypic) characteristics more similar to that of the opposite sex are not discussed here.[1]

I therefore employ the term *sex* rather than *gender*.

Historically, societies have engaged in sex selection for centuries, typically in the wake of a cultural or individual preference for male children. Infanticide, for instance, has been practiced throughout civilization, and is even depicted in the Biblical description of Israelite boys being thrown into the Nile (Exodus 1:22). More recently, we have seen this form of selection against girls in some Asian countries (Dickens, Serour, Cook, & Qiu, 2005). Scientific progress has now made sex selection possible through a range of other means, including selective abortions (aborting the undesired sex), assisted reproductive technology (choosing embryos of the desired sex for implantation), and gamete selection (fertilizing the woman's egg only with sperm carrying either the X or Y chromosome).[2] Such developments in the reproductive realm raise important ethical, legal, and regulatory considerations pertaining to when and how these technologies should be used (see also van den Akker, Chap. 7 in this volume). The decision to allow sex selection under certain circumstances may lead to a reevaluation of existing stereotypes about gender and sexuality in a given society, as well as impact resource allocation in reproductive medicine. On the other hand, a broad prohibition of the use of sex selection might affect the pace of adopting certain innovations, along with the extent of economic investment in reproductive technology. Perhaps most importantly, if and how a society regulates sex selection might be construed as a reflection of the value it places on gender, gender discrimination, women's rights, and parental reproductive autonomy (Dickens et al., 2005).

10.2 The Science Behind Sex Selection

Sex selection that relies on modern assisted reproduction techniques, rather than infanticide or fatal child neglect, can be performed at three distinct, time-sensitive stages: pre-conception, pre-implantation, and pre-natal. *Pre-conception* techniques allow for determination of sex at the earliest stage, before conception/fertilization actually occurs, whereas *pre-natal* techniques (employed after pregnancy has been achieved) inevitably involve selective abortions. An interim option, *pre-implantation*, requires in vitro fertilization (IVF) and chosing pre-embryos of a desired sex using Preimplantation Genetic Diagnosis (PGD).[3] Clearly, this timeline—from pre-

[1]For a discussion of this issue see: Mieszczak, Houk, and Lee (2009); Wherrett (2015).

[2]Gamete denotes a single sperm and/or ovum.

[3]PGD involves removal of one cell from the developing pre-embryo, usually around day 3–6 after fertilization, for genetic testing. Among the tests performed (mainly for medical purposes), sex can be determined. PGD requires substantial expertise, is costly, and may not be available in all fertility clinics.

conception to termination of pregnancy—is apt to arouse a growing scale of controversy. That is, the earlier sex selection occurs, the less likely it is to be controversial.

As the woman has 2 X chromosomes (and thus each egg contains an X chromosome), only the male, with his XY combination, can determine the sex of the embryo by fertilizing the egg with a sperm containing either an X or Y chromosome. The predominant method of pre-conception sex selection is therefore by sorting X from Y chromosome sperm and selectively inseminating the woman (injecting the ejaculate into the uterus) or fertilizing the egg (via IVF) with the sperm more likely to produce a certain gender. MicroSort, a pre-conception sperm sorting service, for instance, reports a 92% success rate in selecting for girls and a 81.5% success rate in selecting for boys.[4]

In pre-implantation sex selection, performed through IVF and PGD, the sex of the embryo is also determined outside the woman's body. Once the clinician identifies the sex of the pre-embryos, only those of the desired sex are re-implanted in the uterus.[5] The PGD procedure results in nearly a 100% success rate of sex selection, with the success rate of pregnancy and live birth approximating that of IVF without PGD.[6] Sex selection may accompany IVF for a variety of reasons (Table 10.1). Some couples require IVF along with PGD to eliminate the risk of a genetic disease that affects a particular sex. In other cases, couples may be undergoing IVF for reasons of infertility or to eliminate the risk of a non-sex specific genetic condition, and take advantage of the opportunity to choose the sex of their child. Finally, some healthy couples might elect to undergo IVF + PGD specifically to enable sex selection. Here, the physical risks associated with IVF, as well as the considerable resources required, are undertaken for the sole purpose of choosing the sex of the child.[7] This might be regarded as a case where high-end medical procedures are used for non-medical purposes (Daar, 2005).[8]

In post-conception sex selection, perhaps the most controversial procedure, the sex of the fetus is determined during pregnancy using ultrasound, amniocentesis, or the newly developed non-invasive prenatal testing (NIPT; a test of blood drawn from the mother that identifies circulating fetal DNA). Parents can then elect to have an abortion to select against sex (Dondorp et al., 2015; Lewis, Hill, & Chitty, 2016; Norton et al., 2015). In a jurisdiction that allows the unfettered right to abortion, where no reason for the procedure has to be given, this practice would appear to be acceptable. However, in countries that regulate abortion it would be likely to arouse a negative knee-jerk reaction (Ivey, 2009). Indeed, an argument can be made

---

[4]This practice has an undetermined risk/benefit ratio. Following an FDA probe, MicroSort relocated its business outside the USA.

[5]This raises the question of the fate of the pre-embryos of the undesired sex. This issue is discussed below.

[6]In other words, PGD does not substantially reduce the chance of pregnancy by IVF.

[7]As PGD for non-medical reasons is expensive and not generally covered by health insurance plans or national health insurance, only wealthy parents are able to enjoy this technology, creating an access inequality.

[8]Examples of similar situations exist in medicine and healthcare, such as reconstructive surgery techniques which became the foundation of elective plastic surgery, a multi-billion dollar industry.

Table 10.1 Options for sex selection during IVF treatments

	IVF	PGD	Comment
Infertility	Yes	Not needed	No control for sex
Infertility and/or risk of genetic condition	Yes	Possible	Eliminate disease + control for sex
Sex selection	Yes	Yes	Control for sex

in favor of pre-conception and pre-implantation sex selection as they may prevent the possibility of more troubling sex-selective abortions. Moreover, while abortion inevitably raises the issue of a woman's rights over her body, the other sex selection methods, which are performed outside the womb, allow for the introduction into the discussion of the interests of the state, the child, and/or the woman's sexual partner (Heyd, 2003).

10.3 Reasons for Sex Selection

Parents cite a variety of motivations for sex selection. Some may be attempting to avoid a disease or disability, others may want to have their child's sex align with social preferences, and still others simply want to fulfill a personal desire, such as having a child of a particular sex, whether it is their only child or because they already have a child or children of the opposite sex (Steinbock, 2002). Intuitively, the motivation for sex selection might influence the ethical considerations, and thus the regulatory response (along the spectrum from disallowing such practices, through being indifferent to them, to objecting morally, with or without sanctions).

Perhaps the least controversial reason for sex selection is to avoid the risk of certain sex-linked diseases, a situation termed "medical sex selection." The American College of Obstetricians and Gynecologists (ACOG) endorses sex selection during assisted reproduction when doing so can prevent the risk of hemophilia or Duchenne muscular dystrophy, both chromosome X-linked diseases that commonly affect only boys (American Society for Reproductive Medicine (ASRM), 2015). However, medical sex selection has its pitfalls, since defining what is "medically indicated" can become fuzzy. Does a higher prevalence of ADHD or autism in boys warrant the medical sex selection of girls in a family with a close relative suffering from ADHD? Or is opting for a boy in a family carrying the BRCA gene, which increases the risk of adult-onset ovarian and breast cancer in females, a treatable disease, justifiably "medical"?

In a 2013 report, the European Society of Human Reproduction and Embryology Task Force on Ethics and Law reviewed similar concerns about the distinction between medical and non-medical sex selection (Dondorp et al., 2013). It concluded that, as long as the motivation can be attributed to health concerns, sex selection is justifiable in principle, as it emerges from the child's physical best interest, as opposed to following stereotypes and cultural preferences for a particular gender. The Task Force ultimately endorsed a broader definition and concept of medical sex selection, noting that the totality of circumstances should be weighed before the decision to allow sex selection can be made, particularly when the risk of the procedure may outweigh any potential benefit (Dondorp et al., 2013). This stance (i.e., the need for a case-by-case assessment) embodies the idea of a review process, a practice not endorsed by all societies that cherish women's autonomy.

When the reason for choosing the sex of a future child is not medical, it is termed appropriately "nonmedical sex selection" (NMSS). As noted above, for example, a family with children of one sex may wish to have a child of the other sex as well, seemingly without any preference for one gender or the other, a justification known as "family balancing" (Pennings, 1996). The notion of balancing can be viewed not only from the technical perspective—having children of both sexes—but also from the perspective of parents' rights, i.e., the desire to have the experience of rearing both sexes. Other cases include families seeking to reproduce the sex of a deceased child in an effort to compensate in some way for their terrible loss, or couples wishing to comply with religious obligations or cultural imperatives. For instance, some Jewish sects believe that one cannot fulfill the religious obligation of procreation without having children of both sexes (Heyd 2003). Finally, a family may wish to select the sex of their first child, or their only child in a one-child society (English & Braude, 2014).

10.4 Arguments For and Against Sex Selection

Ethical issues abound in discussions of NMSS. They pertain to the interests of all parties involved: women (autonomy, equality); parents (reproductive privacy); the conceived children (being of the desired/undesired sex, the burden of parental expectations and the roles to be assumed); and society (ASRM 2015; Heyd 2003; Robertson, 2001; Sureau, 1999). Legislators, regulators, and the courts have explicitly recognized that the reproductive right is not absolute; it can be limited by the countervailing interests of others, such as the state or third parties. Thus, the challenge is formidable: to navigate between what is medically possible and what society deems ethically permissible.

A recurrent fear of the consequences of widespread NMSS is the distortion of a population's gender ratio. Demographic data already suggests a growing imbalance in the male/female ratio in some societies, especially those that practice pre-natal sex selection (Bongaarts & Guilmoto, 2015). It should be noted that IVF and PGD are both expensive and expertise-dependent, and therefore pre-implantation sex selection is not expected to have a dramatic demographic impact. However, even if a hands-off, market-based approach to sex selection were to be universally adopted, it would not have the same effect on all societies (Dickens et al., 2005). Studies from many countries suggest that, if permitted, no sex imbalance would result from NMSS. For instance, parents in Germany and the UK exhibit a general indifference toward a "preferred" gender, although they do display interest in family balancing out of a desire to parent both sexes. One can argue for NMSS as an expression of parental autonomy and the right to choose in a society that does not harbor strong gender biases. In other words, without a social preference for a particular sex, allowing for individual choice would not be expected to have demographic implications (Ivey, 2009). It is important to remember, however, that in many countries, subpopulations retain different traditions, cultural preferences, or customs, so that a nuanced approach might be more sensible, although it is a tremendous challenge from a liberal-democratic legal perspective (Grech, 2017; Puri, Adams, Ivey, & Nachtigall, 2011).

There is also another side to this issue. Even in countries where sex selection might create sex imbalance, is that necessarily a bad thing? If the life expectancy of women is longer than that of men, might a higher birthrate for males not be preferable? Some scholars have suggested that sex imbalance with a surplus of men could lead to the devaluation of women, as society might focus more on their sexuality. But the opposite argument can also be made: a shortage of women might augment their social worth (Mohapatra, 2012).

Clearly, a policy that permits NMSS has the potential to perpetuate, or even increase, inherent gender discrimination in societies, particularly traditional ones, which are predominated by a significant preference for males over females. It has been argued that sex selection might also lead to a larger socioeconomic gap between the genders, as more parents will choose to have first-born sons, and on average, first-born children are more successful than subsequent children (Steinbock, 2002).

Feminist scholars grapple with the idea of NMSS because it uniquely brings two opposing causes face to face: gender equality and reproductive autonomy (Ivey, 2009; Moazam, 2004). While allowing NMSS promotes reproductive autonomy, and therefore women's autonomy, this is primarily true in Western societies. In societies with lesser respect for women's rights, it could subject women to pressure to undergo IVF (with its associated risks) or perpetuate discrimination against women by systematically preferring males over females. As Ivey (2009) maintains, "the liberal position, which espouses a permissive legislative regime, is suitable where there is no empirically measurable demographic impact, but where women's reproductive freedoms remain vulnerable to attack by the state" (p. i).

The interest of the future child also raises intriguing questions. Allowing couples to select the sex of their children could lead to better psychological outcomes, as parents would be less likely to force male gender roles on female children and vice versa. Conversely, parents might expect a daughter to exhibit all the characteristics of the female gender, thus upholding and enforcing gender stereotypes. On the other hand, a child of the undesired gender could be at a severe disadvantage. This suggests a choice between a top-down non-permissive NMSS policy that might result in a child's lifelong neglect, and a policy of parental autonomy allowing for sex selection that would endow a child with an inner sense of desirability.

10.5 The Regulation of Sex Selection and Its Effectiveness: An International Survey

The different stages of sex selection—pre-natal, pre-conception, and pre-implantation—have different regulatory targets and means. Each stage requires its own scope of regulation and/or a specific decision maker (e.g., the legislature, an agency such as the Department of Health, the parents, fertility clinic specialists).

Pre-natal sex selection is regulated by the laws regarding abortion. Thus, imposing regulations on sex selection at this stage is extremely difficult in a country that views abortion (at least at the pre-viability stage) as part of the right to privacy and the prerogative of women, irrespective of their motives. Any attempt at regulation therefore draws heavily on the general abortion debate.[9] In the United States, a handful of states (Arizona, Illinois, Kansas, North Carolina, North Dakota, Oklahoma, Pennsylvania, and South Dakota) specifically ban sex selection at this point in the pregnancy by means of abortion-related legislation. On the other hand, Sweden explicitly permits termination based on the sex of the fetus. India has sought to reduce sex-selective abortions by preventing doctors from revealing the sex of the fetus during pregnancy and by restricting the availability of portable ultrasound devices that can be used for this purpose. For example, the law in the State of Maharashtra stipulates: "No person conducting a prenatal diagnostic procedure shall communicate to the pregnant woman concerned or her relatives the sex of the fetus, by words, signs or in any other manner."[10] In Canada, the Assisted Human Reproduction Act decrees that "it is a crime for anyone, for the purpose of birth of a child, knowingly to perform any procedure or provide, prescribe or administer anything that would ensure or increase the probability that an embryo will be of a particular sex, or that would identify the sex of an in vitro embryo, except to prevent, diagnose or treat a sex-linked disorder or disease."[11]

Pre-conception sex selection is achieved primarily by sperm sorting. In the United States, sperm-sorting technology, such as MicroSort, is classified as a medical device and is regulated by the Food and Drug Administration. Interestingly, MicroSort was banned in the United States, not for reasons of safety or effectiveness, but rather because the FDA concluded that "it had no public health benefit." In the UK, the governmental Human Fertilisation and Embryology Authority (HFEA) recommended that sperm sorting for non-medical reasons be restricted. Similarly, Germany and Italy only permit sperm-sorting for medical sex selection (Kalfoglou, Kammersell, Philpott, & Dahl, 2013).

Pre-implantation sex-selection regulation varies significantly both intra- and internationally. For instance, in the United States the major challenge is the near total absence of effective regulation of reproductive medicine in general, along with the lack of unity in the industry, a situation Birdsall (2010) terms "the American Wild

---

[9]Griswold v. Connecticut, 381 U.S. 479 (1965); Eisenstadt v. Baird, 405 U.S. 438 (1972); Roe v. Wade, 410 U.S. 113 (1973); Planned Parenthood of Southeastern Pa. v. Casey, 505 U.S. 833 (1992).

[10]Available at http://chdslsa.gov.in/right_menu/act/pdf/PNDT.pdf (last visited April 1, 2018).

[11]S. 5(1)(c), 2004.

West of reproductive medicine." While industry groups such as the ACOG have issued somewhat muted recommendations against NMSS, they are just that—recommendations alone. IVF clinics and practitioners do not regularly communicate with each other, nor have they formed any network from which data can be easily gathered.

Thus, while opinions differ as to whether sex selection at the various stages should be permitted, in effect what we have at present in the US is a hands-off self-regulated industry. However, judicial cases, including Griswold, Roe v. Wade, and Eisenstaedt, with their focus on personal autonomy in reproductive decisions, suggest that sex selection for both medical and nonmedical reasons is generally permitted. In 2012, legislation was first introduced in Congress to attempt to regulate sex-selective practices, particularly abortions. Indeed, the bill, titled the Prenatal Nondiscrimination Act, imposed a fine and potential imprisonment for sex-selective abortions. It has recently been reintroduced and referred to the Subcommittee on the Constitution and Civil Justice.[12]

In contrast, the UK, which has a national health system, heavily regulates reproductive technologies through the HFEA, created by the Human Fertilization and Embryology Act of 1990.[13] The HFEA publishes a Code of Practice regulating any technology involving human embryos, and issues licenses for treatment services, nonmedical fertility services, storage, and research involving embryos. After noting the prevalence of NMSS among users of fertility technology, the HFEA recommended that PGD should be permitted only for medical reasons in view of the potential harm to a child should they learn that they were sex selected. Subsequently, sex selection for nonmedical reasons, whether by PGD or sperm-sorting, was officially banned by a 2008 amendment to the HFE Act. Of the other G12 countries, Australia, Belgium, Canada, France, Germany, Italy, Netherlands, Spain, and Switzerland all have laws that specifically regulate NMSS, generally prohibiting it in most situations.[14] Similarly, Article 14 of the EU convention on Human Rights and Biomedicine states: "The use of techniques of medically assisted procreation shall not be allowed for the purpose of choosing a future child's sex, except where serious hereditary sex-related disease is to be avoided" (Council of Europe, 1996).

Israel regulates sex selection by and/or during PGD in a different manner (Pessach, Glasser, Soskolne, Barash, & Lerner-Geva, 2014). Israel is, by its very nature, a unique case: it is a multireligious, multicultural society with a strong pronatal sentiment within a social-democratic system (Landau, 2008). Thus, the innovative solution devised by the government reflects the various factors at work in the country. It provides for a professional committee composed of physicians, lawyers, clergy, and ethicists that can approve NMSS when certain criteria are met:

(1) Harm—Not having a child of a particular sex must create a real and major risk of significant harm to the mental health of one or both of the parents, or to the future child.

---

[12]https://www.congress.gov/bill/115th-congress/house-bill/4660.

[13]Available at https://www.legislation.gov.uk/ukpga/2008/22/contents (last visited April 1, 2018).

[14]https://cbhd.org/content/g12-country-regulations-assisted-reproductive-technologies.

(2) Siblings—The applicants must have at least four children of the same sex (the average family has 3.7 children) and none of the requested sex (a requirement that can be waived in rare cases).
(3) Informed consent—The parents must receive genetic counseling, including a discussion on the ethical dimension of NMSS, and be informed of the process, risks, and costs. The parents must be told that if none of the normal pre-embryos generated by IVF treatment are of the desired gender, no authorization for another cycle of IVF and PGD for sex selection will be granted before the use of all existing embryos for reproduction.
(4) Judgement—The committee must be convinced, based on professional and ethical deliberation, that sex selection is justified in the particular case.

Additional factors to be considered include whether the parents already need IVF for other reasons, whether PGD would be carried out for medical reasons regardless of sex selection, and the nature of the family and social status of the applicants as reflected in peer pressure and cultural differences. A detailed account of the committee's work can be found in Pessach et al. (2014), which reveals that in 2006–2011, the committee reviewed 411 applications (out of some 50,000 eligible families with 4 or more children of one sex).[15] A final decision was handed down in 216 cases, with 21% of the applications approved. In 2012–2014, the approval rate dropped to 12% (30 out of 250 cases).

The diversity of regulatory schemes for sex selection around the world is an indication of the wide range of opinions and ethical stances regarding the issue. It also means that individuals intent on NMMS can simply travel elsewhere for reproductive treatment. This raises the concern that nonmedical IVF, with the potential need to travel across borders to perform it, is available only to couples with means. Thus, not only is the effectiveness of regulation unclear, but it may disproportionately affect the less affluent.

10.6 Conclusion

The different approaches to the regulation of sex selection demonstrate that there is no simple one-size-fits-all prescription for how to regulate sex selection across cultures. The best strategy would seem to be to balance the various arguments, interests, and possible ramifications with the society-specific context. For example, reconciling reproductive autonomy and gender equality remains a key feminist issue. But this concern may be less pressing in Western societies where, on the whole, no real bias for a particular gender is exhibited (although there might be ethnic variations within the country).

In general terms, advances in genetics and medical technology compel us to consider a number of questions. First, is there a distinctive feature that justifies differential

[15] A clear indication of the low interest of the vast majority of Israeli families in sex selection for non-medical reasons.

regulatory treatment of sex selection at different stages of development? If choosing the sex of a child is wrong, doesn't how we achieve it become largely irrelevant? Is there a stronger argument for the regulation of pre-conception sex selection over pre-implantation PGD, especially when a woman has to undergo PGD for medical reasons in any case? Furthermore, the practicality of regulation must be considered. In most countries, intrusive or semi-intrusive legislation will be unacceptable. Thus, in jurisdictions with no impediments on the right to abortion, parents with a strong desire for a child of a particular sex can be expected to choose this means of NMSS. On the other hand, in countries with limited access to abortion or with a regulated market of reproductive services, providers will be forced to answer to the regulator in respect to sex-selection practices.

In addition, although nonmedical and medical sex selection are almost always treated differently, the definition of medical sex selection can be both over- and under-inclusive. What diseases are sufficiently severe to justify "medical sex selection," and who decides what conditions make that list? Finally, and paradoxically, the US and other Western countries do not endorse pre-conception sex selection despite the fact that social opinion suggests that permissive sex selection would not lead to any significant gender preference. Perhaps it is the declarative function of the law that is its raison d'être, that is, officially discouraging sex selection reflects a moral stance on gender equality and worthiness.

Acknowledgements I would like to thank Aisha Haley JD, UVA Law School for her superb research assistance, and Saralee Glasser MA, from the Gertner Institute, for her constructive comments.

References

American Society for Reproductive Medicine, Ethics Committee. (2015). Use of reproductive technology for sex selection for nonmedical reasons. *Fertility and Sterility, 103*(6), 1418–1422.

Archer, J., & Lloyd, B. (2002). *Sex and gender*. Cambridge, UK: Cambridge University Press.

Birdsall, M. L. (2010). An exploration of "the 'Wild West' of reproductive technology": Ethical and feminist perspectives on sex-selection practices in the United States. *William & Mary Journal of Women and the Law, 17*(1), 223–247.

Bongaarts, J., & Guilmoto, C. Z. (2015). How many more missing women? Excess female mortality and prenatal sex selection, 1970–2050. *Population and Development Review, 41*(2), 241–269.

Council of Europe. (1996). Convention for the protection of human rights and dignity of the human being with regard to the application of biology and medicine: Convention on human rights and biomedicine. Strasbourg: Council of Europe, Directorate of Legal Affairs.

Daar, J. F. (2005). ART and the search for perfectionism: On selecting gender, genes, and gametes. *Journal of Gender, Race & Justice, 9,* 241–272.

Dickens, B. M., Serour, G. I., Cook, R. J., & Qiu, R. Z. (2005). Sex selection: Treating different cases differently. *International Journal of Gynecology & Obstetrics, 90*(2), 171–177.

Dondorp, W., de Wert, G., Bombard, Y., Bianchi, D. W., Bergmann, C., Borry, P. … Cornel, M. C. (2015). Non-invasive prenatal testing for aneuploidy and beyond: Challenges of responsible innovation in prenatal screening. *European Journal of Human Genetics, 23*(11), 1438–1450.

Dondorp, W., de Wert, G., Pennings, G., Shenfield, F., Devroey, P., Tarlatzis, B. ... Diedrich, K. (2013). ESHRE task force on ethics and Law 20: Sex selection for non-medical reasons. *Human Reproduction, 28*(6), 1448–1454.

English, V., & Braude, P. (2014). Regulation of PGD in the UK and Worldwide. In T. El-Toukhy & P. Braude (Eds.), *Preimplantation genetic diagnosis in clinical practice* (pp. 187–195). London: Springer.

Grech, V. (2017). Further evidence of male offspring preference for certain subgroups in the United States (2007–2015). *Early Human Development, 110,* 9–12.

Heyd, D. (2003). Male or female, we will create them: The ethics of sex selection for nonmedical reasons. *Ethical Perspectives, 10*(3–4), 204–214.

Ivey, R. (2009). Resolving the feminist dilemma: Is regulation of non-medical pre-implantation and pre-fertilization sex selection technologies necessary? *Journal of Health Law and Bioethics, 2,* i–xxxiv.

Kalfoglou, A. L., Kammersell, M., Philpott, S., & Dahl, E. (2013). Ethical arguments for and against sperm sorting for non-medical sex selection: A review. *Reproductive Biomedicine Online, 26*(3), 231–239.

Landau, R. (2008). Sex selection for social purposes in Israel: Quest for the "perfect child" of a particular gender or centuries old prejudice against women? *Journal of Medical Ethics, 34*(9), e10.

Lewis, C., Hill, M., & Chitty, L. S. (2016). Women's experiences and preferences for service delivery of non-invasive prenatal testing for aneuploidy in a public health setting: A mixed methods study. *PLoS ONE, 11*(4), e0153147.

Mieszczak, J., Houk, C. P., & Lee, P. A. (2009). Assignment of the sex of rearing in the neonate with a disorder of sex development. *Current Opinion in Pediatrics, 21*(4), 541–547.

Moazam, F. (2004). Feminist discourse on sex screening and selective abortion of female foetuses. *Bioethics, 18*(3), 205–220.

Mohapatra, S. (2012). Global legal responses to prenatal gender identification and sex selection. *Nevada Law Journal, 13*(3), 690–721.

Norton, M. E., Jacobsson, B., Swamy, G. K., Laurent, L. C., Ranzini, A. C. Brar, H. ... Wapner, R. J. (2015). Cell-free DNA analysis for noninvasive examination of trisomy. *New England Journal of Medicine, 372*(17), 1589–1597.

Oakley, A. (2016). *Sex, gender and society*. New York: Routledge.

Pennings, G. (1996). Ethics of sex selection for family balancing: Family balancing as a morally acceptable application of sex selection. *Human Reproduction, 11*(11), 2339–2342.

Pessach, N., Glasser, S., Soskolne, V., Barash, A., & Lerner-Geva, L. (2014). The Israeli National Committee for sex selection by pre-implantation genetic diagnosis: A novel approach (2005–2011). *Israel Journal of Health Policy Research, 3,* 33.

Puri, S., Adams, V., Ivey, S., & Nachtigall, R. D. (2011). "There is such a thing as too many daughters, but not too many sons": A qualitative study of son preference and fetal sex selection among Indian immigrants in the United States. *Social Science and Medicine, 72*(7), 1169–1176.

Robertson, J. (2001). Preconception sex selection. *American Journal of Bioethics, 1*(1), 2–9.

Steinbock, B. (2002). Sex selection: Not obviously wrong. *The Hastings Center Report, 32*(1), 23–28.

Sureau, C. (1999). Sex selection: A crime against humanity or the exercise of a fundamental right? *Human Reproduction, 14*(4), 867–868.

Wherrett, D. K. (2015). Approach to the infant with a suspected disorder of sex development. *Pediatric Clinics, 62*(4), 983–999.

Chapter 11
From Cradle to Grave: A Terror Management Theory Analysis of Parenthood

Sheldon Solomon

> *The cradle rocks above an abyss, and common sense tells us that our existence is but a brief crack of light between two eternities of darkness.*
>
> Vladimir Nabokov, *Speak, Memory: A Memoir*

11.1 Terror Management Theory

> Integral parts of the human whole: the necessity of destruction to procure alimentary sustenance: the painful character of the ultimate functions of separate existence, the agonies of birth and death: the monotonous menstruation of simian and (particularly) human females extending from the age of puberty to the menopause: inevitable accidents at sea, in mines and factories: certain very painful maladies and their resultant surgical operations, innate lunacy and congenital criminality, decimating epidemics: catastrophic cataclysms which make terror the basis of human mentality ...
>
> James Joyce, *Ulysses*

Terror management theory (TMT; Solomon, Greenberg, & Pyszczynski, 1991) was originally derived from cultural anthropologist Becker's (1971, 1973, 1975) efforts to develop a comprehensive account of human motivation and social behavior. TMT posits that humans, like all forms of life, are biologically predisposed toward self-preservation in the service of survival and reproduction. We are however, unique in our capacity for abstract symbolic thought (Deacon, 1997), mental time travel (i.e. to explicitly reflect on the past and anticipate the future; Varki & Brower, 2013), and self-consciousness (Rank, 1945). This is an extraordinarily adaptive suite of cognitive tools, that when juxtaposed with our visual acuity and manual dexterity, enable humans to transform the products of their imagination into reality and transfer knowledge (explicitly and implicitly) across generations (i.e. cultural evolution; Henrich,

S. Solomon (✉)
Skidmore College, Saratoga Springs, NY, USA
e-mail: ssolomon@skidmore.edu

O. Taubman – Ben-Ari (ed.), *Pathways and Barriers to Parenthood*,
https://doi.org/10.1007/978-3-030-24864-2_11

2016). Moreover, self-consciousness renders us, in our finest moments, sublimely appreciative of life: it is wonderful and awe-inspiring to be alive and to know it.

However, self-consciousness, combined with the propensity to ponder the future, also invariably engenders the unsettling and unwelcome realization that, like all other living entities, our lives are of finite duration and we too will inevitably die. We also recognize that we are each susceptible to unexpected and premature deaths for unforeseeable and uncontrollable reasons: perpetually vulnerable embodied creatures who, from a biological or cosmological perspective, are fleeting specks of respiring, defecating, fornicating carbon-based dust unwillingly and unwittingly born in an unfathomably large universe that is blithely indifferent to our fate.

According to Becker and TMT, the explicit awareness of one's mortality, ongoing susceptibility to death, and discomfort with our corporeal nature engenders existential terror manifested as persistent anxiety and/or despair, and this in turn could undermine the capacity to engage in effective instrumental behaviors and thereby reduce one's prospects for survival and reproduction. Humans "manage" existential terror by embracing cultural worldviews[1]: humanly constructed beliefs about reality shared by individuals in a group that afford a sense that one is a valuable member of a meaningful universe that includes the possibility of attaining literal and/or symbolic immortality (Lifton, 1979). Literal immortality consists of the heavens, souls, afterlives, and reincarnations common to many of the world's great religions. Symbolic immortality consists of the belief that a remnant of one's existence will persist in perpetuity, by e.g., having children, amassing huge fortunes, being part of a great and enduring tribe or nation, producing great works of science or art, or performing heroic acts of public service.

Self-esteem is the belief that one is a person of *value* in a world of *meaning*; and the primary function of self-esteem, as well as the cultural worldviews from which self-esteem is derived, is to minimize anxiety in general and death anxiety in particular. Self-esteem acquires its anxiety-buffering qualities in the context of infant socialization. According to attachment theory (Bowlby, 1969), long before babies have the physical, emotional and intellectual capabilities to survive on their own or have any awareness of death, anxiety in response to unmet needs or physical danger instigates the formation of physical and psychological attachments to primary caretakers who nurture and protect their offspring. These attachments in turn provide infants with a pervasive and unconditional sense of safety and security.

Children must however, eventually be fully incorporated into their social milieus by learning the language, beliefs and customs of their culture. Toward this end, parental affection becomes increasingly contingent on children behaving in accord with cultural dictates. When children behave appropriately, they are showered with

---

[1] Although TMT posits that mitigating death anxiety is a central function of cultural worldviews, it does not claim that this is their sole function. Some evolutionary theorists propose that cultural worldviews (particularly religions) foster social coordination and cohesion, which enables large groups of genetically unrelated individuals to coexist peacefully (Sloan-Wilson, 2002). Others propose that cultural worldviews contain explicit and implicit practical knowledge necessary survival and reproduction in particular environments (Henrich, 2016). TMT theorists take no issue with these assertions, except to insist that cultural worldviews also serve to manage existential terror.

parental praise, which produce the same feelings of psychological well-being previously associated with secure attachment. Inappropriate behavior begets very different parental reactions, ranging from punishment to rebuke to frowning indifference, all of which involve a distinct absence of affection. This produces anxiety and insecurity (perhaps linked to a fear of abandonment). Over time, children come to associate being "good" with being safe (good = safe = alive) and being "bad" with being helpless and vulnerable (bad = insecure = dead) and in this fashion, self-esteem becomes a potent anxiety buffer.

Subsequently, the anxiety-buffering qualities of self-esteem, initially obtained from pleasing parents during socialization come to depend on adhering to prevailing cultural standards. Throughout socialization, children learn the ways of the world by way of their culture's history, religion and folklore. The transition begins as children become increasingly aware of the personal implications of the inevitability of death. In *Existential Psychotherapy*, Yalom (1980) presents clinical and empirical evidence suggesting this happens as early as two years of age and is often of considerable concern by age nine or ten. Children now begin to find the promises of security and death transcendence afforded by the culture as (or more) compelling and reassuring than even the best efforts of their parents, who children realize, like all humans, are fallible and mortal. Self-esteem is now obtained by meeting or exceeding the culturally prescribed standards associated with specific social roles afforded by their culture. Throughout their lives, people are fundamentally motivated to maintain faith in their culturally acquired belief systems, confidence in their self-worth, and close relationships with significant others (Mikulincer, Florian, & Hirschberger, 2003) as a psychological bulwark against existential terror, and will consequently respond defensively when their cherished cultural beliefs, self-esteem, or close relationships is undermined.

11.2 Empirical Evaluation of TMT

Three independent lines of empirical inquiry provide compelling convergent support for the basic tenets of TMT.

Anxiety-buffer hypothesis: if self-esteem buffers anxiety, then situationally increased or dispositionally high self-esteem should reduce anxiety in response to subsequent threats. Consistent with this claim, Greenberg et al. (1992) had participants view graphic depictions of death or a neutral film after giving them positive or neutral feedback on a personality inventory to increase their self-esteem or leave it unaltered. Although neutral self-esteem participants showed a significant increase in self-reported anxiety in response to the death-related video, those who received a self-esteem boost did not. A second study employed different manipulations of self-esteem (high scores on a supposed IQ test) and threat (anticipating painful electric shocks) and produced the same effect on a physiological measure of autonomic arousal associated with anxiety (skin conductance). Subsequent studies demonstrated that both manipulated and chronically high levels of self-esteem reduced defensive reactions to death reminders (e.g., Harmon-Jones et al., 1997). Taken together, these experiments (and others reviewed by Pyszczynski, Greenberg, Solomon, Arndt, & Schimel, 2004) confirm that self-esteem buffers anxiety and that this effect extends beyond self-esteem-related threats.

Mortality salience hypothesis: if cultural worldviews, self-esteem, and close relationships serve to mitigate existential terror, then asking people to ponder their own mortality (*mortality salience*; MS) should increase the need for the protection provided by them. This should result in vigorous agreement with and affection for those who share our cherished beliefs (or are similar to us) and equally vigorous hostility and disdain for those who are opposed to our beliefs or merely different from us, as well as efforts to bolster self-esteem and fortify close relationships. To test the mortality salience hypotheses, TMT researchers make mortality momentarily salient by having people write about their death; specifically, by responding to two open ended questions: "Please briefly describe the emotions that the thought of your own death arouse in you."; and, "Jot down, as specifically as you can, what you think will happen to you as you physically die.". Other manipulations of MS include: completing death anxiety scales; viewing graphic depictions of death; being interviewed in front of a funeral parlor; or, subliminal exposure to the word "dead" or "death".

Findings confirm that MS intensifies cultural worldview defense, self-esteem striving, and desire for close relationships. For example, Greenberg et al. (1990) found that Christian participants had more favorable reactions to fellow Christians and less favorable reactions to Jewish targets in response to MS; Taubman – Ben-Ari, Florian, and Mikulincer (1999) found that, after a MS induction, Israeli soldiers who derived self-esteem from their driving skills drove faster and more recklessly in a driving simulator; and Mikulincer and Florian (2000; Study 5) found that MS increased the desire for intimacy in close relationships among securely attached participants (see Burke, Martens, & Faucher, 2010, for a meta-analysis of MS studies).

Death thought accessibility hypothesis: threats to cherished aspects of cultural worldviews, self-esteem, or close attachments should increase the accessibility of non-conscious death-related thoughts (*death thought accessibility*; DTA). The number of incomplete word stems completed with death-related words (e.g., C O F F _ _ could be COFFEE or COFFIN; G R _ V E could be GROVE OR GRAVE) is generally used to measure DTA. For example, Christian fundamentalists confronted with logical inconsistencies in the bible (Friedman & Rholes, 2007), Americans asked to ponder undesired aspects of themselves (Ogilvie, Cohen, & Solomon, 2008), and Israelis asked to think about problems they have experienced in their current romantic relationship (Florian, Mikulincer, & Hirschberger, 2002) showed increased DTA (see Hayes, Schimel, Arndt, & Faucher, 2010 for a meta-analysis of DTA research).

Moreover, conditions that increase DTA also increase cultural worldview defense, self-esteem striving, and desire for close relationships (e.g., Greenberg, Pyszczynski, Solomon, Simon, & Breus, 1994). Additionally, defending one's worldview, bolstering one's self-esteem, or thinking about close relationships decreases DTA (Hart, Shaver, & Goldenberg, 2005).

11.3 A Terror Management Theory Analysis of Parenthood

> It was the best of times, it was the worst of times.
>
> *A Tale of Two Cities*, Charles Dickens

One need not be a practicing clinician or developmental psychologist to discern that having a child constitutes a major life transition rife with generally positive, but also occasionally negative, psychological and interpersonal consequences; indeed, just becoming a parent will typically suffice to produce these insights! From a TMT perspective, parenthood can serve to assuage existential anxieties by bolstering every component of the terror management system: literal and symbolic immortality, cultural worldviews, self-esteem, and close relationships (see also Morse and Steger, Chap. 1 in this volume).

People can accept their own transience more graciously knowing that they live on through their children. Children afford a touch of literal immortality as ambulatory vehicles for 50% of each parent's genetic contribution to their offspring, often reflected in the child's appearance, disposition, and predilections. It is surely uplifting to find that your daughter is a "spitting image" of you; and, that she shares your good cheer, your gregarious sense of humor, as well as your fondness for reggae music and sour pickles. Symbolically, children carry on the family name and family traditions, thus serving as a corporeal conduit between generations of venerable ancestors going back to a distant past, as well as extending forward to infinite future generations.

Children also reinforce their parents' faith in the prevailing cultural worldview by adopting the core beliefs and values of the culture. Parents stress their beliefs and values to their children in hopes that they will adopt them and pass them on to future generations. Some parents disown, abandon, or even murder offspring who do not adhere their beliefs, suggesting that passing on cultural worldviews can be more important than passing on genes. For example, in 2014 a Malaysian father shouted "*Aku tak mengaku anak*" (I disown you), when his son came home for lunch wearing a badge of support for a rival political party (from Solomon, Greenberg, & Pyszczynski, 2015, p. 104). And in 2017, when Stanzin Saldon, from a Buddhist family, married Murtaza Agha, who is a Muslim, her father locked her in the family home, spat in her face, summoned shamans to erase her memory of Mr. Agha, and shouted, "Why did you not die no sooner than you were born?" (Raj & Gettleman, 2017).

Additionally, being a mother or father can be a potent source of self-esteem to the extent that parenting is valued by their culture, and parents perceive themselves as successful in this regard; i.e. that they are "good" parents. Tribal, religious, and interdependent cultures generally value parenthood because producing children is viewed as critical to maintaining the vitality of the group over time. In more secular, individualistic (i.e. western and westernized) cultures, becoming a parent may afford a welcome psychological respite from social roles associated with relatively unattainable standards of value. Specifically, in media saturated market driven cultures, males are judged by their wealth, based on the assumption that anyone can be as wealthy as Bill Gates or Donald Trump if they are sufficiently intelligent and industrious. Females are judged by their youth and beauty, based on the assumption that all women should be inordinately thin and perpetually young. It is simply not possible however, for all males to be fantastically wealthy, or for all females to be young and nubile forever. It is therefore not surprising that many young adults in such societies have low self-esteem and suffer physically and psychologically as a result. Yet one need not be a successful hedge fund manager or a beauty queen to be a fine parent.

Finally, parents generally develop close relationships with their children. During infancy, such affiliations are somewhat one-sided in that they consist primarily of parents caring for their strikingly helpless and needy offspring. Over time, parent-child relationships are elaborated and enriched. Children become more than endearing dependents as they mature, providing their parents with an invaluable source of friendship, comradery, and psychosocial support.

Existing empirical evidence is consistent with the proposition that parenting can serve a variety of terror management functions. One way to acquire symbolic immortality (perhaps with a touch of perceived literal immortality), is namesaking; i.e. to name your children after yourself. For example, the former heavyweight boxing champion George Foreman named five of his children George, George, George, George, and Georgetta! To determine if namesaking confers a sense of symbolic immortality, after a MS or aversive control induction (i.e. failing an exam), Vicary (2011) had American participants imagine they were having a child in the next 5 years. Participants then reported the likelihood giving the child their own first name, a middle name the same as their first name, a middle name the same as their middle name, or a variant of their own name (e.g. Peter naming his son Pete). They also responded to parallel questions regarding the likelihood of naming the child after their mothers, fathers, grandmothers, and grandfathers. Composite scores were generated for each set of questions (naming after oneself; naming after a family member), and results indicated that MS increased participant's intentions to name their child after themselves, but not their family members.

Another line of inquiry is based on the notion that just having children, regardless of their names, is also an effective bulwark against existential terror. To the extent that this is true, death reminders should increase the desire to have children. Zhou, Liu, Chen, and Yu (2008) reminded Chinese university students of their mortality via a word-completion task where 10 of 30 words could only be completed with death-related words (e.g. funeral, tomb, coffin, dead body; in the control condition all 30 words were neutral). All participants then read a statement of the birth control policy in China—"The Chinese government introduced the one-child policy in 1979 to alleviate the overpopulation, social, and environmental problems of China. The one-child policy promotes one couple having only one child. Additional children will result in monetary penalties"—and rated their attitudes toward the one-child policy. As predicted, participants in the MS condition reported less support for the one-child policy, which the authors interpreted as reflecting an enhanced desire for children.

More direct evidence that MS increases the desire for children was obtained by Fritsche et al. (2007, Study 1). German university students were asked to write the first sentence that came to mind when they thought about their own death, or the first sentence that came to mind when they thought about dental pain. Participants who wrote about death subsequently reported a greater desire to have children, and to have them sooner, than those who wrote about pain. In light of this finding, Fritsche et al. (2007, Study 3) hypothesized that thinking about having children would diminish the cultural worldview defense that typically occurs in response to a mortality salience induction. To test this hypothesis, they had East Germans write about their thoughts and feelings about either having their own children or watching television. Next participants wrote about their thoughts and feelings about dying, or being in pain. Finally, everyone rated the degree to which 16 positive and 16 negative adjectives appropriately described East Germans and West Germans. Although the East Germans had less favorable impressions of West Germans when reminded of death than watching television, this did not happen when participants wrote about having their own children first (see Wisman & Goldenberg, 2005, Study 2 for a similar finding with Dutch participants). Death is thus apparently not so troubling when the prospect of children is on one's mind.

Additional research has replicated and extended these findings. After a MS or control induction, Wisman and Goldenberg (2005) predicted and found that Dutch men, but not women, reported a desire for more children (see also Mathews & Sear, 2008). This prediction was based on the possibility of a gender difference regarding the potential conflict between becoming a parent and maintaining one's professional aspirations. Specifically, having a career and children is compatible for men given that they do not generally perform caregiving tasks that could undermine professional advancement; however, women often find themselves in an implicit or explicit psychological bind to the extent that they perceive becoming a parent as antithetical to furthering their professional ambitions.

Consistent with this view, in Study 1, after a MS or neutral control induction, men and women completed a measure of death thought accessibility (DTA), and then reported how many children they would like to have as well as if they were currently in a committed relationship. Results indicated a main effect for MS on the DTA measure, demonstrating that DTA increased in response to a death reminder for both men and women. However, there was a MS X Gender interaction on the dependent measure due to men, but not women, reporting wanting to have more children in response to MS; and, this effect was independent of relationship status.

Study 3 replicated this finding, and demonstrated directly that the MS induced increase of the number of desired children was moderated by career striving (while ruling out the possibility that this effect could be accounted for in terms of participants' desire for sexuality). Dutch men and women first completed a measure of career striving (e.g., "I would never give up my career for my family", "If I had to choose between a career and having children, I would choose having children" (reverse scored). They then wrote about their mortality or being in intense pain, reported how many children they would like to have, and their current desire for sex. The predicted significant MS X gender interaction on the measure of how many children one wanted was unaffected by desire for sex. There was however, a three-way MS X Gender X Career Striving interaction on the primary dependent measure. MS increased the number of children men desired regardless of career striving (i.e. there was just a main effect for MS). However, for women, there was a MS X Career Striving interaction, such that whereas women with high career striving reported desiring fewer children in response to MS, the MS induction had no effect for women with low career strivings.

Wisman and Goldenberg (2005) then conducted a final study (Study 4) to confirm that women's concerns about motherhood being antithetical to their career aspirations inhibits the increased desire for children in response to MS. After writing about their mortality or watching television, young Dutch women read a reputed newspaper article claiming that motherhood was either incompatible or compatible with having a career (Wisman & Goldenberg, 2005, p. 56):

"Almost 84% of women that have children are *more* satisfied with their jobs and earn *more* than comparable childless colleagues of the same age … "We think it a matter of priority," suggests Professor Dr. Bernard Schafely, one of the researchers of the University of Utrecht … "the switch from raising a child to good functioning on the job floor, appear to be a *smaller* leap then one would expect." Anyway, it is very *good* news for women who have children … There may be also *disadvantages* associated with having children, but overall having children is definitely *compatible* with achieving a career." (Antonyms of the italicized words were used in the career is incompatible with children condition.)

In accord with predictions (and replicating the finding of Study 1–3), MS had no effect on women's reported desire for children when they were primed with the notion that motherhood is incompatible with having a successful career. But MS increased women's reported desire for children when motherhood was described as being compatible with career success.

Although these experiments demonstrate that arousing existential concerns increases the desire for children (either in general or when motherhood is perceived as compatible with professional aspirations), Yaakobi, Mikulincer, and Shaver (2014) argued that these findings do not directly demonstrate that parenting per se serves an anxiety-buffering function. To provide such evidence, married Israeli undergraduates who did not have children (and who, if female, were not pregnant at the time of the study) completed a Hebrew version of the Experiences in Close Relationships scale (Brennan, Clark, & Shaver, 1998) in order to assess attachment anxiety and avoidance. Participants returned to lab two weeks later and were randomly assigned to think about death, eating food, or physical pain (i.e. neutral and aversive control inductions respectively). Afterwards, they completed a 14-item questionnaire on parenthood-related cognitions on the importance (e.g., "I'm looking forward to becoming a parent") and vividness (e.g., "I can vividly imagine feeding my child") of becoming a parent. Yaakobi et al. (2014) predicted and found that the MS induction increased participants' reports of the importance and vividness of parenthood for participants low in avoidant attachment orientation. [The attachment orientation prediction was based on prior research demonstrating that insecure attachment is associated with decreased interest in having children (e.g., Nathanson & Manohar, 2012), and that insecure parents report being less likely to have joyous and pleasant interactions with their children and have positive views of them (e.g., Impett, English, & John, 2011).]

After replicating this finding (Study 2), Yaakobi et al. (2014; Study 3) demonstrated that the prospect of becoming a parent buffered death anxiety in securely attached individuals. After a MS or control induction, securely and insecurely attached participants were asked to imagine either becoming a parent ("Describe, in as much detail as you can, what you think will happen to you after the birth.") or parallel questions about a desirable vacation. All participants then completed a Hebrew version of a word-stem completion task to measure death thought accessibility. Results indicated the predicted three-way interaction between MS, parenthood thoughts, and avoidant attachment; specifically, that a death reminder increased death-thought accessibility in all conditions except for low avoidance participants primed with parenthood thoughts. This finding was conceptually replicated in Study 4, where MS increased the desire for romantic intimacy (a well-documented TMT defense; Mikulincer et al., 2003) in all conditions except for low avoidance participants primed with parenthood thoughts. Then in Study 5, Yaakobi et al. (2014) reversed this effect by having secure and insecure participants think about obstacles to becoming a parent (i.e. an inability to have children because of infertility problems), an upcoming exam, or watching television, followed by a measure of death-thought accessibility. Consistent with predictions, thinking about infertility increased death-thought accessibility, but only for low avoidance (i.e. securely attached) participants.

According to Yaakobi et al. (2014) people with high avoidance attachment orientations are unlikely to employ parenthood-related cognitions to mitigate existential anxieties because they (implicitly or explicitly) view the demands of parenthood as conflicting with their personal strivings for autonomy and professional success. To explore this possibility directly, in Study 6, after a MS or neutral control induction, participants read a modification of Wisman and Goldenberg's (2005, Study 4) purported newspaper article claiming that parenthood was either compatible or incompatible with having a successful career, and then completed a scale to assess parenthood-related cognitions. Consistent with predictions, when parenthood was described as incompatible with a successful career, parenthood-related cognitions increased in response to MS only for participants low in avoidance attachment orientation (replicating the finding of Studies 1–2). However, all participants (i.e. high and low avoidance attachment) had increased parenthood-related cognitions in response to MS when parenthood was depicted as quite compatible with professional aspirations.

In sum, the studies described above provide convergent empirical support for the terror management function of parenthood. Specifically, death reminders increased intentions to name children after oneself (namesaking), opposition to laws limiting having more than one child, and the desire to have more children and to have them sooner. Moreover, making the prospect of having children or becoming a parent salient reduced death-thought accessibility and worldview defenses in response to a mortality salience induction.

However, the fact that women with high career ambitions do not desire to have more children in response to mortality salience (unless primed with the notion that having children is compatible with having a successful career), and that parenthood-related cognitions do not buffer death anxiety for those with high avoidance attachment orientation (unless also primed with the notion that having children is compatible with having a successful career), suggests that there are situational and dispositional factors that could mitigate the effectiveness of parenthood as a means to manage existential terror.

Indeed, from a TMT perspective, while parenthood can serve as a potent form of terror management, it can also magnify existential anxieties by undermining every component of the terror management system: literal and symbolic immortality, cultural worldviews, self-esteem, and close relationships.

Becoming a parent can be a source of psychological ambivalence or despair for those who derive a sense of meaning and value (i.e. self-esteem) from being successful professionally, particularly in globalized multi-national market-based cultural milieus where people are judged, and judge themselves, in proportion to their vocational and fiscal stature. The time and resources (be they physical, cognitive, emotional, economic) devoted to bearing and caring for children can be at the expense of career pursuits, which can ultimately reduce one's prospects for professional advancement. Additionally, the loss of self-esteem associated with relinquishing professional success and aspirations is often compounded by the fact that in such cultural settings, caring for, and in some instances even bearing, children is viewed as a menial activity best performed by poorly educated and poorly compensated minorities.

Becoming a parent can also serve to make one's mortality implicitly or explicitly salient in a variety of ways. For some people, having children marks an irrevocable transition from youth to adulthood, perhaps with the vague or not so vague sense of the inevitable passage of time leading to one's aging and ultimate mortality. For others, bearing and caring for children is a grim reminder of our corporeal nature: that we are defecating, urinating, fornicating, menstruating, lactating, ejaculating, projectile vomiting animals; and this in turn produces intimations of mortality. In accord with this notion, research has shown that death-thought accessibility increased after viewing pictures of urine, mucus, feces, and vomit (Cox, Goldenberg, Pyszczynski, & Weise, 2007), reminding people that they are animals (Goldenberg et al., 2001), or having them think about physical aspects of sex (and this effect was particularly pronounced in participants high in neuroticism; Goldenberg, Pyszczynski, McCoy, Greenberg, & Solomon, 1999).

Existential concerns aroused by the heightened salience of humankind's corporeal nature are apt to be particularly prominent for women, given the visible physical changes and effusions of bodily fluids associated with pregnancy, breast-feeding, and diapering (see Magid, 2017, for an extended discussion of how pregnancy and parenthood can increase mortality salience for mothers). This in turn can have deleterious interpersonal as well as intrapsychic consequences for mothers.

In 2015, for example, Donald Trump famously halted a legal proceeding when a lawyer for the opposition asked for a medical break to pump breast milk for her infant daughter, declaring "You're disgusting" as he stormed out of the room (Barbaro & Eder, 2015). Research confirms that existential anxieties magnify hostility and disdain toward pregnant and lactating women. Participants reminded of the similarities between humans and animals subsequently had more negative reactions to a *Vanity*

Fair magazine cover with actress Demi Moore as pregnant, compared to participants who viewed another *Vanity Fair* magazine cover of Moore when she was not pregnant (Goldenberg, Goplen, Cox, & Arndt, 2007). A second study by Goldenberg et al. (2007) then found that participants reminded of the similarities between humans and animals rated actress Gwyneth Paltrow as less competent when they viewed a color photo of her when she was pregnant, compared to participants who viewed another image where she was similarly clad but was not pregnant. Additionally, Cox, Goldenberg, Arndt, and Pyszczynski (2007) found that, after a mortality salience induction, participants had more negative reactions to a vignette describing a woman breastfeeding her infant in public (Study 1), and sat further away from a potential partner who they believed was breastfeeding an infant in the next room (Study 2).

Mothers are also apt to harbor existential anxieties about their health and their infant's health, both during and after pregnancy; this is quite understandable given that for much of human history, and in many communities to this day, it was (and is) quite common for women to die during childbirth and for there to be high rates of infant mortality. Moreover, because of the profound helplessness and dependence of human infants, for mothers (as well as other primary caretakers), even momentary separation from their progeny could elicit intimations of mortality. To assess the merits of this hypothesis, Taubman – Ben-Ari and Katz - Ben-Ami (2008) asked first-time Israeli mothers, after measuring their attachment orientation, to imagine being separated from their baby and to describe the thoughts and feelings this image arouses in them, or to imagine watching a television show and to describe their subsequent thoughts and feelings. All participants then completed a word-stem completion task to measure death-thought accessibility. Mothers who pondered the prospect of being separated from their babies had higher death-thought accessibility, regardless of their attachment orientation.

Irrespective of its origin—be it loss of self-esteem, mortality salience, reminders of sex or animality, or separation anxiety—heightened death-thought accessibility engendered by various experiences associated with parenting could in turn exacerbate other psychological difficulties. Specifically, studies have shown that in response to a MS induction, spider phobics become more fearful of spiders, individuals with obsessive-compulsive disorder use more soap and water to wash their hands, and socially anxious individuals spend more time by themselves rather than mingling with their peers (Strahan et al., 2007). Additional research (reviewed in Solomon et al., 2015) finds that death reminders increase smoking, alcohol consumption, and risky decision-making. All of these affections likely undermine positive experiences associated with parenthood, as well as the quality of parenting provided to their children.

11.4 Summary and Conclusion

Terror management theory posits that humans manage the existential terror engendered by the awareness of death by embracing cultural worldviews that afford a sense that one is a person of value in a world of meaning, and hence eligible for literal and/or symbolic immortality, as well as forging and maintaining close relationships with significant others. Viewed from a TMT perspective, parenthood can be a potent bulwark against existential terror, by conferring a sense of symbolic immortality (with a touch of literal immortality for those comforted by having their genes extended to future generations); by infusing one's life with meaning and value; and, by developing close and enduring relationships with one's children. Having children can however, also magnify existential anxieties by reminding parents that they are no longer young; by undermining self-esteem to the extent that parenthood is viewed as antithetical to professional and fiscal aspirations; and, by a host of activities associated with bearing and caring for children that are vivid reminders that we are embodied animals.

Existing research is consistent with a TMT account of parenthood. Specifically, in response to mortality salience, people are more likely to intend to name their children after themselves; they report wanting to have more children and to have them sooner; and, child and parenthood-related thoughts come more readily to mind. Moreover, thinking about having children or becoming a parent reduces death-thought accessibility and defensive reactions to a mortality salience induction; and, young mothers who imagine a separation from their infants have increased death-thought accessibility. Nevertheless, additional research is clearly in order to provide a more comprehensive account of how parenthood can serve to manage or magnify existential anxieties, including examining the mediating and moderating role of various dispositional, situational, and cultural factors.

Ideally, understanding the benefits and pitfalls associated with parenthood from a TMT perspective will be helpful to therapists working with parents who have existential concerns (see Spinelli, 1997, for some interesting case studies). Political and economic efforts to alter cultural values to hold parenthood in higher regard in order to fortify the meaning and significance that one can derive from being a parent are also in order. Finally, parents themselves (myself included!) would be well served to recognize existential ups and downs of having children; this will hopefully make them better parents, and better people.

References

Barbaro, M., & Eder, S. (2015, July 28). Under Oath, Donald Trump shows his raw side. *New York Times*. Retrieved from https://www.nytimes.com/2015/07/29/us/politics/depositions-show-donald-trump-as-quick-to-exaggerate-and-insult.html?ref=politics&_r=0.

Becker, E. (1971). *The birth and death of meaning; An interdisciplinary perspective on the problem of man* (2nd ed.). New York: Free Press.

Becker, E. (1973). *The denial of death*. New York: Free Press.

Becker, E. (1975). *Escape from evil*. New York: Free Press.

Bowlby, J. (1969). *Attachment and Loss: Vol. 1. Attachment*. New York, NY: Basic Books.

Brennan, K. A., Clark, C. L., & Shaver, P. R. (1998). Self-report measurement of adult attachment: An integrative overview. In J. A. Simpson & W. S. Rholes (Eds.), *Attachment theory and close relationships* (pp. 46–76). New York, NY, US: Guilford Press.

Burke, B. L., Martens, A., & Faucher, E. H. (2010). Two decades of terror management theory: A meta-analysis of mortality salience research. *Personality and Social Psychology Review, 14*(2), 155–195.

Cox, C. R., Goldenberg, J. L., Arndt, J., & Pyszczynski, T. (2007). Mother's milk: An existential perspective on negative reactions to breast-feeding. *Personality and Social Psychology Bulletin, 33*(1), 110–122.

Cox, C. R., Goldenberg, J. L., Pyszczynski, T., & Weise, D. (2007). Disgust, creatureliness and the accessibility of death-related thoughts. *European Journal of Social Psychology, 37*(3), 494–507.

Deacon, T. W. (1997). *The symbolic species: The co-evolution of language and the brain*. New York: W.W. Norton & Company Inc.

Florian, V., Mikulincer, M., & Hirschberger, G. (2002). The anxiety-buffering function of close relationships: Evidence that relationship commitment acts as a terror management mechanism. *Journal of Personality and Social Psychology, 82*(4), 527–542.

Friedman, M., & Rholes, W. S. (2007). Successfully challenging fundamentalist beliefs results in increased death awareness. *Journal of Experimental Social Psychology, 43*(5), 794–801.

Fritsche, I., Jonas, E., Fischer, P., Koranyi, N., Berger, N., & Fleischmann, B. (2007). Mortality salience and the desire for offspring. *Journal of Experimental Social Psychology, 43*(5), 753–762.

Goldenberg, J. L., Goplen, J., Cox, C. R., & Arndt, J. (2007). "Viewing" pregnancy as an existential threat: The effects of creatureliness on reactions to media depictions of the pregnant body. *Media Psychology, 10*(2), 211–230.

Goldenberg, J. L., Pyszczynski, T., Greenberg, J., Solomon, S., Kluck, B., & Cornwell, R. (2001). I am not an animal: Mortality salience, disgust, and the denial of human creatureliness. *Journal of Experimental Psychology: General, 130*(3), 427–435.

Goldenberg, J. L., Pyszczynski, T., McCoy, S. K., Greenberg, J., & Solomon, S. (1999). Death, sex, love, and neuroticism: Why is sex such a problem? *Journal of Personality and Social Psychology, 77*(6), 1173–1187.

Greenberg, J., Pyszczynski, T., Solomon, S., Rosenblatt, A., Veeder, M., Kirkland, S., & Lyon, D. (1990). Evidence for terror management theory II: The effects of mortality salience on reactions to those who threaten or bolster the cultural worldview. *Journal of Personality and Social Psychology, 58*(2), 308–318.

Greenberg, J., Pyszczynski, T., Solomon, S., Simon, L., & Breus, M. (1994). Role of consciousness and accessibility of death-related thoughts in mortality salience effects. *Journal of Personality and Social Psychology, 67*(4), 627–637.

Greenberg, J., Solomon, S., Pyszczynski, T., Rosenblatt, A., Burling, J., Lyon, D. ... Pinel, E. (1992). Why do people need self-esteem? Converging evidence that self-esteem serves an anxiety-buffering function. *Journal of Personality and Social Psychology, 63*(6), 913–922.

Harmon-Jones, E., Simon, L., Greenberg, J., Pyszczynski, T., Solomon, S., & McGregor, H. (1997). Terror management theory and self-esteem: Evidence that increased self-esteem reduces mortality salience effects. *Journal of Personality and Social Psychology, 72*(1), 24–36.

Hart, J., Shaver, P. R., & Goldenberg, J. L. (2005). Attachment, self-esteem, worldviews, and terror management: Evidence for a tripartite security system. *Journal of Personality and Social Psychology, 88*(6), 999–1013.

Hayes, J., Schimel, J., Arndt, J., & Faucher, E. H. (2010). A theoretical and empirical review of the death-thought accessibility concept in terror management research. *Psychological Bulletin, 136*(5), 699–739.

Henrich, J. (2016). *The secret of our success: How culture is driving human evolution, domesticating our species, and making us smarter*. Princeton, NJ: Princeton University Press.

Impett, E. A., English, T., & John, O. P. (2011). Women's emotions during interactions with their grown children in later adulthood. *Social Psychological and Personality Science, 2*(1), 42–50.

Lifton, R. J. (1979). *The broken connection: On death and the continuity of life*. New York: Simon and Schuster.

Magid, L. (2017). *Mortality salience and motherhood* (Unpublished doctoral dissertation). Long-Island University-Post, Brookville, New York.

Mathews, P., & Sear, R. (2008). Life after death: An investigation into how mortality perceptions influence fertility preferences using evidence from an internet-based experiment. *Journal of Evolutionary Psychology, 6*(3), 155–172.
Mikulincer, M., & Florian, V. (2000). Exploring individual differences in reactions to mortality salience: Does attachment style regulate terror management mechanisms? *Journal of Personality and Social Psychology, 79*(2), 260–273.
Mikulincer, M., Florian, V., & Hirschberger, G. (2003). The existential function of close relationships: Introducing death into the science of love. *Personality and Social Psychology Review, 7*(1), 20–40.
Nathanson, A. I., & Manohar, U. (2012). Attachment, working models of parenting, and expectations for using television in childrearing. *Family Relations, 61*(3), 441–454.
Ogilvie, D., Cohen, F., & Solomon, S. (2008). The undesired self: Deadly connotations. *Journal of Research in Personality, 42*(3), 564–576.
Pyszczynski, T., Greenberg, J., Solomon, S., Arndt, J., & Schimel, J. (2004). Why do people need self-esteem? A theoretical and empirical review. *Psychological Bulletin, 130*(3), 435–468.
Raj, S., & Gettleman, J. (2017, October 12). On the run for love: Couple bridges a Buddhist-Muslim divide. *New York Times*. Retrieved from https://www.nytimes.com/2017/10/12/world/asia/india-buddhist-muslim-marriage.html?_r=0.
Rank, O. (1945). *Will therapy/truth and reality*. New York: Alfred A. Knopf.
Sloan-Wilson, D. (2002). *Darwin's cathedral: Evolution, religion, and the nature of society*. Chicago, IL: University of Chicago Press.
Solomon, S., Greenberg, J., & Pyszczynski, T. (1991). A terror management theory of social behavior: The psychological functions of self-esteem and cultural worldviews. *Advances in Experimental Psychology, 24*, 93–159.
Solomon, S., Greenberg, J., & Pyszczynski, T. (2015). *The worm at the core: On the role of death in life*. New York, NY: Random House.
Spinelli, E. (1997). *Tales of un-knowing: Eight stories of existential therapy*. New York, NY: New York University Press.
Strachan, E., Schimel, J., Arndt, J., Williams, T., Solomon, S., Pyszczynski, T., & Greenberg, J. (2007). Terror mismanagement: Evidence that mortality salience exacerbates phobic and compulsive behaviors. *Personality and Social Psychology Bulletin, 33*(8), 1137–1151.
Taubman – Ben-Ari, O., Florian, V., & Mikulincer, M. (1999). The impact of mortality salience on reckless driving: A test of terror management mechanisms. *Journal of Personality and Social Psychology, 76*(1), 35–45.
Taubman – Ben-Ari, O., & Katz - Ben-Ami, L. (2008). Death awareness, maternal separation anxiety, and attachment style among first-time mothers: A terror management perspective. *Death Studies, 32*(8), 737–756.
Varki, A., & Brower, D. (2013). *Denial: Self-deception, false beliefs, and the origins of the human mind*. New York: Twelve.
Vicary, A. M. (2011). Mortality salience and namesaking: Does thinking about death make people want to name their children after themselves? *Journal of Research in Personality, 45*(1), 138–141.
Wisman, A., & Goldenberg, J. L. (2005). From the grave to the cradle: Evidence that mortality salience engenders a desire for offspring. *Journal of Personality and Social Psychology, 89*(1), 46–61.
Yaakobi, E., Mikulincer, M., & Shaver, P. R. (2014). Parenthood as a terror management mechanism: The moderating role of attachment orientations. *Personality and Social Psychology Bulletin, 40*(6), 762–774.
Yalom, I. (1980). *Existential psychotherapy*. New York, NY: Basic Books.
Zhou, X., Liu, J., Chen, C., & Yu, Z. (2008). Do children transcend death? An examination of the terror management function of offspring. *Scandinavian Journal of Psychology, 49*(5), 413–418.

Chapter 12
The Impact of Birth on Women's Health and Wellbeing

Susan Ayers and Alexandra Sawyer

12.1 Introduction

Being pregnant, giving birth and becoming a parent is a time of great change and adjustment which for some women can exacerbate existing mental health problems or lead to the development of new mental health problems. It has been estimated that 15–20% of women develop some form of mental health problem in pregnancy or after birth and the cost of this to society is substantial. For example, in the UK it has been estimated that perinatal mental health disorders cost £8.1 billion per annual cohort of women, with a substantial proportion of this cost (72%) being due to long term impacts on the child (Bauer, Parsonage, Knapp, Lemmi, & Adelaja, 2014).

Until recently, research on birth largely focused on risk factors associated with negative outcomes such as maternal and infant mortality or morbidity, negative birth experiences, and traumatic births. However, birth can also be a positive and empowering experience for women. Even when birth is complicated and potentially traumatic, research suggests the majority of women are resilient (Dikmen Yildiz, Ayers, & Phillips, 2018) and many report positive personal growth (e.g. Sawyer & Ayers, 2009; Sawyer, Ayers, Bradley, Young, & Smith, 2012; Sawyer, Nakić Radoš, Ayers, & Burn, 2015; Taubman – Ben-Ari, Ben-Shlomo, Sivan, & Dolizki, 2009; see also Taubman – Ben-Ari, Chap. 16 in this volume).

In this chapter we look at the importance of birth events in the health and wellbeing of women and infants. We consider a range of birth experiences from traumatic to positive, and examine the impact different types of birth experiences have on women's health and wellbeing and subsequently their infant's health and wellbeing.

S. Ayers (✉)
Centre for Maternal and Child Health Research, City, University of London, Northampton Square, London, UK
e-mail: Susan.Ayers@city.ac.uk

A. Sawyer
School of Health Sciences, University of Brighton, Brighton, UK
e-mail: A.Sawyer@brighton.ac.uk

O. Taubman – Ben-Ari (ed.), *Pathways and Barriers to Parenthood*,
https://doi.org/10.1007/978-3-030-24864-2_12

The implications of this research for maternity care and supporting women to have positive births are considered.

12.2 The Importance of Birth Events in the Health and Wellbeing of Women and Infants

The importance of birth events in the health and wellbeing of women and their infants is obvious in cases where severe complications arise, such as women suffering life threatening complications or the baby being born preterm. For example, preterm birth is associated with increased mortality and morbidity in infants and increased psychological problems in women. Very preterm births before 32 weeks gestation account for 1.4% of live births but 51% of infant deaths (Chow, Dattani, Hilder, Macfarlane, & Moser, 2007). Morbidity amongst children born very preterm who survive is also high: of very preterm infants who survive, 5–10% develop cerebral palsy and those without severe disability have a 2 times increased risk for developmental, cognitive and behavioural difficulties (Bhutta, Cleves, Casey, Cradock, & Anand, 2002; Zeitlin et al., 2008). Having a preterm baby can also have a negative psychosocial and emotional impact on women and their families. It can be a stressful and potentially traumatic time with women reporting increased symptoms of depression, posttraumatic stress and poorer mother-infant interaction or attachment in the immediate postpartum period (Elkit, Hartvig, & Christiansen, 2007; Forcada-Guex, Borghini, Pierrehumbert, Ansermet, & Muller-Nix, 2011; Karatzias, Chouliara, Maxton, Freer, & Power, 2007; Vigod, Villegas, & Dennis, 2010).

Birth events that are not life threatening can also be important in the health and wellbeing of women and their infants, particularly women's psychological wellbeing. For example, a survey of 1500 women with self-identified perinatal mental health problems found that when women were asked about the causes of their symptoms 40% said it was due to a traumatic birth (Boots Family Trust Alliance, 2013). This is far higher than the prevalence of actual life-threatening complications (or 'near miss' events) for women which occur in 0.6–15% of births (Tunçalp, Hindin, Souza, Chou, & Say, 2012).

This disparity between the prevalence of actual life-threatening complications and women's perceptions of birth as traumatic is supported by evidence that *subjective* birth experiences are more important than medical complications in whether women find birth traumatic and develop posttraumatic stress disorder (PTSD) (Garthus-Niegel, von Soest, Vollrath, & Eberhard-Gran, 2013). Hence, although women who have operative births (e.g. assisted vaginal or caesarean sections) are at increased risk of finding birth traumatic, there will be many women who have caesarean births who will be fine psychologically, and conversely some women whose births are medically straightforward who experience birth as traumatic.

There is evidence that women's physical and mental health during pregnancy and after birth affect the developing foetus and infant (see also Ungar et al., Chap. 8 in this volume). Research on the developmental origins of health and disease finds associations between pregnancy/birth outcomes and adult disease in offspring, thought to occur through epigenetic processes (Wadhwa, Buss, Entringer, & Swanson, 2009). This effect is most established in terms of physical health, such as poor nutrition during pregnancy and low birthweight being associated with a greater risk of the infant developing cardiovascular disease as an adult (Kelishadi & Poursafa, 2014). However, evidence also indicates that psychological factors during pregnancy can affect the developing foetus with the strongest evidence for links between stress and anxiety in pregnancy and greater risk of a range of adverse outcomes for the child (Talge, Neal, & Glover, 2007). The way in which an infant is born may also affect the child's later health and wellbeing. This evidence suggests that caesarean birth may be associated with increased risk of autoimmune diseases in infants, such as asthma and allergies. This is thought to be due to protective microbiome 'seeding' of the infants' gastrointestinal microbiota when they pass through the vaginal canal (Neu & Rushing, 2011).

In contrast, positive birth events may result in better outcomes for women and their infants. Far less research has examined positive births and those studies that have been done mostly focus on factors associated with positive birth, rather than the impact of positive birth on women and their infants. Of the available evidence, qualitative research suggests positive births can be empowering and increase women's confidence through overcoming pain and trusting their body (Nilsson, Thorsell, Hertfelt Wahn, & Ekström, 2013). Quantitative studies suggest positive birth is associated with enhanced maternal attachment, higher postnatal functioning, and a more positive birth experience in the future (Green, Coupland, & Kitzinger, 1990; Michels, Kruske, & Thompson, 2013). Evidence on factors associated with positive and traumatic births and the impact of these on women and infants is outlined in more detail in the following sections.

12.3 Traumatic Births

There is now substantial evidence that a proportion of women find birth traumatic. Evidence from cohorts in Western countries suggests 20–33% of women appraise birth as traumatic (Ayers, Joseph, McKenzie-McHarg, Slade, & Wijma, 2008; Creedy, Shochet, & Horsfall, 2000; Soet, Brack, & Dilorio, 2003). Many of these women report symptoms of PTSD but not all fulfil the diagnostic criteria for PTSD. Posttraumatic stress disorder was outlined by the Diagnostic Statistical Manual 5th Revision (DSM-5) of the American Psychiatric Association as occurring after an event in which: (1) there is actual or threatened death; (2) actual or threatened serious injury; or (3) actual or threatened sexual violence (American Psychiatric Association, 2013). It is possible for birth to fill these criteria if a women thinks her or her baby will die or be severely injured. Birth may also involve actual or threatened violence. In law the term 'obstetric violence' has been defined as "...the appropriation of a woman's body and reproductive processes by health personnel, in the form of dehumanizing treatment, abusive medicalization and pathologization of natural processes, involving a woman's loss of autonomy and of the capacity to freely make her own decisions about her body and her sexuality, which has negative consequences for a woman's quality of life." (Belém do Pará Convention, 2012). The World Health Organisation has subsequently called for the prevention and elimination of disrespect and abuse in childbirth (WHO, 2015).

An example of a traumatic birth which involves both physical injury and disrespect was reported by Ballard, Stanley, and Brockington (1995) in a case study of a woman who had an emergency caesarean section without effective anaesthesia in which "she experienced excruciating pain during an operation which took 10 min. She was screaming, shouting, and struggling to get off the operating table during the procedure, and was held down by attendants while the anaesthetist attempted to supplement the epidural" (p. 526). The evidence supports the importance of the way women are treated and supported during birth. For example, Harris and Ayers (2012) surveyed 675 women who had traumatic births and asked women to write about their worst moment during birth, or trauma 'hotspot'. This study found that the worst hotspots were due to obstetric complications and pain (36%), complications or separation from the baby (27%), but also interpersonal difficulties such as feeling abandoned, ignored or not supported (37%).

Symptoms of PTSD fall into four clusters: (1) re-experiencing, (2) avoidance, (3) hyperarousal and (4) negative cognitions and mood. For a diagnosis, symptoms need to be evident for at least one month and cause significant disability and impairment to a woman's life. It should be noted that PTSD is also highly comorbid with depression, with up to 72% of women reporting both PTSD and depression (Dikmen Yildiz, Ayers, & Phillips, 2017). It is important to distinguish between PTSD where diagnostic criteria are fulfilled, appraisal of birth as traumatic, and a traumatic stress response. Appraisal of birth as traumatic is when women consciously label their experience of birth as 'traumatic' although they may not have any psychological symptoms associated with this. A traumatic stress response is where women experience symptoms but do not fulfil all the diagnostic criteria for PTSD. Although a traumatic stress response can be severe it does not necessarily develop into PTSD. Research on traumatic stress responses in other samples has shown that the majority of people who have symptoms after a traumatic event recover spontaneously during the first five months after the event (Morina, Wicherts, Lobbrecht, & Priebe, 2014).

PTSD symptoms may have unique consequences when birth is the triggering trauma because of the involvement of the baby. If women associate the baby with the trauma they may want to avoid contact with the baby to avoid being reminded about the event. Qualitative research suggests this may be the case for some women but not all (Ayers, Eagle, & Waring, 2006). Another unique aspect is that, unlike other traumatic events, giving birth and having a baby is viewed positively in most societies. This means there can be a lack of acknowledgement by society and friends and family that birth can be traumatic. Women may feel isolated and not able to talk about birth trauma. There may also be pressure for women to have another baby and therefore revisit the trauma. However, this is speculative at this stage because there is little empirical evidence examining these factors.

Reviews suggest between 3 and 5% of women will develop PTSD after birth (Dekel, Stuebe, & Dishy, 2017; Dikmen Yildiz et al., 2017; Grekin & O'Hara, 2014) with increased prevalence (15–18%) in high-risk groups such as women who have severe complications or a preterm or stillborn baby. There is some indication that PTSD may be more prevalent in the first 3 months after birth with a prevalence of 5–8% (Dekel et al., 2017). This higher prevalence immediately after the event is consistent with the evidence in other populations mentioned above where spontaneous resolution of symptoms occurs during the first 5 months after a traumatic event (Morina et al., 2014).

12.4 Risk and Resilience

A number of risk factors make it more likely women will develop perinatal mental health problems. Some of these risk factors are remarkably consistent across different disorders and cultures. For example, mental health problems are more likely to occur if women live in circumstances of social adversity (e.g. deprivation, low socio-economic status), have a history of psychological problems, have experienced childhood or current adversity (e.g. domestic violence, child sexual abuse), and do not have much support available to them (e.g. isolated, single parent, poor family support). In addition, if women are anxious or depressed during pregnancy this is likely to continue or worsen postpartum (Bayrampour, Tomfohr, & Tough, 2016; Denckla et al., 2018).

Models of birth trauma and PTSD have to account for the fact that the causes of maternal mental health problems are multifactorial and include individual factors, event factors, and social factors. Conceptual frameworks of the aetiology of postpartum PTSD draw together key vulnerability, risk and maintaining factors thought to be important in the development of birth-related PTSD (Ayers, Bond, Bertullies, & Wijma, 2016; Slade, 2006; van Son, Verkerk, van der Hart, Komproe, & Pop, 2005). These usually draw on psychological approaches such as the diathesis-stress model which explains health outcomes as an interaction between an individual's predispositional vulnerability and stressful experiences.

A recent review and meta-analysis of 50 studies (N = 21,429) from 15 countries used the diathesis-stress model to summarise those factors most strongly associated with postpartum PTSD. These were examined according to whether they were vulnerability factors already present in pregnancy, risk factors during birth, or maintaining factors after birth. The key vulnerability factors were fear of childbirth, depression, poor health or complications in pregnancy, and a history of PTSD or counselling for pregnancy or birth-related factors. These vulnerability factors were proposed to interact with birth events to determine whether women appraised birth as traumatic, and subsequently had traumatic stress responses. Risk factors during birth were having negative subjective birth experiences, an operative birth (assisted vaginal or caesarean birth), lack of support, and dissociating during birth. Postpartum factors that maintained PTSD symptoms were additional stress, poor coping, and comorbid depression (Ayers et al., 2016).

These factors are broadly consistent with the wider literature on factors associated with PTSD in other populations (Brewin, Andrews, & Valentine, 2000; Ozer, Best, Lipsey, & Weiss, 2003), and with similar reviews of postpartum PTSD (Andersen, Melvaer, Videbech, Lamont, & Joergensen, 2012; Grekin & O'Hara, 2014). Thus there is a substantial body of evidence identifying the main risk factors for birth trauma and PTSD, as well as models proposing how these factors may interact to cause postpartum PTSD. However, a few issues need to be considered when evaluating these. First, the evidence and models that have been proposed are mainly psychosocial in their approach and do not consider possible underlying physiological mechanisms or social and environmental influences on trauma. For example, there is increasing evidence from populations such as Holocaust survivors and refugees that vulnerability to trauma can be transmitted from one generation to the next (e.g. Sangalang & Vang, 2017). This intergenerational transmission of vulnerability is not completely attributable to increased exposure to trauma but also likely to involve epigenetic mechanisms where offspring are more likely to develop PTSD in response to severe events (Cunliffe, 2016). There is also the possibility that hormones which are elevated in labour and birth, such as cortisol and oxytocin, affect women's responses to stressful and potentially traumatic events (Bell, Erickson, & Carter, 2014). Similarly, although the importance of social factors in birth trauma is evident in terms of the evidence that support during birth is associated with less PTSD symptoms (Ayers et al., 2016), broader social and environmental factors such as healthcare systems organisational culture or societal views of birth have not been considered.

Thus there are likely to be other factors important in birth trauma that have not been researched (such as environmental factors), or not been researched enough to be included in meta-analyses and models (Ayers et al., 2016). Examples of the latter are maladaptive cognitive appraisals after birth (Ford, Ayers, & Bradley, 2010; Vossbeck-Elsebusch, Freisfeld, & Ehring, 2014), anxiety sensitivity (Keogh, Ayers, & Francis, 2002; Verreault et al., 2012), and insomnia (Garthus-Niegel, Ayers, von Soest, Torgersen, & Eberhard-Gran, 2014) which are promising in that they are associated with the onset or maintenance of postpartum PTSD in the few studies that have examined them.

The focus to date on risk factors for birth trauma and PTSD is embedded within, and influenced by, the wider healthcare culture of risk avoidance. It is therefore understandable that researchers have concentrated on this. However, this overlooks the contrasting but potentially complementary perspective of examining positive factors that may play a protective or preventative role. Positive psychology is a field of research which broadly looks at what enables people to flourish and thrive. It encompasses many different theoretical and research areas which have a common focus on positive human functioning, health, and adaptation to adversity (Aspinwall & Tedeschi, 2010). Similarly, in midwifery, researchers have called for a salutogenic health-promoting approach to care rather than a pathogenic approach (Magistretti, Downe, Lindstrøm, Berg, & Schwarz, 2016). For events to be salutogenic, theorists propose they need to be comprehensible, manageable, and for people to find meaning in them (Antonovsky, 1979, 1987).

In the PTSD literature, research taking this perspective has focused on resilience and post-traumatic growth. Whilst this literature is very advanced for PTSD in other populations, far less research has looked at resilience and personal growth in perinatal women. Understanding resilience and personal growth during the perinatal period could provide a more nuanced and comprehensive understanding of postpartum PTSD. It may also enable us to identify ways to enhance women's capacity to adapt and thrive, and therein inform changes to maternity care services in ways that increase resilience as well as reduce risk.

Resilience has been conceptualized on a number of dimensions. The two main dimensions are the ability for people to recover from stressful or adverse events i.e. 'bounce back'; and the ability to have sustainability i.e. the capacity to continue in the face of adversity (Reich, Zautra, & Hall, 2010). Evidence from other populations suggests the majority of people are resilient. For example, trauma and adversity are experienced by 50–60% of people in Europe at some point in their lifetime (Horn, Charney, & Feder, 2016). However, the lifetime prevalence of PTSD in the general population in Europe is approximately 10%, suggesting most people who experience a traumatic event recover (Horn et al., 2016).

In postpartum PTSD, a longitudinal study of 226 women who had a traumatic birth (defined as meeting diagnostic criteria for a traumatic event) found that 62% of women were resilient and did not have diagnostic PTSD one month or six months postpartum. Another 18% of women had PTSD at one month but had recovered by six months. Chronic PTSD was only observed in 14% of women; and a further 6% had delayed onset PTSD at six months. This suggests around 80% of women who have traumatic births will recover in terms of not meeting diagnostic criteria, although they still may have symptoms. Women who were in the resilient group reported more social support and satisfaction with healthcare professionals, as well as less depression, fear of childbirth, and less additional traumas since birth (Dikmen Yildiz et al., 2018).

Resilience is associated with many positive factors. A review of resilience in adult populations found it was associated with greater positive emotion, optimism, active coping, cognitive reappraisal, altruism, mastery, social support, facing fears, and having a sense of purpose or meaning (Horn et al., 2016). There are also genetic, epigenetic and environmental factors associated with resilience. For example, developmental studies have shown that children vary in how responsive they are to stress. Unsurprisingly, children who are more responsive to stress have the worst health outcomes if raised in a negative environment. What is surprising, however, is that most responsive children have the best outcomes if raised in a positive environment (see also Ungar et al., Chap. 8 in this volume). This effect has been found for both physical and psychological health outcomes (Del Giudice, Ellis, & Shirtcliff, 2011). One could hypothesise from this that if women are in a birth environment which enables positive births they will flourish—and this may be particularly the case for women who are highly responsive to stress.

To date very little research has examined factors associated with resilience in perinatal women. One study of over 1300 women in the USA examined what characterised women with a resilient, moderate or vulnerable psychosocial profile. This found that women who were resilient were characterised by low depression and stress and high support and self-efficacy. These women also had less risky health correlates in pregnancy and were likely to have better birth outcomes. In contrast, vulnerable women were characterised by high depression and stress and poor support and self-efficacy. Vulnerable women were more likely to have an unintended pregnancy, risky health behaviours and deliver preterm (Maxson, Edwards, Valentiner, & Miranda, 2016).

This research on resilience suggests that increasing women's positive emotions, mastery/control, active coping and encouraging a sense of purpose or meaning during pregnancy, birth and postpartum may increase resilience and therein prevent or reduce postpartum PTSD. One factor that is highly associated with both risk and resilience is support (Ayers et al., 2016; Horn et al., 2016). There is a lot of evidence that continuous support during labour is important in birth outcomes (Bohren, Mofmeyr, Sakala, Fukuzawa, & Cuthbert, 2017) and conversely that poor support or interpersonal difficulties during birth are a risk factor for postpartum PTSD (Ayers et al., 2016; Harris & Ayers, 2012). Prospective studies show support can potentially buffer women against traumatic birth events and is particularly important for women with previous histories of trauma or who have complications or high levels of intervention during birth (Ford & Ayers 2011). Support during labour and birth is therefore likely to be critical in terms of both reducing risk and increasing resilience.

12.5 Personal Growth After Birth

Similar to resilience, mechanisms involved in positive psychological outcomes such as personal growth after birth have been relatively ignored. Personal growth is defined as a positive change in one's belief or functioning as a result of the struggle with highly challenging life circumstances (Tedeschi, Park, & Calhoun, 1998). Within the general growth literature three common categories of personal growth outcomes have been identified (Tedeschi et al., 1998). These are changes in interpersonal relationships (e.g. increased compassion or altruism, or a greater sense of closeness in relationships), changes in self-perception (e.g. a greater sense of personal strength, resilience, or self-reliance, coupled with developing a new path or opportunities), and changes in philosophy of life (e.g. a greater appreciation for each day, changes in religious or spiritual/existential beliefs).

It is now acknowledged that developmental events which are not necessarily traumatic or negative also have the potential to promote personal growth (Aldwin & Levenson, 2004). This is consistent with theories of personal growth which recognise that it is the characteristics of the subjective experience of the event and disruption of a person's assumptive beliefs that are important, rather than the event itself

(Calhoun, Cann, & Tedeschi, 2010; Linley & Joseph, 2004). Thus even more normative or stressful events may promote personal growth.

Evidence shows that women can experience personal growth following childbirth. Several qualitative studies provide support for this. For example, a qualitative study with 15 mothers in the USA who had experienced a traumatic birth found four themes of personal growth which included *"Opening oneself up to a new present"*, *"Achieving a new level of relationship nakedness"*, *"Fortifying spiritual-mindedness"*, and *"Forging new paths"* (Beck & Watson, 2016). A meta-ethnographic review of qualitative studies conducted in New Zealand, the USA, the UK, and Australia also found a theme of "*strength of purpose*", such as determination to succeed as a mother, was reported by women following a traumatic birth (Elmir, Schmied, Wilkes, & Jackson, 2010). Quantitative studies also provide evidence that a proportion of women experience personal growth after birth. Three studies in the UK found that a moderate amount of personal growth is reported by between 44 and 50% of women after birth (Sawyer & Ayers, 2009; Sawyer et al., 2012; Sawyer et al., 2015). The most common areas of personal growth were greater appreciation of life and personal strength (Sawyer & Ayers, 2009; Sawyer et al., 2012). Similar findings have been found in postpartum women in other countries such as Japan (Nishi & Usuda, 2017) and Israel (Taubman – Ben-Ari et al., 2009). In Israel, a study found that women experienced both positive and negative outcomes in the transition to motherhood (Taubman – Ben-Ari et al., 2009), and women did not need to perceive the birth as traumatic in order to experience personal growth.

Research has also explored personal growth following childbirth in more stressful circumstances such as preterm birth. Studies in Israel have found that women who had preterm infants reported more personal growth than women with full-term infants (Noy, Taubman – Ben-Ari, & Kuint, 2015; Porat-Zyman, Taubman – Ben-Ari, & Spielman, 2017; Taubman – Ben-Ari, Findler, & Kuint, 2010; Taubman – Ben-Ari & Spielman, 2014; see also Taubman – Ben-Ari, Chap. 16 in this volume). A study in Turkey showed that women with babies admitted to a neonatal intensive care reported similar levels of personal growth to studies with cancer survivors (Boztepe, Inci, & Tanhan, 2015).

Various theoretical models have been proposed to conceptualise the process through which personal growth occurs (e.g. Joseph & Linley, 2005; Tedeschi & Calhoun, 2004). Although there is some variation, most models suggest that the experience of a stressful event violates an individual's basic belief system and that some type of meaning making or cognitive processing to rebuild these beliefs occurs, resulting in perceptions that one has grown through the process (Horowitz, 1986; Janoff-Bulman, 2004). Such models also provide a framework for understanding individual differences in reports of personal growth. Tedeschi and Calhoun's (2004) cognitive processing model of personal growth emphasises the importance of pre-trauma variables (e.g. personality, demographic variables), event-related variables (e.g. objective severity, perceived threat or stress), and post-event variables (e.g. social support, coping strategies, distress) in the development of personal growth. However, factors associated with personal growth following childbirth vary between studies. There is some indication that women who have more adverse experiences show more growth. This includes experiences such as operative birth (Sawyer et al., 2012), preterm birth (Noy et al., 2015; Porat-Zyman et al., 2017; Taubman – Ben-Ari et al., 2010) and women with symptoms of PTSD (Sawyer et al., 2012; Sawyer et al., 2015). However, it should be noted that other indicators of birth stress such as pain during labour, perceiving birth as traumatic, or childbirth meeting DSM criteria for a traumatic stressor, have inconsistent associations with personal growth (Sawyer & Ayers, 2009; Sawyer et al., 2012). There is also indication that personal growth is associated with approach coping (Sawyer & Ayers, 2009; Sawyer et al., 2015) and more likely in women with lower levels of education (Noy et al., 2015; Taubman – Ben-Ari et al., 2010) or young women (Sawyer et al., 2015; Taubman – Ben-Ari et al., 2010).

The evidence surrounding the relationship between support and personal growth after childbirth is mixed. Several studies in Israel found that support is related to higher levels of personal growth, particularly support from women's mothers (Noy et al. 2015; Rozen, Taubman – Ben-Ari, Straus, & Morag, 2018). In comparison, two studies in the UK found that personal growth was not related to support from healthcare professionals during birth or support from family and friends after birth. One explanation for these contradictory results is that different types of support play a different role in the development of personal growth. Schroevers, Helgeson, Sanderman, and Ranchor (2010) examined three different types of social support (perceived availability of social support, actual emotional support received, and satisfaction with actual emotional support received) and their relationship to personal growth in cancer patients. They found that actual received emotional support from family and friends predicted higher levels of personal growth, and in comparison perceived availability of emotional support was not significantly related to positive outcomes. This finding is consistent with cognitive processing theories of personal growth as talking to others may facilitate cognitive processes and coping responses that promote positive change, whereas perceiving that others are available is not sufficient to stimulate these processes.

There have been very few studies looking at the role of personal growth following childbirth in women's long term health outcomes. However, longitudinal studies and reviews of personal growth in other populations indicate that growth has adaptive significance and does seem to be predictive of better emotional adjustment long term (e.g. Barskova & Oesterreich, 2009; Ickovics et al., 2006; Sawyer, Ayers, & Field, 2010). Therefore personal growth may be useful to incorporate into clinical interventions which could be re-conceptualised to include personal growth and not just the alleviation of distress symptoms (Ayers et al., 2008; Joseph & Linley, 2005).

In summary, it is important to recognise that even more normative or stressful events may promote personal growth. Examining both positive and negative psychological outcomes following childbirth allows a more comprehensive account of psychological adjustment to be developed. Joseph and Linley (2008) maintain that posttraumatic stress and personal growth should be considered as two elements of a more integrative conceptualisation of both positive and negative change following challenging events. Nonetheless, considering the unique characteristics of childbirth, it would be interesting to investigate the similarities and differences between personal growth following birth and growth following more "traditional" traumatic events. For example, events such as childbirth may involve more incremental change in comparison to traumatic stressors that have a rapid or unpredictable onset (Aldwin & Levenson, 2004).

12.6 Positive Births

The value of examining factors associated with a positive birth experience is increasingly recognised. Learning from women's birth stories and adapting care during birth based on what women themselves consider important will likely enhance the birth experience and promote normality in the context of what is often a medicalised birth environment (Downe, Finlayson, Oladapo, Bonet, & Gülmezoglu, 2018; Karlström, Nystedt, & Hildingsson, 2015). The importance of supporting women and encouraging a positive birth experience is reflected in health policy undertaken by many European countries and the World Health Organisation about respectful, women-centred care during birth (Ministry of Health and Care Services, 2009; National Institute for Health and Clinical Excellence [NICE], 2010; WHO, 2015).

However, what is meant by a positive birth has not been clearly defined or conceptualised in the literature. A focus group study in Sweden with women who reported having a very positive birth found that women used a range of expressions to describe their positive experiences. Primarily, women reported the birth as a significant moment in their lives associated with joy and happiness. This is consistent with work by Crowther, Smythe, and Spence (2014) who explored the experience of joy at birth from a hermeneutic perspective and concluded that there was a need to explore experiential aspects of birth, rather than just the outcome. More research is needed to provide a clear understanding and conceptualisation of what is meant by a positive birth.

Despite the lack of an agreed definition or concept of positive birth, research has examined the prevalence of positive births and factors associated with it. Several survey studies have explored the prevalence of women who report a positive birth experience. For example, a large-scale survey study in Sweden reported that the percentage of women who described that birth as positive or very positive two months later was 29.2 and 32.7%, respectively (Hildingsson, Johansson, Karlström, & Fenwick, 2013). Women's assessment of birth also changed over time with 22% of the women becoming more positive and 15% more negative after one year. This overall prevalence is slightly lower than another study in the Netherlands, which found that over half of women were "very happy" with their birth when asked after 3 years (Rijnders et al., 2008).

It is clear that the experience of birth is subjective and multi-dimensional. Factors associated with positive birth experiences include support and preparedness for birth. A review and meta-analysis of 20 randomised controlled trials of interventions to increase positive birth experiences found that more positive births were associated with greater support for women during birth (risk ratio 1.35), minimal intervention

(RR 1.29), and being prepared for birth and readiness for complications. Interestingly, relaxation and pain relief strategies were not effective in terms of increasing positive birth experiences (Taheri, Takian, Taghizadeh, Jafari, & Sarafraz, 2018).

This is broadly consistent with non-randomised evidence. For example, studies have found that prenatal factors, such as positive feelings about the birth in pregnancy, are associated with positive birth experiences (Hildingsson et al., 2013; Kringeland, Daltveit, & Møller, 2010). Characteristics of the birth, including minimal intervention, have also been associated with a positive birth experience, such as a quick birth (Nilsson et al., 2013), non-operative birth (Hildingsson et al., 2013), and less pain (Goodman, Mackey, & Tavakoli, 2004). However, the experience of pain during labour does not prevent a positive birth experience (Hildingsson et al., 2013).

In addition, numerous studies suggest that feeling in control is associated with a positive birth experience (Bryanton, Gagnon, Johnston, & Hatem, 2008; Goodman et al., 2004; Hildingsson et al., 2013; Karlström et al., 2015). Control is a subjective experience and Green and Baston (2003) distinguish between the control the woman has over her body (internal) and the control she has over medical staff and decisions made in relation to her labour (external). It is important to some women that they maintain control over their behaviour and body and these women may be more likely to perceive the birth as positive if they are satisfied with their own performance (Hildingsson et al., 2013; Karlström et al., 2015). External control is also important in influencing perceptions of birth. For example, a study with 293 Swedish first-time mothers found that those who felt involved in decisions were more likely to have a positive birth experience (Waldenström, Borg, Olsson, Sköld, & Wall, 1996).

In keeping with the importance of support during birth, good communication from midwives is associated with a positive birth experience. A qualitative study in the UK found that when women felt midwives were advocates and had open communication styles which clearly outlined birthing choices this led to a trusting relationship (Hallam, Howard, Locke, & Thomas, 2016). A trusting relationship between woman and midwife is also associated with positive birth experiences (Dahlberg & Aune, 2013; Dahlberg et al., 2016). Support also seems to be a significant factor in a positive birth experience, with support from midwives playing an important role in positive birth experiences (Dahlberg et al., 2016; Hildingsson et al., 2013). For example, a study in Sweden found that women who were provided with individualised emotional support were more likely to report positive birth experiences, even if the birth was challenging and/or if there were medical complications (Nilsson et al., 2013). This suggests support may act as a buffer against the impact of negative birth events. In addition, the father of the child may have a significant role in positive birth experiences (Karlström et al., 2015; Nilsson et al., 2013). For example, a qualitative study in Sweden found that it was essential to women to have the father close to provide encouragement and reassurance (Karlström et al., 2015).

There is limited research examining the impact of a positive birth on the mother and child. Available studies suggest that a positive birth experience is associated with a positive attitude towards motherhood, which can lead to feelings of enhanced self-esteem and accomplishment (Simkin, 1991). Furthermore, a mother's positive perception of her birth experience has been linked to enhanced maternal attachment and competence (Green et al., 1990; Mercer & Ferketich, 1994). More recently, a study with 664 women in Australia found that women who stated that they were looked after very well and had a very positive birth experience were significantly more likely to experience high postnatal functioning (Michels et al., 2013). A positive birth experience has also been associated with a more positive birth experience in the future (Goodman et al., 2004).

12.7 Implications for Healthcare

Focusing on women's experiences of birth has both practical and political relevance in healthcare systems in terms of guiding practice, policy, and research. We have seen how negative and/or traumatic birth experiences are associated with a range of adverse consequences for the health and wellbeing of mothers and infants; and conversely that positive births are associated with positive outcomes for women. This has implications for healthcare utilisation. Studies show that women experiencing distress following birth are more likely to use healthcare services postpartum. For example, a study in Australia found that women with high levels of distress were more likely to have lower long-term health related quality of life and higher health-care utilisation compared to women with no birth distress. This effect was still significant one year after birth (Turkstra et al., 2015).

Interventions during the transition to parenthood are important to reduce negative impacts on women, children, and families. However, progress in this regard is patchy for several reasons. First, only a small proportion of women with perinatal mental health problems come to the attention of health services, and fewer of these women receive treatment (Khan, 2015). This is due to a range of factors which include lack of (or ineffective) screening, barriers to women seeking help during this time, clinical barriers to diagnosis and treatment, lack of perinatal psychology services, and limited evidence on effective treatments. In terms of treatment there is most evidence for the treatment of postnatal depression with cognitive behaviour therapy or interpersonal therapy. Clinical guidelines are available that recommend treatments on the basis of current evidence (NICE, 2014; Scottish Intercollegiate Guidelines Network: SIGN 2012). Despite this, recent reviews of diagnosis and treatment of perinatal affective disorders by physicians suggest anti-depressants are often the first line of treatment, for many of the reasons listed above (Ford, Lee, Shakespeare, & Ayers, 2017; Ford, Shakespeare, Elias, & Ayers, 2017).

Thus, more research is needed on ways to improve the identification and treatment of women with perinatal mental health problems in primary care and other services. In order to ensure appropriate and effective care pathways and services are provided it is important that policy makers, researchers, clinicians, and women and families who have experienced perinatal mental illness work together (Ayers & Shakespeare, 2015).

Finally, the importance of supporting women to have a positive birth is clear, although there is no agreed definition of positive birth, or a simple solution to ensuring women have positive birth experiences. Salutogenesis theory (Antonovsky, 1979, 1987) provides a framework to examine this by focusing on the generation and maintenance of health. Applying a salutogenic approach to maternity care services could help shift the current focus on risk and adversity to one of resilience, personal growth and wellbeing. As most women and babies are healthy at the outset of pregnancy and throughout the childbearing process, the key task of maternity care should be to maintain and enhance this healthy state (Perez-Botella, Downe, Magistretti, Lindstrom, & Berg, 2015).

12.8 Conclusion

To understand the impact of birth on women and infants' health and wellbeing it is important to examine both positive and negative births, as well as risk, resilience and personal growth in response to birth. All of these offer a different perspective on the same phenomena and enable the development of interventions that tackle both the reduction of risk and increase of resilience and positive experiences to ensure women adapt and thrive. More research is needed to determine how specific risk and resilience factors interact to determine whether women experience birth as positive or traumatic. This means not having a singular focus on one or the other but examining both risk and resilience factors, including how they interact over time and the many pathways through which they may influence how women experience birth and the impact of this on them and their babies. It is also important to recognise individual, organisational, social and cultural influences on women's experiences and the impact of birth on them and their children.

References

Aldwin, C. M., & Levenson, M. (2004). Post-traumatic growth: A developmental perspective. *Psychological Inquiry, 15*(1), 19–22.

American Psychiatric Association. (2013). *Diagnostic and statistical manual of mental disorders* (5th ed.). Arlington, VA: American Psychiatric Publishing.

Andersen, L. B., Melvaer, L. B., Videbech, P., Lamont, R. F., & Joergensen, J. S. (2012). Risk factors for developing post-traumatic stress disorder following childbirth: A systematic review. *Acta Obstetrica et Gynecologica Scandinavia, 91*(11), 1261–1272.

Antonovsky, A. (1979). *Health, stress and coping*. San Francisco: Jossey-Bass.

Antonovsky, A. (Ed.). (1987). *Unraveling the mystery of health: How people manage stress and stay well*. San Francisco, CA, US: Jossey-Bass.

Aspinwall, L. G., & Tedeschi, R. G. (2010). The value of positive psychology for health psychology: Progress and pitfalls in examining the relation of positive phenomena to health. *Annals of Behavioral Medicine, 39*(1), 4–15.

Ayers, S., Bond, R., Bertullies, S., & Wijma, K. (2016). The aetiology of post-traumatic stress following childbirth: A meta-analysis and theoretical framework. *Psychological Medicine, 46*(6), 1121–1134.

Ayers, S., Eagle, A., & Waring, H. (2006). The effects of postnatal PTSD on women and their relationships: A qualitative study. *Psychology, Health & Medicine, 11*(4), 389–398.

Ayers, S., Joseph, S., McKenzie-McHarg, K., Slade, P., & Wijma, K. (2008). Post-traumatic stress disorder following childbirth: Current issues and recommendations for research. *Journal of Psychosomatic Obstetrics and Gynaecology, 29*(4), 240–250.

Ayers, S., & Shakespeare, J. (2015). Should perinatal mental health be everyone's business? *Primary Health Care Research and Development, 16*(4), 323–325.

Ballard, C. G., Stanley, A. K., & Brockington, I. F. (1995). Posttraumatic stress disorder (PTSD) after childbirth. *British Journal of Psychiatry, 166*(4), 525–528.

Barskova, T., & Oesterreich, R. (2009). Post-traumatic growth in people living with a serious medical condition and its relations to physical and mental health: A systematic review. *Disability and Rehabilitation, 31*(21), 1709–1733.

Bauer, A., Parsonage, M., Knapp, M., Lemmi, V., & Adelaja, B. (2014). *The costs of perinatal mental health problems*. Retrieved from https://www.centreformentalhealth.org.uk/costs-of-perinatalmh-problems.

Bayrampour, H., Tomfohr, L., & Tough, S. (2016). Trajectories of perinatal depressive and anxiety symptoms in a community cohort. *Journal of Clinical Psychiatry, 77*(11), e1467–e1473.

Beck, C. T., & Watson, S. (2016). Posttraumatic growth after birth trauma: I was broken, now I am unbreakable. *MCN American Journal of Maternal and Child Nursing, 41*(5), 264–271.

Belém do Pará Convention (2012). *Second hemispheric report on the implementation of the Belém do Pará Convention*. Washington, USA. Retrieved from http://www.oas.org/en/mesecvi/docs/MESECVI-SegundoInformeHemisferico-EN.pdf.

Bell, A. F., Erickson, E. N., & Carter, C. S. (2014). Beyond labor: The role of natural and synthetic oxytocin in the transition to motherhood. *Journal of Midwifery & Women's Health, 59*(1), 35–42.

Bhutta, A. T., Cleves, M. A., Casey, P. H., Cradock, M. M., & Anand, K. J. S. (2002). Cognitive and behavioral outcomes of school-aged children who were born preterm: A meta-analysis. *JAMA, 288*(6), 728–737.

Bohren, M. A., Mofmeyr, G., Sakala, C., Fukuzawa, R. K., & Cuthbert, A. (2017). Continuous support for women during childbirth. *Cochrane Database of Systematic Reviews, 7,* Art. No.: CD003766.

Boots Family Trust Alliance. (2013). *Perinatal mental health: Experiences of women and health professionals*. Retrieved from https://www.tommys.org/sites/default/files/Perinatal_Mental_Health_Experiences%20of%20women.pdf.

Boztepe, H., Inci, F., & Tanhan, F. (2015). Posttraumatic growth in mothers after infant admission to neonatal intensive care unit. *Paediatria Croatica, 59*(1), 14–18.

Brewin, C. R., Andrews, B., & Valentine, J. D. (2000). Meta-analysis of risk factors for posttraumatic stress disorder in trauma-exposed adults. *Journal of Consulting and Clinical Psychology, 68*(5), 748–766.

Bryanton, J., Gagnon, A. J., Johnston, C., & Hatem, M. (2008). Predictors of women's perceptions of the childbirth experience. *Journal of Obstetric, Gynecologic, and Neonatal Nursing, 37*(1), 24–34.

Calhoun, L. G., Cann, A., & Tedeschi, R. G. (2010). The posttraumatic growth model: Sociocultural considerations. In T. Weiss & R. Berger (Eds.), *Posttraumatic growth and culturally competent practice: Lessons learned from around the globe* (pp. 1–14). Hoboken, NJ: John Wiley & Sons.

Chow, Y., Dattani, N., Hilder, L., Macfarlane, A., & Moser, K. (2007). Introducing new data on gestation-specific infant mortality among babies born in 2005 in England and Wales. Presents analyses of infant mortality by gestational age and social and biological factors. *Health Statistics Quarterly, 35,* 13–27.

Creedy, D. K., Shochet, I. M., & Horsfall, J. (2000). Childbirth and the development of acute trauma symptoms: Incidence and contributing factors. *Birth, 27*(2), 104–111.

Crowther, S., Smythe, E., & Spence, D. (2014). The joy at birth: An interpretive hermeneutic literature review. *Midwifery, 30*(4), e157–e165.

Cunliffe, V. T. (2016). The epigenetic impacts of social stress: How does social adversity become biologically embedded? *Epigenomics, 8*(12), 1653–1669.

Dahlberg, U., & Aune, I. (2013). The woman's birth experience—The effect of interpersonal relationships and continuity of care. *Midwifery, 29*(4), 407–415.

Dahlberg, U., Persen, J., Skogås, A.-K., Selboe, S.-T., Torvik, H. M., & Aune, I. (2016). How can midwives promote a normal birth and a positive birth experience? The experience of first-time Norwegian mothers. *Sexual and Reproductive Health, 7,* 2–7.

Dekel, S., Stuebe, C., & Dishy, G. (2017). Childbirth induced posttraumatic stress syndrome: A systematic review of prevalence and risk factors. *Frontiers in Psychology, 8,* 560.

Del Giudice, M., Ellis, B. J., & Shirtcliff, E. A. (2011). The adaptive calibration model of stress responsivity. *Neuroscience and Biobehavioral Reviews, 35*(7), 1562–1592.

Denckla, C. A., Mancini, A. D., Consedine, N. S., Milanovic, S. M., Basu, A., Seedat, S., et al. (2018). Distinguishing postpartum and antepartum depressive trajectories in a large population-based cohort: The impact of exposure to adversity and offspring gender. *Psychological Medicine, 48*(7), 1139–1147.

Dikmen Yildiz, P., Ayers, S., & Phillips, L. (2017). The prevalence of posttraumatic stress disorder in pregnancy and after birth: A systematic review and meta-analysis. *Journal of Affective Disorders, 208,* 634–645.

Dikmen Yildiz, P., Ayers, S., & Phillips, L. (2018). Longitudinal trajectories of post-traumatic stress disorder (PTSD) after birth and associated risk factors. *Journal of Affective Disorders, 229,* 377–385.

Downe, S., Finlayson, K., Oladapo, O., Bonet, M., & Gü lmezoglu, A. M. (2018). What matters to women during childbirth: A systematic qualitative review. *PLoS ONE, 13*(4), e0194906.

Elkit, A., Hartvig, T., & Christiansen, M. (2007). Psychological sequalae in parents of extreme low and very low birth weight infants. *Journal of Clinical Psychology in Medical Settings, 14*(3), 238–247.

Elmir, R., Schmied, V., Wilkes, L., & Jackson, D. (2010). Women's perceptions and experiences of a traumatic birth: A meta-ethnography. *Journal of Advanced Nursing, 66*(10), 2142–2153.

Forcada-Guex, M., Borghini, A., Pierrehumbert, B., Ansermet, F., & Muller-Nix, C. (2011). Prematurity, maternal posttraumatic stress and consequences on the mother–infant relationship. *Early Human Development, 87*(1), 21–26.

Ford, E., & Ayers, S. (2011). Support during birth interacts with trauma history and birth intervention to predict postnatal post-traumatic stress symptoms. *Psychology & Health, 26*(12), 1553–1570.

Ford, E., Ayers, S., & Bradley, R. (2010). Exploration of a cognitive model to predict post-traumatic stress symptoms following childbirth. *Journal of Anxiety Disorders, 24*(3), 353–359.

Ford, E., Lee, S., Shakespeare, J., & Ayers, S. (2017a). Diagnosis and management of perinatal depression and anxiety in general practice: A meta-synthesis of qualitative studies. *British Journal of General Practice, 67*(661), e538–e546.

Ford, E., Shakespeare, J., Elias, F., & Ayers, S. (2017b). Recognition and management of perinatal depression and anxiety by general practitioners: A systematic review. *Family Practice, 34*(1), 11–19.

Garthus-Niegel, S., Ayers, S., von Soest, T., Torgersen, L., & Eberhard-Gran, M. (2014). Maintaining factors of posttraumatic stress symptoms following childbirth: A population-based, 2 year follow-up study. *Journal of Affective Disorders, 172,* 146–152.

Garthus-Niegel, S., von Soest, T., Vollrath, M. E., & Eberhard-Gran, M. (2013). The impact of subjective birth experiences on post-traumatic stress symptoms: A longitudinal study. *Archives of Women's Mental Health, 16*(1), 1–10.

Goodman, P., Mackey, M. C., & Tavakoli, A. S. (2004). Factors related to childbirth satisfaction. *Journal of Advanced Nursing, 46*(2), 212–219.

Green, J. M., & Baston, H. A. (2003). Feeling in control during labor: Concepts, correlates, and consequences. *Birth, 30*(4), 235–247.

Green, J. M., Coupland, V. A., & Kitzinger, J. V. (1990). Expectations, experiences, and psychological outcomes of childbirth: A prospective study of 825 women. *Birth, 17*(1), 15–24.

Grekin, R., & O'Hara, M. W. (2014). Prevalence and risk factors of postpartum posttraumatic stress disorder: A meta-analysis. *Clinical Psychology Review, 34*(5), 389–401.

Hallam, J. L., Howard, C. D., Locke, A., & Thomas, M. (2016). Communicating choice: An exploration of mothers' experiences of birth. *Journal of Reproductive and Infant Psychology, 34*(2), 175–184.

Harris, R., & Ayers, S. (2012). What makes labour and birth traumatic? A survey of intrapartum 'hotspots'. *Psychology & Health, 27*(10), 1166–1177.

Hildingsson, I., Johansson, M., Karlström, A., & Fenwick, J. (2013). Factors associated with a positive birth experience: An exploration of Swedish women's experiences. *International Journal of Childbirth, 3*(3), 153–164.

Horn, S. R., Charney, D. S., & Feder, A. (2016). Understanding resilience: New approaches for preventing and treating PTSD. *Experimental Neurology, 284*(Pt B), 119–132.

Horowitz, M. (1986). *Stress response syndromes*. New York: Aronson.

Ickovics, J., Meade, C., Kershaw, T., Milam, S., Lewis, J., & Ethier, K. (2006). Urban teens: Trauma, posttraumatic growth, and emotional distress among female adolescents. *Journal of Consulting and Clinical Psychology, 74*(5), 841–850.

Janoff-Bulman, R. (2004). Posttraumatic growth: Three explanatory models. *Psychological Inquiry, 15*(1), 30–34.

Joseph, S., & Linley, P. A. (2005). Positive adjustment to threatening events: An organismic valuing theory of growth through adversity. *Review of General Psychology, 9*(3), 262–280.

Joseph, S., & Linley, P. A. (2008). Reflections on theory and practice in trauma, recovery, and growth: A paradigm shift for the field of traumatic stress. In S. Joseph & P. A. Linley (Eds.), *Trauma, recovery and growth: Positive psychological perspectives on posttraumatic stress* (pp. 339–356). Hoboken, NJ: Wiley.

Karatzias, T., Chouliara, Z., Maxton, F., Freer, Y., & Power, K. (2007). Post-traumatic symptomatology in parents with premature infants: A systematic review of the literature. *Journal of Prenatal and Perinatal Psychology & Health, 21*(3), 249–260.

Karlström, A., Nystedt, A., & Hildingsson, I. (2015). The meaning of a very positive birth experience: Focus groups discussions with women. *BMC Pregnancy Childbirth, 15*, 251.

Kelishadi, R., & Poursafa, P. (2014). A review on the genetic, environmental, and lifestyle aspects of the early-life origins of cardiovascular disease. *Current Problems in Pediatric & Adolescent Health Care, 44*(3), 54–72.

Keogh, E., Ayers, S., & Francis, H. (2002). Does anxiety sensitivity predict posttraumatic stress symptoms following childbirth? A preliminary report. *Cognitive Behaviour Therapy, 31*(4), 145–155.

Khan, L. (2015). *Falling through the gaps: Perinatal mental health and general practice*. Retrieved from https://www.centreformentalhealth.org.uk/falling-through-the-gaps.

Kringeland, T., Daltveit, A. K., & Møller, A. (2010). What characterizes women who want to give birth as naturally as possible without painkillers or intervention? *Sexual & Reproductive Healthcare, 1*(1), 21–26.

Linley, P. A., & Joseph, S. (2004). Positive change following trauma and adversity: A review. *Journal of Traumatic Stress, 17*(1), 11–21.

Magistretti, C. M., Downe, S., Lindstrøm, B., Berg, M., & Schwarz, K. T. (2016). Setting the stage for health: Salutogenesis in midwifery professional knowledge in three European countries. *International Journal of Qualitative Studies on Health and Well-being, 11*(1), ISSN 1748-2623.

Maxson, P. J., Edwards, S. E., Valentiner, E. M., & Miranda, M. L. (2016). A multidimensional approach to characterizing psychosocial health during pregnancy. *Maternal and Child Health Journal, 20*(6), 1103–1113.

Mercer, R., & Ferketich, S. (1994). Predictors of maternal role competence by risk status. *Nursing Research, 43*(1), 38–43.

Michels, A., Kruske, S., & Thompson, R. (2013). Women's postnatal psychological functioning: The role of satisfaction with intrapartum care and the birth experience. *Journal of Reproductive and Infant Psychology, 31*(2), 172–182.

Ministry of Health and Care Services. (2009). *White Paper 12. A happy event—A continuous pregnancy, birth and post natal care*. Oslo.
Morina, N., Wicherts, J. M., Lobbrecht, J., & Priebe, S. (2014). Remission from post-traumatic stress disorder in adults: A systematic review and meta-analysis of long term outcome studies. *Clinical Psychology Review, 34*(3), 249–255.
National Institute for Health and Clinical Excellence. (2010). *Pregnancy and complex social factors: A model for service provision for pregnant women with complex social factors. NICE guidelines* [CG110]. Retrieved from https://www.nice.org.uk/guidance/cg110/chapter/Woman-centred-care.
National Institute for Health and Clinical Excellence. (2014). *Antenatal and postnatal mental health: The NICE Guideline on clinical management and service guidance*. Retrieved from http://www.nice.org.uk/guidance/cg192.
Neu, J., & Rushing, J. (2011). Cesarean versus vaginal delivery: Long term infant outcomes and the hygiene hypothesis. *Clinics in Perinatology, 38*(2), 321–331.
Nilsson, L., Thorsell, T., Hertfelt Wahn, E., & Ekström, A. (2013). Factors influencing positive birth experiences of first-time mothers. *Nursing Research and Practice,* 349124.
Nishi, D., & Usuda, K. (2017). Psychological growth after childbirth: An exploratory prospective study. *Journal of Psychosomatic Obstetrics & Gynecology, 38*(2), 87–93.
Noy, A., Taubman – Ben-Ari, O., & Kuint, J. (2015). Well-being and personal growth in mothers of full-term and pre-term singletons and twins. *Stress & Health, 31*(5), 365–372.
Ozer, E. J., Best, S. R., Lipsey, T. L., & Weiss, D. S. (2003). Predictors of posttraumatic stress disorder and symptoms in adults: A meta-analysis. *Psychological Bulletin, 129*(1), 52–73.
Perez-Botella, M., Downe, S., Magistretti, C. M., Lindstrom, B., & Berg, M. (2015). The use of salutogenesis theory in empirical studies of maternity care for healthy mothers and babies. *Sexual & Reproductive Healthcare, 6*(1), 33–39.
Porat-Zyman, G., Taubman – Ben-Ari, O., & Spielman, V. (2017). Dyadic transition to parenthood: A longitudinal assessment of personal growth among parents of pre- and full-term infants. *Stress & Health, 33*(1), 24–34.
Reich, J. W., Zautra, A. J., & Hall, J. S. (Eds.). (2010). *Handbook of adult resilience*. New York: The Guilford Press.
Rijnders, M., Baston, H., Schönbeck, Y., Van Der Pal, K., Prins, M., Green, J., et al. (2008). Perinatal factors related to negative or positive recall of birth experience in women 3 years postpartum in the Netherlands. *Birth, 35*(2), 107–116.
Rozen, G., Taubman – Ben-Ari, O., Straus, T., & Morag, I. (2018). Personal growth of mothers of preterms—Objective severity of the event, subjective stress, personal resources, and maternal emotional support. *Journal of Happiness Studies, 19*(7), 2167–2186.
Sangalang, C. C., & Vang, C. (2017). Intergenerational trauma in refugee families: A systematic review. *Journal of Immigrant and Minority Health, 19*(3), 745–754.
Sawyer, A., & Ayers, S. (2009). Post-traumatic growth in women after childbirth. *Psychology & Health, 24*(4), 457–471.
Sawyer, A., Ayers, S., Bradley, R., Young, D., & Smith, H. (2012). Posttraumatic growth after childbirth: A prospective study. *Psychology and Health, 27*(3), 362–377.
Sawyer, A., Ayers, S., & Field, A. P. (2010). Posttraumatic growth and adjustment among individuals with cancer or HIV/AIDS: A meta-analysis. *Clinical Psychology Review, 30*(4), 436–447.
Sawyer, A., Nakić Radoš, S., Ayers, S., & Burn, E. (2015). Personal growth in UK and Croatian women following childbirth: A preliminary study. *Journal of Reproductive and Infant Psychology, 33*(3), 294–307.
Schroevers, M. J., Helgeson, V. S., Sanderman, R., & Ranchor, A. V. (2010). Type of social support matters for prediction of posttraumatic growth among cancer survivors. *Psycho-Oncology, 19*(1), 46–53.
Scottish Intercollegiate Guidelines Network (SIGN). (2012). *Management of perinatal mood disorders*. Edinburgh: SIGN; (SIGN publication no. 127). Retrieved from http://www.sign.ac.uk.

Simkin, P. (1991). Just another day in a woman's life? Women's long term perception of their first birth experience. *Birth, 18*(4), 203–210.

Slade, P. (2006). Towards a conceptual framework for understanding post-traumatic stress symptoms following childbirth and implications for further research. *Journal of Psychosomatic Obstetrics & Gynecology, 27*(2), 99–105.

Soet, J. E., Brack, G. A., & Dilorio, C. (2003). Prevalence and predictors of women's experience of psychological trauma during childbirth. *Birth, 30*(1), 36–46.

Taheri, M., Takian, A., Taghizadeh, Z., Jafari, N., & Sarafraz, N. (2018). Creating a positive perception of childbirth experience: Systematic review and meta-analysis of prenatal and intrapartum interventions. *Reproductive Health, 15*(1), 73.

Talge, N. M., Neal, C., & Glover, V. (2007). Antenatal maternal stress and long-term effects on child neurodevelopment: How and why? *Journal of Child Psychology and Psychiatry, 48*(3–4), 245–261.

Taubman – Ben-Ari, O., Ben-Shlomo, S., Sivan, E., & Dolizki, M. (2009). The transition to motherhood: A time for growth. *Journal of Social and Clinical Psychology, 28*(8), 943–970.

Taubman – Ben-Ari, O., Findler, L., & Kuint, J. (2010). Personal growth in the wake of stress: The case of mothers of pre-term twins. *The Journal of Psychology: Interdisciplinary and Applied, 144*(2), 185–204.

Taubman – Ben-Ari, O., & Spielman, V. (2014). Personal growth following the first child's birth: A comparison of parents of pre- and full-term babies. *Social Work Research, 38*(2), 91–106.

Tedeschi, R. G., & Calhoun, L. G. (2004). Posttraumatic growth: Conceptual foundations and empirical evidence. *Psychological Inquiry, 15*(1), 1–18.

Tedeschi, R. G., Park, C., & Calhoun, L. G. (1998). *Posttraumatic growth: Positive changes in the aftermath of crisis*. Mahwah, NJ: Erlbaum.

Tunçalp, O., Hindin, M. J., Souza, J. P., Chou, D., & Say, L. (2012). The prevalence of maternal near miss: A systematic review. *BJOG, 119*(6), 653–661.

Turkstra, E., Creedy, D. K., Fenwick, J., Buist, A., Scuffham, P. A., & Gamble, J. (2015). Health services utilization of women following a traumatic birth. *Archives of Women's Mental Health, 18*(6), 829–832.

van Son, M. J. M., Verkerk, G., van der Hart, O., Komproe, I., & Pop, V. (2005). Prenatal depression, mode of delivery and perinatal dissociation as predictors of postpartum posttraumatic stress: An empirical study. *Clinical Psychology and Psychotherapy, 12*(4), 297–312.

Verreault, N., Da Costa, D., Marchand, A., Ireland, K., Banack, H., Dritsa, M., et al. (2012). PTSD following childbirth: A prospective study of incidence and risk factors in Canadian women. *Journal of Psychosomatic Research, 73*(4), 257–263.

Vigod, S. N., Villegas, L., & Dennis, C. L. (2010). Prevalence and risk factors for postpartum depression among women with preterm and low-birth-weight infants: A systematic review. *BJOG, 117*(5), 540–550.

Vossbeck-Elsebusch, A. N., Freisfeld, C., & Ehring, T. (2014). Predictors of posttraumatic stress symptoms following childbirth. *BMC Psychiatry, 14*, 200.

Wadhwa, P. D., Buss, C., Entringer, S., & Swanson, J. M. (2009). Developmental origins of health and disease: Brief history of the approach and current focus on epigenetic mechanisms. *Seminars in Reproductive Medicine, 27*(5), 358–368.

Waldenström, U., Borg, I. M., Olsson, B., Sköld, M., & Wall, S. (1996). The childbirth experience: A study of 295 new mothers. *Birth, 23*(3), 144–153.

World Health Organisation. (2015). *The prevention and elimination of disrespect and abuse during facility-based childbirth.* World Health Organisation Statement, WHO 2015. Retrieved from http://apps.who.int/iris/bitstream/handle/10665/134588/WHO_RHR_14.23_eng.pdf;jsessionid=0716EA2AB35D11E752EEC654599DCC90?sequence=1.

Zeitlin, J., Draper, E. S., Kollée, L., Milligan, D., Boerch, K., Agostino, R., et al. (2008). Differences in rates and short-term outcome of live births before 32 weeks of gestation in Europe in 2003: Results from the MOSAIC cohort. *Pediatrics, 121*(4), e936–e944.

Chapter 13
Resolution of Difficult Experiences and Future Parenting

Miri Scharf, Pnina Isenberg-Borenstein and Rachel Marcow Rosenberg

13.1 Attachment Theory and Resolution of Difficult Experiences

Attachment theory explains people's reactions to difficult experiences and individual differences in their coping. Attachment representations are said to guide expectations, feelings, and information processing, as well as emotion regulation, in situations that are attachment-related (Bretherton & Munholland, 2016; see also Mikulincer & Shaver, Chap. 18 in this volume), and attachment relationships influence regulation of emotion and the use of intra- and interpersonal resources when coping with stressful situations (Field, Gao, & Paderna, 2005; see also Rholes & Paetzold, Chap. 17 in this volume). Whereas adverse experiences can tax individuals' resources, they can also promote hardiness and influence how people handle subsequent negative experiences (Seery, Holman, & Silver, 2010). It is most likely the interplay between the experiences and individuals' perceptions and emotions that shapes their responses and coping.

When faced with stressful situations, securely attached individuals tend to openly express distress and mobilize problem-solving strategies. Furthermore, based on their past experiences with close others, they may turn to such people for support in the effort to overcome stressful situations (Mikulincer & Shaver, 2016). In contrast, individuals with high levels of attachment avoidance tend to use deactivating strategies, restrict accessibility to and suppress expressivity of their vulnerability, and are less likely to turn to others for support in coping with difficulties (Kobak, Cole,

M. Scharf (✉) · P. Isenberg-Borenstein · R. Marcow Rosenberg
Department of Counseling and Human Development, University of Haifa, 3498838 Haifa, Israel
e-mail: Scharfm@edu.haifa.ac.il

P. Isenberg-Borenstein
e-mail: pnina.isenberg@gmail.com

R. Marcow Rosenberg
e-mail: rachelros79@gmail.com

O. Taubman – Ben-Ari (ed.), *Pathways and Barriers to Parenthood*,
https://doi.org/10.1007/978-3-030-24864-2_13

Ferenz-Gillies, Fleming, & Gamble, 1993; Mikulincer & Shaver, 2016). Those with high levels of attachment anxiety tend to use hyperactivating strategies, expressed in intensification and exaggeration of threats, in order to draw and maintain the attention of close others (Mikulincer & Shaver, 2016). Not only do these strategies intensify negative emotions, but their effectiveness for maintaining the support of close others has been questioned. In some studies, anxiously attached individuals have shown ineffective use of support-seeking strategies for maintaining proximity to close others, and in others, no association has been found between anxious attachment and support-seeking strategies (Cantazaro & Wei, 2010; Collins & Feeney, 2000; Fraley & Shaver, 1998).

Stressful experiences might threaten individuals' sense of meaning, mastery, and self-esteem, and increase the risk of difficulties in their daily functioning, including parenting. However, it appears that it is the lack of resolution of the experiences, rather than the adversities themselves, that is associated with subsequent problems (Fraley & Bonanno, 2004; Ho, Chan, Ma, & Field, 2013). Research on stressful life events has focused mostly on their negative implications for adjustment. But such events can also promote stress-related growth if the consequent disruption of individuals' core beliefs about themselves causes them to reprioritize their goals and rebuild their self-schemas and worldviews (Helgeson, Reynolds, & Tomich, 2006; Tedeschi & Calhoun, 1996; see also Taubman – Ben-Ari, Chap. 16 in this volume). Coping and the process of growth may take time, and perceiving that only good things have emerged from a difficult experience might indicate an attempt to deny the negative implications of the adverse experience. But some people are able to resolve adversity after a period of time, reorientating themselves to the present and future and achieving a balanced view of the impact of the experience on their life.

Below we describe in detail two studies of women coping with difficult and challenging experiences. The first relates to stillbirth and the second to the normative experience of labor and early parenting.

13.1.1 Study 1: Stillbirth and Its Implications

For many couples, pregnancy is a period of anticipation and excitement. An infant may represent the fulfillment of dreams and fantasies, a way to start over, or the embarking on one of life's most significant roles (Robinson, Baker, & Nackerud, 1999). Not surprisingly, therefore, stillbirth, the birth of a fetus that has died in the womb or during delivery after week 20 of pregnancy, arouses reactions that are similar to, or even more severe than, those generated by other forms of bereavement (Scheidt et al., 2012; Shreffler, Greil, & McQuillan, 2011; Wijngaards-de Meij et al., 2007). Our study focused on the experience of this loss as a formative event in the life of women and mothers-to-be. We sought to shed light on the relationship between the attachment dimensions of anxiety and avoidance and the unresolved loss or trauma of women who experienced stillbirth, as well as on the women's intimacy with their partners and their perceptions of future parenthood.

Stillbirth can have a profound adverse impact on the psychological, social, and financial status of parents and their close family. Its effects can persist long-term, influencing subsequent pregnancies and parenthood (Armstrong, Hutti, & Myers, 2009; Cacciatore, 2013). Previous studies have shown that following a stillbirth, 25% of women developed depression, anxiety (Scheidt, Waller, Wangler, Hasenburg, & Kersting, 2007; Toffol, Koponen, & Partonen, 2013), or posttraumatic stress disorder during a subsequent pregnancy or after the birth of a healthy baby (Armstrong et al., 2009; Turton, Hughes, Evans, & Fainman, 2001). Perinatal loss has also been linked to marital relationship difficulties, including divorce, as well as feelings of failure as a mother/wife or of a father as provider and protector (Tseng, Cheng, Chen, Yang, & Cheng, 2017).

Grieving and resolution of the experience of stillbirth can be complicated. First, parental grief following a stillbirth may not be culturally acceptable. There is usually no funeral or public ritual of mourning for a perinatal death, and therefore parents often feel that they cannot openly express their grief because it is not socially recognized (Kelley & Trinidad, 2012). Doka (1989) uses the term *disenfranchised grief* to describe a loss that is unrecognized by society. Furthermore, if grieving does not follow the expected societal rules with regard to duration and intensity, the parents' grief can be disenfranchised by their support system as well (Corr, 2002).

Nevertheless, stillbirth can also engender personal growth. Making meaning can play a critical role in the grieving process and influence the resolution of the experience and subsequent distress (Gold, Leon, Boggs, & Sen, 2016). Following a stillbirth, some parents were found to feel more caring and compassionate, and less likely to take anything for granted. Some couples felt a greater closeness and a special bond in response to the loss they had experienced. Moreover, the quality of the marital relationship (Cacciatore, DeFrain, Jones, & Jones, 2008; Kersting & Wagner, 2012; Scheidt et al., 2012) and social support (Cacciatore, 2013; Scheidt et al., 2012) were found to predict the differing severity of couples' grief after a perinatal loss.

In our study, we employed quantitative and qualitative methods to examine these issues. The participants consisted of 30 pregnant women (over 20 gestation weeks) aged 25–35, without children, who had experienced a stillbirth after at least 20 weeks of pregnancy within 3–12 months prior to the study (the research group), and 30 pregnant women in their first pregnancy (a paired sample) with the same background variables who had not lost a fetus (the control group). No differences were found between the groups in level of education (about 90% had more than a high school education), length of marriage, or duration of pregnancy. There was, however, a small difference in the mean age of the two groups ($M = 31.0$, $SD = 3.7$; $M = 28.6$, $SD = 2.5$, in the research group and the control group, respectively) which probably stemmed from the fact that the women in the research group had had a previous pregnancy.

The women completed a number of self-report questionnaires: the Experience in Close Relationships Questionnaire (ECR-Short form; Brennan, Clark, & Shaver, 1998; Wei, Russell, Mallinckrodt, & Vogel, 2007), to examine attachment avoidance and anxiety (Cronbach $\alpha = .70$ and .61, respectively); the Berkeley-Leiden Adult Attachment Questionnaire (BLAAQ-U; Main, van IJzendoorn, & Hesse, 1993), to examine the level of unresolved loss and unusual beliefs (α = .90 and .86, respectively); and the Personal Assessment of Intimacy in Relationships (PAIR; Olson & Schaefer, 1981), to examine emotional, social, sexual, intellectual, and recreational intimacy in their relationships (α = .91 for the total scale). Their perception of future parenthood was examined by means of several additional questionnaires: the Ability to Relate to Children (Rholes, Simpson, Blakely, Lanigan, & Allen, 1997; α = .90); Parental Attitudes Towards Childrearing (PACR; Easterbrooks & Goldberg, 1984), comprising warmth, encouragement of independence, strictness, and aggravation (α = .63, .64, .77, and .65 respectively); the Maternal Separation Anxiety Scale (MSAS; Hock, McBride, & Gnezda, 1989; α = .92); and the Short Health Anxiety Inventory (SHAI; Warwick & Salkovskis, 1989; α = .75), assessing the mother's anxiety regarding the future health of the child. In addition, 10 of the women who experienced stillbirth were interviewed using semi-structured clinical interviews to gain a deeper understanding of their coping.

A series of MANOVAs was conducted, with group (research versus control) as the independent variable and the scores on the various questionnaires as the dependent variables. The MANOVAs for attachment dimensions and unresolved loss and trauma yielded significant effects: [F (2,57) = 6.75, $p < .01$, $\eta^2 = .19$] and [F (2,57) = 12.08, $p < .001$, $\eta^2 = .30$], respectively. As hypothesized, women who had experienced stillbirth displayed higher levels of attachment anxiety and avoidance and higher levels of unresolved loss than the control group. The results for unusual beliefs were only marginally significant (see Table 13.1), and no differences emerged for any of the dimensions of couple intimacy or perceptions of future parenthood (these examinations, therefore, are not presented in the table).

Because of the study design, we cannot rule out the possibility that the differences found on the personality-emotional characteristics of attachment and resolution of mourning existed before the experience of stillbirth. It is reasonable to assume, however, that this traumatic event at least temporarily harmed the women's psychosocial characteristics. The higher levels of attachment avoidance and anxiety may reflect a

Table 13.1 Differences between the Groups: Attachment and Unresolved Loss or Trauma

	Stillbirth (n = 30)		Control group (n = 30)		F group	η^2
	M	SD	M	SD		
Attachment avoidance	2.59	1.27	1.94	.49	6.96**	.11
Attachment anxiety	3.46	1.07	2.73	.74	9.25**	.14
Unresolved loss	2.54	.73	1.78	.41	25.44***	.30
Unresolved trauma	2.03	.74	1.72	.57	3.34+	.05

+$p < .10$; ** $p < .01$; ***$p < .001$

need for distancing while still needing close support, along with the worry that such support would not be adequately and consistently provided. The higher levels of unresolved loss may result from the fact that the traumatic loss had been experienced relatively recently, no more than one year prior to the study.

We also examined whether the stillbirth experience moderated the associations between attachment orientation or unresolved loss or trauma and the variables of couple intimacy and imagined future parenting. To test the moderations, a moderation models were examined employing the SPSS Macro for multiple regressions following Preacher, Rucker, and Hayes (2007) moderation model (model 1) testing the assumption that the relationship between the independent variable (i.e., attachment avoidance, attachment anxiety, and unresolved loss or trauma) and the dependent variable (couple intimacy and imagined future parenting) is contingent on the level of the moderator (i.e., the stillbirth or the control group). The regression analyses revealed one significant interaction. Specifically, as can be seen in Fig. 13.1 women's attachment avoidance positively predicted strictness among women in the control group ($B = .501$, $SE = .220$, $p = .026$, 95% CI .060, .942), but not among women of the research group.

Surprisingly, therefore, the results suggest that even though the experience of the loss of a fetus is a difficult, perhaps even traumatic, event, in some cases it may buffer women from the negative implications of their perception of their imagined relationship with a future child. Moreover, it does not appear to harm couple intimacy. The stillbirth experience might lessen the distancing tendencies of women with higher levels of avoidance, causing them to relax control over their emotions and behaviors and act in a manner contrary to their tendency to keep distant and aloof in close relationships (Mayseless & Scharf, 2007). It is important to note, however, that the women in our study reported on their imagined parenting. The results should also be examined in the context of actual parenting.

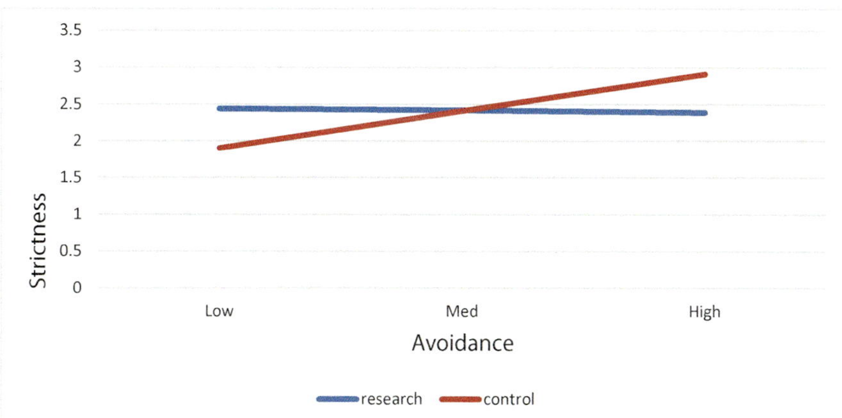

Fig. 13.1 Impact of attachment avoidance on strictness according to study's groups

The qualitative analysis shed light on women's experience following a stillbirth. Various aspects of this experience were also expressed in their responses in the interviews, as demonstrated below.

Ayelet described difficulties related to unrecognized loss:

> The environment doesn't understand anything you're going through. They want to help but they don't have the tools, and some people just don't have tact. I had a girlfriend whose pregnancy was a month longer than mine. The first time we talked [after the stillbirth], she said: At least you didn't have to suffer the eighth and ninth month. It's like, listen, I would have been very happy to suffer those months, really happy. I had friends at work who completely ignored the loss even when they saw me. As if it didn't happen. It was mostly men. They didn't know what to do with it and just walked by. There were all kinds of girlfriends with children who started to develop ideas about how I was supposed to feel about them having a healthy child. There was no connection between their inventions and reality.

The interviews revealed that despite the tendency of the women who had experienced stillbirth to distance themselves from their spouses, express anxiety regarding the next pregnancy, and perceive themselves as having a "damaged" maternal identity, they also saw their distancing behavior as part of a natural processing and resolution of the loss. They described it as an event that strengthened them and made them better women and mothers. Indeed, most women related to the stillbirth as contributing to the creation of their unique identity as experienced, understanding mothers who had suffered from the tragic pain of loss but come out of it stronger. Daphne explained it as follows:

> How did it change me? I think it calmed me in some way. I feel I've changed, but I don't know if I can define it. I let go more easily today. I accept reality as it is. Also, when I don't feel good about something, I don't obsess about it because there's nothing I can do. I don't make things into a drama. I don't get obsessive about it. I mean, if something happens and I don't like it, I don't jump through hoops to make it suit me. I'm talking about things that are irreversible….And I'm taking care of myself. I read more books, I play in the garden more because it makes me happy, I play with my dogs more. I really enjoy it….There is a lot of change. It changes you.

Another woman stated:

> As far as I was concerned, it was a sign of life in general and not necessarily something that relates to stillbirth….That's not the point. I'm not worried about that. I'll be a mother. I'll adopt if I need to. I'm not dealing with it now. I just want to be a better person. That's what I got from it….What kind of a mother will I be? That's also a fear. I don't know. I can't say that I'll be a good mother. I hope not to be an impatient mother. I work on myself. I'm impatient despite my profession [clinical professional] and…so of course my job in life will be to develop patience with my child. That's it. It's the only thought that worries me. That I not find myself like all the parents who yell at their children, even though I know it's not a good way to bring them up.

Finally, in the words of another mother, "I believe that the moment I become a mother, I'll be a different mother, better than I would have been if I had given birth on time."

Thus the narratives demonstrate growth deriving from the traumatic experience. The interviews revealed that the mothers had an optimistic, yet balanced and realistic, view of themselves and their future parenting.

13.1.2 Study 2: The Childbirth Experience

The experience of labor and delivery has a special and emotional place in the lives of many parents. Nevertheless, according to a recent meta-analysis (Grekin & O'Hara, 2014), the prevalence of postpartum PTSD ranges between 3.1% among community samples and 15.7% among risk samples. Furthermore, 20 to 48% of women perceive childbirth as traumatic and report a number of PTSD symptoms (Alcorn, O'Donovan, Patrick, Creedy, & Devilly, 2010; see also Ayers & Sawyer, Chap. 12 in this volume). It is most likely the interplay between the events and women's perceptions and emotions during the delivery that is the determining factor in the onset of PTSD. Women mention several issues as contributing to the distress of the experience, including: medical interventions; pain; negative subjective experiences; dissatisfaction with the care received during delivery or the feeling they were treated unsympathetically; lack of support; a sense of being powerless and not in control; and a flooding of emotions (Ayers, Bond, Bertullies, & Wijma 2016; Cigoli, Gilli, & Saita, 2006; DeGroot & Vik, 2017; Elmir, Schmied, Wilkes, & Jackson, 2010). Unlike other traumatic events, however, birth is a normative and common experience, and talking about it is routine and culturally acceptable. Furthermore, the opportunity to retell the birth story may facilitate a coherent perception and narrative of it (Ayers, Radoš, & Balouch, 2015).

An unresolved traumatic childbirth experience can interfere with the development of the mother's bond with her baby. Nevertheless, few studies to date have examined the emotional and cognitive processes related to the way the birth experience is resolved (Waldenström, 2003; Wilson, Rholes, Simpson, & Tarn, 2007). Our second study therefore sought to employ a longitudinal design to examine the associations between attachment security and the experience of support during childbirth on the one hand, and the resolution of the labor experience and quality of the interaction with the baby three months later on the other. The mother–baby interaction was examined by means of analysis of the mother's emotional availability. This observation allowed for assessment of the interaction as expressed by the ability of both parties to respond to feelings, desires, motivations, and aims in a mutually adapted manner (Biringen, 2000; Biringen et al., 2000).

The participants in this study were women who had recently delivered their first child, having given birth vaginally to a full-term, live baby between three and three-and-a-half months earlier. Pregnant women were recruited through ads published throughout the university, on the Internet and in forums dealing with pregnancy and childbirth, and via the snowball method. Sixty-six women agreed to take part in the study. Of these, 18 delivered by caesarean section and were excluded from the sample. Another 14 women were excluded because they did not return the questionnaires in the first stage, and one participant was excluded due to premature birth. The final sample therefore consisted of 33 who met all the criteria and completed both stages of the assessment. Mean age was 28; 97% had an academic education; 70.6% had participated in a preparatory course for the birth with their partner; 72% received an epidural during delivery; and 18% were supported by a doula during birth. Thirty-three percent of the women reported special difficulties during labor, such as intense pain, fetal distress, or vacuum birth.

The first assessment was conducted during the third trimester of pregnancy. The women completed several self-report instruments, including: a demographic questionnaire; the Experience in Close Relationships Questionnaire (ECR; Brennan et al., 1998), to examine attachment anxiety and avoidance (Cronbach $\alpha = .92$ and .88 respectively); the Berkeley-Leiden Adult Attachment Questionnaire (BLAAQ-U; Main et al., 1993), to examine past resolution of loss ($\alpha = .86$) prior to the childbirth experience; and the Enacted Support Questionnaire (ESQ; Barrera, 1986; Barrera & Baca, 1990; Barrera et al., 1981), to examine the perception of support from partners, friends, mothers, and fathers ($\alpha = .91$, .81, .89, and .85 respectively).

For the second assessment, when the babies were three to three-and-a-half months old, a three-hour meeting was scheduled with each of the mothers at their home. The meeting began with an interview to gain an in-depth understanding of the mother's perception and resolution of the childbirth experience and her relationship with her infant. The mother–baby interaction was then observed using the emotional availability scales (Biringen & Robinson, 1991). First, the mothers were asked to play a structured game with the baby, selecting from three available toys: an activity mat, a rattle, and a mirror. In the second part of the observation, they were asked to play freely, choosing what to do with the baby on their own. Following the observation, the mothers were asked to complete the questionnaire relating to support during childbirth (Enacted Support Questionnaire—ESQ; Barrera, 1986; Barrera & Baca, 1990; Barrera, Sandler, & Ramsay, 1981) a second time, along with a childbirth questionnaire (Traumatic Event Scale—TES; Wijma, Soderouist, & Wijma, 1997; $\alpha = .73$) aimed at identifying women suffering from trauma as a result of the childbirth experience.

The following findings emerged. No significant associations were found between high levels of anxious attachment and support during childbirth. However, mothers characterized by high anxious or avoidant attachment tended to have a more traumatic perception of the childbirth experience. The qualitative analysis revealed additional variables that appear to be associated with the traumatic perception of childbirth. More than half of the mothers (18 of 33) described the experience as very difficult, referring in the interviews to lack of control during the birth, fear of their own and their baby's death, and a profusion of negative feelings (anger, frustration, despair) regarding the birth and the attitude of the medical team. These feelings may therefore be significant contributors to the perception of the birth as a difficult event.

Furthermore, among mothers characterized by high levels of avoidant attachment, there was a positive association between support during the birth and their maternal feelings and sensitive response to the baby. This use of support is uncustomary for people high on avoidant attachment. It might reflect changes the women underwent during their pregnancy that enabled them to turn to others and effectively take advantage of their help. Alternatively, having supportive close others might have helped them revise their perceptions regarding the trustworthiness of others and the importance of closeness and support. It is also possible that the stress they experienced during labor disrupted their automatic responses, facilitating modifications to their usual way of coping. Their enhanced ability to turn to others and use their support might have persisted after the baby was born, helping them adapt during a time that is often challenging, especially for first-time mothers. Thus, whether due to a new capacity the mothers developed or to the qualities and support of close others, support during childbirth appears to serve as a buffer in the relations of avoidantly attached mothers and their babies, promoting their sensitivity to the infant.

Analysis of the participants' narratives in the interviews enabled us to differentiate between three groups that correspond to the three main categories of attachment patterns. The first, displaying secure attachment, can be characterized by a statement made by one of the mothers, Lilach: "I have learned about myself and grown stronger from the experience." Mothers in this group reflectively evaluated their experience during childbirth, relating to both positive and negative emotions. In general, they were able to recognize the best and worst parts of the experience, even when it was difficult and did not match their expectations. For these women, the event of giving birth was meaningful and empowering.

Hannah, for example, described a difficult birth that did not quite coincide with her expectations. Despite her painful memories, she was able to focus on the positive aspects of her labor, including a sense of strength derived from her ability to cope with it. She described it as follows:

> I really felt like the queen of the world…I felt like the queen of the world in the whole process, as if from the moment the labor pains began until the baby was lying on me, I really felt like I was a queen, that I could stand it and could do it. Here I am doing this. It's a bit painful, uncomfortable - actually it doesn't hurt a little, it hurts a lot - it's uncomfortable and it's difficult, but here I am doing it and here comes another labor pain. Today, in retrospect, I can say I was going to get the biggest prize I could ask for….This was a very important time in my life. It's the kind of an event…I can say it was a formative event in my life, nothing less, truly a formative event….As I said before, I learned a lot about myself. It really made me strong. It put me in a place where I also softened a lot, because of this place, this event.

When speaking of her child, she said:

> I believe that my child came to soften me a little, and that's okay. It's not terrible if I didn't finish something to the end or I told him he's like that….I don't have to do everything by the book. From my point of view, the fact that I'm here gives him the feeling that mother is right here and you'll always have somewhere to return to, you'll always have a home, if you want it….Mother will always be there for you.

In reference to her daughter, another mother said:

> She's a pure pleasure, a pure pleasure. She's an amazing girl, just amazing. She's so communicative and deep, she has such a look. I don't know how to explain it. She smiles and she's sweet….It's very, very easy to love her, very easy, and she's really placid….Even if she cries, you pick her up and she calms down immediately….We're connected. It's a very great love. It's falling in love. I think I'm in love with her….She's so responsive, you know, she's cute, she gives a lot of feedback….She smiles and she's happy to see me and my husband….She knows very well what she wants, in a gentle way. [She laughs.]

In contrast, the second group corresponded to anxious attachment and was characterized by ambivalent perceptions of pregnancy, parenthood, and the child. In the words of one participant: "Whether it's good or it's bad, there's no way back." As Shani put it:

> Of course I explained [my feelings] to my partner, but as long as he was not in a place where he really wanted a child, he could listen and say ok when I told him about my fears and where I am. But I knew that once he was in a place where he really wanted to be [pregnant] now, that would become my job then and there, and if we wait, then maybe we won't succeed, all kinds of things like that. And what do you mean I don't want [to get pregnant], what kind of woman [doesn't want a child].

Yuval related how the discovery of her pregnancy was followed by negative emotions. She described difficulties in accepting the pregnancy, fear of loss of autonomy in her life, and fear that the future baby would harm her relationship with her partner:

> As if once you have this [the pregnancy] there is no way back, then there's such a feeling of…really? This is really happening? [She laughs.] That, no, there's no other way, no way back. So, from there on all that's left is to understand that…there are going to be changes and…to accept that…and that I will not be only with my husband and it's difficult….Up to now I could be free and do what I want….It'll be together, just a different kind of together. And…I'll have to be entirely committed to the little creature….It's hard to understand that from the point that…I'm the center of my world, or my couple relationship is the center of my world…my child is now the center. That's the difficulty.

The mothers in this group described their relationship with their baby mainly in negative terms, such as distance, anger, and guilt. Yuval described caring for the child as instrumental, and expressed feelings of alienation and distance:

> It was matter of fact from the start. You're the baby girl, I'll be the mother. I have to change your diapers, feed you, change your diaper again, help you burp, change your clothes. At first she was really a piece of nothing, she just was there, she did what I wanted. I wanted to change her clothes, I changed her clothes. She wanted to sleep, she slept. She wanted to eat, she ate. As if it was very, very, very laconic…not thrilling or exciting.

Another woman described her baby boy in a similar manner, saying: "until now he was a lump, like a potato that eats and sleeps, food, diaper." The difficulties of breastfeeding also made her feel negative and resentful toward her baby:

> I gave up breastfeeding because I felt I was starting to develop [she hesitates]…I suffered terribly from the pump, and it hurt, and it took time I didn't have anyway… It hurt me terribly, and…I started to have bad feelings toward him, like…look what I have to do because of you, not for you.

The tumultuous emotions and ambivalence in the narratives of the women in this group are evident. This hyperactivation contributes to vague and incoherent perceptions of the self, the pregnancy, and the child, expressed in negative emotions directed toward the child who was born before the mother had made up her mind that she really wanted a child now. The indecisiveness resulted in a less smooth transition to pregnancy and parenthood in view of the lack of preparation for the necessary investment in developing a parent identity, learning the child's traits, and developing a unique bond with the baby, and not just providing for its physical needs.

The third group corresponded to the attachment avoidance dimension, characterized by the phrase: "I know he's mine, but I don't feel it." Mothers in this group offered a limited description of their experience of childbirth, answering in few words. They lacked emotional expression and were emotionally disconnected from the process they had undergone. In fact, it was difficult to understand their experience from their narratives. Noa, for example, gave only brief answers throughout the interview, and sometimes resisted answering at all. She found it hard to recall the process of childbirth, and focused mainly on her current experience. Her emotional detachment was obvious in all her answers:

> Throughout my pregnancy, I lived my life exactly the same [as always]....In retrospect, I don't remember myself pregnant, as if I went through it quickly. I didn't feel anything, I had no side effects during pregnancy....I didn't feel a change or anything...really... a completely normal life...the entire period of pregnancy.... I can't tell you there was an amazing change. I can't tell you there was any change in my body, except that my belly was big. I didn't feel it, I didn't understand. Even today, I think I didn't understand what it meant that I was pregnant. Nothing, nothing, nothing. I lived my life, it was exactly the same....

> Even today I can't tell you a million percent...he [her baby] is mine....I know he's mine but I don't feel it. As if sometimes I say, hey, I have a child. As if I take hold of myself and say, hey, I'm a mother. It's not real. Certainly not after three months, at least not for me....Our house...you know, people keep coming in and going out. We grew up together, in this neighborhood, me and my partner. I just made lunch, and a good friend of ours came in....My partner came out from [working on] the computer, [and asked] where's the child? [She laughs.] I told him I don't know. [She giggles.] I didn't notice. Maybe someone took him for a walk. After half an hour they came back. [She giggles.] Do you understand? Like we live our life and he lives it with us. No, I don't feel like suddenly I can't do things because...so it's like there's no feeling of a fundamental...change.

When Noa was asked to describe her son's character, she had a very difficult time and could not really do it: "I can't tell you, except that I can say I think he will be, that he is stubborn, but no, no, I can't tell you. I don't...I can't point to any personality traits." Her description of her parenthood and her child reflects detachment and alienation. She was neither familiar with her child, nor interested in getting to know him better. This distancing not only limited access to negative emotions, but also precluded positive emotions and enjoyment.

To conclude, according to attachment theory, people characterized by insecure attachment tend to recall less positive memories from attachment-related experiences (Dykas & Cassidy, 2011; Simpson, Rholes, & Winterheld, 2010). Moreover, women with an avoidant attachment style who underwent operative births showed the greatest risk of developing PTSD symptoms (Ayers, Jessop, Pike, Parfitt, & Ford, 2014; see also Ayers & Sawyer, Chap. 12 in this volume). It is not surprising, therefore, that mothers displaying high levels of anxious or avoidant attachment tended to have a more negative and traumatic perception of the childbirth experience three months later. In addition, support in general, and during childbirth in particular, was associated with more sensitive parenting. Individual differences in attachment patterns were also revealed in the way the women perceived themselves as mothers and the way they perceived their children, and thus might shape the emerging mother-child relationship.

13.2 Summary and Conclusions: Are Difficult Experiences Destructive or Constructive?

The experience of stillbirth, as well as delivery of a healthy child, can be stressful and even traumatic for the mother. It may act as a trigger, turning individuals' vulnerabilities into actual difficulties and generating stressful reactions, such as mourning, anxiety, and anger, which must be resolved. In the present studies, the resolution of difficult experiences was examined from the perspective of attachment theory. A healthy resolution process is indicated by a successful effort to accept the fact that there has been a change in the individual's external world and to rearrange their inner world accordingly. Whereas a disordered mourning process might be expressed in particularly intense and long-lasting emotional reactions to the event (Bowlby, 1980, 1988), the healthy resolution of difficult experiences is reflected in reorientation to the present and future and a balanced view of the impact of the loss on oneself. Thus, acknowledgement of the changes following stillbirth or a stressful childbirth experience promotes successful coping. Lack of resolution might leave mothers with negative feelings and hamper future parental functioning.

Our studies highlight both the risk and the protective factors in the normative stressful life event of the transition to parenthood, pointing to factors that promote positive change and increased strength in the face of adversity. It was found that attachment security can buffer the adverse implications of mothers' stressful experiences. Based on their past experience, securely attached individuals are more likely to openly communicate their distress, mobilize problem-solving strategies, and seek social support than are insecurely attached individuals (Mikulincer & Shaver, 2016; see also Mikulincer & Shaver, Chap. 18 in this volume). In contrast, high levels of attachment anxiety, attachment avoidance, and prior unresolved loss appear to make mothers more vulnerable when encountering the stressful circumstance of the transition to parenthood (Simpson, Rholes, Campbell, Tran, & Wilson, 2003; see also Rholes & Paetzold, Chap. 17 in this volume).

The studies reveal the protective role of support and closeness, especially when facing difficult experiences. This is particularly beneficial in cases where individuals' characteristics make them more vulnerable from the outset. Intimacy with one's partner and support from a close other during childbirth might offset the negative implications of the difficult or traumatic experience. It has also been suggested that health professionals involved in childbirth need to emotionally support mothers, who often experience a traumatic birth regardless of their child's survival or health (Üstündağ Budak, Harris, & Blissett, 2016). Other researchers (Kendall-Tackett, 2014) have suggested examining women's attitudes toward pregnancy, labor, and delivery, their fear of childbirth, and their interactions with the medical team in order to better understand the variables that contribute to mothers' adjustment or maladjustment and the best way to facilitate their coping.

The sociocultural context also plays an important role and can influence the chances that stillbirth or a difficult labor will develop into disenfranchised grief. The strong value of family, together with an almost universal desire to marry and have children (Scharf & Mayseless, 2010), make these childbirth-related experiences especially sensitive. In the case of stillbirth, in Israel the process of mourning may be complicated by the traditional Jewish burial of the fetus in a mass grave whose site is not revealed to the parents, as well as the lack of established mourning customs. Furthermore, because of the high value placed on children in the country, stillbirth may be perceived as a failure to fulfill an essential societal expectation (Golan & Leichtentritt, 2016). The same sociocultural climate might also restrict openness to expressing difficulties with regard to the delivery.

The interviews enabled in-depth observation of women's experiences from their point of view, providing insight into their difficulties and strengths. However, as the study samples were small, these issues warrant further investigation in larger and more heterogeneous samples (e.g., less educated women, different cultural backgrounds, etc.).

Finally, the studies provide evidence of women's resilience and growth despite significant risk or adversity. Previous research has also shown that adverse experiences can promote hardiness and resilience and facilitate coping with similar experiences in the future (Seery et al., 2010). For example, parents of premature babies reported a greater level of personal growth than parents of full-term infants, which might be the result of their successful coping with prior difficult experiences (Taubman – Ben-Ari & Spielman, 2014; see also Taubman – Ben-Ari, Chap. 16 in this volume). People who have overcome adversity in the past may be better at appreciating life's small pleasures, as demonstrated in the women's narratives in our studies. In addition, a recent study of individuals' mindsets with regard to stress found that those who hold a "stress-is-enhancing mindset" reveal more adaptive physiological responses and more approach-oriented behavioral responses when coping with stress (Crum, Salovey, & Achor, 2013). The authors demonstrated that a short intervention can be successful in changing mindsets, and that a stress-is-enhancing mindset is associated with positive changes in self-reported psychological symptoms and work performance. Thus, incorporating such elements into existing pre-birth courses might alter people's perceptions of the malleability of stress and facilitate their coping if and when they are faced with stressful events and situations.

References

Alcorn, K. L., O'Donovan, A., Patrick, J. C., Creedy, D., & Devilly, G. J. (2010). A prospective longitudinal study of the prevalence of post-traumatic stress disorder resulting from childbirth events. *Psychological Medicine, 40*(11), 1849–1859.

Armstrong, D. S., Hutti, M. H., & Myers, J. (2009). The influence of prior perinatal loss on parents' psychological distress after the birth of a subsequent healthy infant. *Journal of Obstetric, Gynecologic, and Neonatal Nursing, 38*(6), 654–666.

Ayers, S., Bond, R., Bertullies, S., & Wijma, K. (2016). The aetiology of post-traumatic stress following childbirth: A meta-analysis and theoretical framework. *Psychological Medicine, 46*(6), 1121–1134.

Ayers, S., Jessop, D., Pike, A., Parfitt, Y., & Ford, E. (2014). The role of adult attachment style, birth intervention and support in posttraumatic stress after childbirth: A prospective study. *Journal of Affective Disorders, 155*, 295–298.

Ayers, S., Radoš, S. N., & Balouch, S. (2015). Narratives of traumatic birth: Quality and changes over time. *Psychological Trauma: Theory, Research, Practice, and Policy, 7*(3), 234–242.

Barrera, M. (1986). Distinctions between social support concepts, measures, and models. *American Journal of Community Psychology, 14*(4), 413–445.

Barrera, M., & Baca, L. M. (1990). Recipient reactions to social support: Contributions of enacted support, conflicted support and network orientation. *Journal of Social and Personal Relationships, 7*(4), 541–551.

Barrera, M., Sandler, I. N., & Ramsay, T. B. (1981). Preliminary development of a scale of social support: Studies on college students. *American Journal of Community Psychology, 9*(4), 435–447.

Biringen, Z. (2000). Emotional availability: Conceptualization and research finding. *American Journal of Orthopsychiatry, 70*(1), 104–114.

Biringen, Z., Brown, D., Donaldson, L., Green, S., Krcmarik, S., & Lovas, G. (2000). Adult attachment interview: Linkages with dimensions of emotional availability for mothers and their pre-kindergarteners. *Attachment and Human Development, 2*(2), 188–202.

Biringen, Z., & Robinson, J. (1991). Emotional availability in mother-child interaction: A reconceptualization for research. *American Journal of Orthopsychiatry, 61*(2), 258–271.

Bowlby, J. (1980). *Attachment and loss, Vol. 3: Loss*. New York, NY: Basic Books.

Bowlby, J. (1988). *A secure base: Clinical applications of attachment theory*. London: Routledge.

Brennan, K. A., Clark, C. L., & Shaver, P. R. (1998). Self-report measurement of adult attachment. In J. A. Simpson & W. S. Rholes (Eds.), *Attachment theory and close relationships* (pp. 46–76). New York, NY: Guilford.

Bretherton, I., & Munholland, K. A. (2016). The internal working model in light of contemporary neuroimaging research. In J. Cassidy & P. R. Shaver (Eds.), *Handbook of attachment: Theory, research, and clinical applications* (3rd ed., pp. 63–88). New York: Guilford Press.

Cacciatore, J. (2013). Psychological effects of stillbirth. *Seminars in Fetal & Neonatal Medicine, 18*(2), 76–82.

Cacciatore, J., DeFrain, J., Jones, K., & Jones, H. (2008). Stillbirth and the couple: A gender-based exploration. *Journal of Family Social Work, 11*(4), 351–372.

Cantazaro, A., & Wei, M. (2010). Adult attachment, dependence, self-criticism, and depressive symptoms: A test of a mediational model. *Journal of Personality, 78*(4), 1135–1162.

Cigoli, V., Gilli, G., & Saita, E. (2006). Relational factors in psychopathological responses to childbirth. *Journal of Psychosomatic Obstetrics & Gynecology, 27*(2), 91–97.

Collins, N. L., & Feeney, B. C. (2000). A safe haven: An attachment theory perspective on support seeking and caregiving in intimate relationships. *Journal of Personality and Social Psychology, 78*(6), 1053–1073.

Corr, C. (2002). Rethinking the concept of disenfranchised grief. In K. Doka (Ed.), *Disenfranchised grief: New directions, challenges, and strategies for practice* (pp. 39–60). Champaign, IL: Research Press.

Crum, A. J., Salovey, P., & Achor, S. (2013). Rethinking stress: The role of mindsets in determining the stress response. *Journal of Personality and Social Psychology, 104*(4), 716–733.

DeGroot, J. M., & Vik, T. A. (2017). Disenfranchised grief following a traumatic birth. *Journal of Loss and Trauma, 22*(4), 346–356.

Doka, K. J. (1989). *Disenfranchised grief: Recognizing hidden sorrow*. Lexington, MA, England: Lexington Books/D.C. Heath and Com.

Dykas, M. J., & Cassidy, J. (2011). Attachment and the processing of social information across the life span: Theory and evidence. *Psychological Bulletin, 137*(1), 19–46.

Easterbrooks, M. A., & Goldberg, W. A. (1984). Toddler development in the family: Impact of father involvement and parenting characteristics. *Child Development, 55*(3), 740–752.

Elmir, R., Schmied, V., Wilkes, L., & Jackson, D. (2010). Women's perceptions and experiences of a traumatic birth: A meta-ethnography. *Journal of Advanced Nursing, 66*(10), 2142–2153.

Field, N. P., Gao, B., & Paderna, L. (2005). Continuing bonds in bereavement: An attachment theory based perspective. *Death Studies, 29*(4), 277–299.
Fraley, R. C., & Bonanno, G. A. (2004). Attachment and loss: A test of three competing models on the association between attachment-related avoidance and adaptation to bereavement. *Personality and Social Psychology Bulletin, 30*(7), 878–890.
Fraley, R. C., & Shaver, P. R. (1998). Airport separations: A naturalistic study of adult attachment dynamics in separating couples. *Journal of Personality and Social Psychology, 75*(5), 1198–1212.
Golan, A., & Leichtentritt, R. D. (2016). Meaning reconstruction among women following stillbirth: A loss fraught with ambiguity and doubt. *Health and Social Work, 41*(3), 147–154.
Gold, K. J., Leon, I., Boggs, M. E., & Sen, A. (2016). Depression and posttraumatic stress symptoms after perinatal loss in a population-based sample. *Journal of Women's Health, 25*(3), 263–269.
Grekin, R., & O'Hara, M. W. (2014). Prevalence and risk factors of postpartum posttraumatic stress disorder: A meta-analysis. *Clinical Psychology Review, 34*(5), 389–401.
Helgeson, V. S., Reynolds, K. A., & Tomich, P. L. (2006). A meta-analytic review of benefit finding and growth. *Journal of Consulting and Clinical Psychology, 74*(5), 797–816.
Ho, S. Y., Chan, I. F., Ma, E. W., & Field, N. P. (2013). Continuing bonds, attachment style, and adjustment in the conjugal bereavement among Hong Kong Chinese. *Death Studies, 37*(3), 248–268.
Hock, E., McBride, S., & Gnezda, M. T. (1989). Maternal separation anxiety: Mother-infant separation from the maternal perspective. *Child Development, 60*(4), 793–802.
Kelley, M. C., & Trinidad, S. B. (2012). Silent loss and the clinical encounter: Parents' and physicians' experiences of stillbirth—A qualitative analysis. *BMC Pregnancy and Childbirth, 12,* 137.
Kendall-Tackett, K. (2014). Birth trauma: The causes and consequences of childbirth-related trauma and PTSD. In D. Barnes (Ed.), *Women's reproductive mental health across the lifespan* (pp. 177–191). Cham, Switzerland: Springer International Publishing.
Kersting, A., & Wagner, B. (2012). Complicated grief after perinatal loss. *Dialogues in Clinical Neuroscience, 14*(2), 187–194.
Kobak, R. R., Cole, H. E., Ferenz-Gillies, R., Fleming, W. S., & Gamble, W. (1993). Attachment and emotion regulation during mother-teen problem solving: A control theory analysis. *Child Development, 64*(1), 231–245.
Main, M., van IJzendoorn, M. H., & Hesse, E. (1993). *Unresolved/unclassifiable responses to the adult attachment interview: Predictable from unresolved state and anomalous beliefs in the Berkeley-Leiden adult attachment questionnaire.* Unpublished manuscript, Department of Psychology, University of California at Berkeley.
Mayseless, O., & Scharf, M. (2007). Attachment representations of adolescents and their capacity for intimacy in close relationships. *Journal of Research on Adolescence, 17*(1), 23–50.
Mikulincer, M., & Shaver, P. (2016). *Attachment in adulthood: Structure, dynamics, and change* (2nd ed.). NY: The Guilford Press.
Olson, D. H., & Schaefer, M. T. (1981). Assessing intimacy: The pair inventory. *Journal of Marital and Family Therapy, 7*(1), 47–60.
Preacher, K. J., Rucker, D. D., & Hayes, A. F. (2007). Addressing moderated mediation hypotheses: Theory, methods, and prescriptions. *Multivariate Behavioral Research, 42*(1), 185–227.
Rholes, W. S., Simpson, J. A., Blakely, B. S., Lanigan, L., & Allen, E. A. (1997). Adult attachment styles, the desire to have children, and working models of parenthood. *Journal of Personality, 65*(2), 357–385.
Robinson, M., Baker, L., & Nackerud, L. (1999). The relationship of attachment theory and perinatal loss. *Death Studies, 23*(3), 257–270.
Scharf, M., & Mayseless, O. (2010). Finding the authentic self in a communal culture: Developmental goals in emerging adulthood. In S. Shulman & J. Nurmi (Eds.), *The role of goals in navigating individual lives during emerging adulthood* (pp. 83–95). San Francisco, CA, US: Jossey-Bass.
Scheidt, C. E., Hasenburg, A., Kunze, M., Waller, E., Pfeifer, R., Zimmermann, P., et al. (2012). Are individual differences of attachment predicting bereavement outcome after perinatal loss? A prospective cohort study. *Journal of Psychosomatic Research, 73*(5), 375–382.

Scheidt, C. E., Waller, N., Wangler, J., Hasenburg, A., & Kersting, A. (2007). Mourning after perinatal death—Prevalence symptoms and treatment—A review of the literature. *Psychotherapie, Psychosomatik, Medizinische Psychologie, 57*(1), 4–11.

Seery, M. D., Holman, E. A., & Silver, R. C. (2010). Whatever does not kill us: Cumulative lifetime adversity, vulnerability, and resilience. *Journal of Personality and Social Psychology, 99*(6), 1025–1041.

Shreffler, K. M., Greil, A. L., & McQuillan, J. (2011). Pregnancy loss and distress among U.S. women. *Family Relations: An Interdisciplinary Journal of Applied Family Studies, 60*(3), 342–355.

Simpson, J. A., Rholes, W. S., Campbell, L., Tran, S., & Wilson, C. L. (2003). Adult attachment, the transition to parenthood, and depressive symptoms. *Journal of Personality and Social Psychology, 84*(6), 1172–1187.

Simpson, J. A., Rholes, W. S., & Winterheld, H. A. (2010). Attachment working models twist memories of relationship events. *Psychological Science, 21*(2), 252–259.

Taubman – Ben-Ari, O., & Spielman, V. (2014). Personal growth following the first child's birth: A comparison of parents of pre- and full-term babies. *Social Work Research, 38*(2), 91–106.

Tedeschi, R. G., & Calhoun, L. G. (1996). The posttraumatic growth inventory: Measuring the positive legacy of trauma. *Journal of Traumatic Stress, 9*(3), 455–472.

Toffol, E., Koponen, P., & Partonen, T. (2013). Miscarriage and mental health: Results of two population-based studies. *Psychiatry Research, 205*(1–2), 151–158.

Tseng, Y., Cheng, H., Chen, Y., Yang, S., & Cheng, P. (2017). Grief reactions of couples to perinatal loss: A one-year prospective follow-up. *Journal of Clinical Nursing, 26*(23–24), 5133–5142.

Turton, P., Hughes, P., Evans, C. H., & Fainman, D. (2001). Incidence, correlates and predictors of post-traumatic stress disorder in the pregnancy after stillbirth. *The British Journal of Psychiatry, 178,* 556–560.

Üstündağ Budak, A. M., Harris, G., & Blissett, J. (2016). Perinatal trauma with and without loss experiences. *Journal of Reproductive and Infant Psychology, 34*(4), 413–425.

Waldenström, U. (2003). Women's memory of childbirth at two months and one year after the birth. *Birth: Issues in Perinatal Care, 30*(4), 248–254.

Warwick, H. M. C., & Salkovskis, P. M. (1989). Cognitive and behavioral characteristics of primary hipochondriasis. *Scandinavian Journal of Behavior Therapy, 18*(2), 85–92.

Wei, M., Russell, D. W., Mallinckrodt, B., & Vogel, D. L. (2007). The experiences in close relationship scale (ECR)-short form: Reliability, validity, and factor structure. *Journal of Personality Assessment, 88*(2), 187–204.

Wijma, K., Soderouist, J., & Wijma, B. (1997). Posttraumatic stress disorder after childbirth: A cross sectional study. *Journal of Anxiety Disorder, 11*(6), 587–597.

Wijngaards-de Meij, L., Stroebe, M., Schut, H., Stroebe, W., van den Bout, J., van der Heijden, P. G. M., et al. (2007). Patterns of attachment and parents' adjustment to the death of their child. *Personality and Social Psychology Bulletin, 33*(4), 537–548.

Wilson, C. L., Rholes, W. S., Simpson, J. A., & Tran, S. (2007). Labor, delivery, and early parenthood: An attachment theory perspective. *Personality and Social Psychology Bulletin, 33*(4), 505–518.

Chapter 14
Confronting Existential Concerns in the Transition to Parenthood: A Theoretical and Therapeutic Model

Noga Levin-Keini and Shirley Ben Shlomo

14.1 Introduction

Examining the confrontation with stressful traumatic events through an existentialist prism has been common practice since the early 20th century (Frankl, 1984). However, it is only in the past 20 years, with the development of the theoretical approach of positive psychology (Seligman & Csikszentmihalyi, 2000), that this prism has been used to examine the transition to parenthood. Positive psychology holds that the impact of stressful life events should be considered not only in terms of mental health, but also in terms of the individual's ability to grow and develop beyond the level at which they functioned prior to the event, or what is known as posttraumatic growth (Tedeschi & Calhoun, 2004). Initial studies adopting this approach focused mainly on traumatic events such as terminal illnesses (Widows, Jacobsen, Booth-Jones, & Fields, 2005), bereavement (Bonanno, Papa, Moskowitz, & Folkman, 2005), and the birth of a child with special needs (King & Patterson, 2000), rather than on normative stressful events in the life cycle.

Studies describing the possibility of growth and development as a result of normative events, among them the transition to motherhood, were first published in Israel and England in 2009 (Sawyer & Ayers, 2009; Taubman – Ben-Ari, Ben Shlomo, Sivan, & Dolizki, 2009; see also Ayers & Sawyer, Chap. 12; Taubman – Ben-Ari, Chap. 16 in this volume). Some continued to use the term "posttraumatic growth," while others preferred "personal growth" or "psychological growth." Since then, many studies have been carried out in the context of the transition to parenthood in general, and motherhood in particular, examining, for example, growth and meaning

N. Levin-Keini (✉)
The School of Social Work, Ashkelon Academic College, Ashkelon, Israel
e-mail: Keini_e@walla.co.il

S. Ben Shlomo
The Louis and Gabi Weisfeld School of Social Work, Bar Ilan University, Ramat Gan, Israel
e-mail: Shirley.ben@biu.ac.il

O. Taubman – Ben-Ari (ed.), *Pathways and Barriers to Parenthood*,
https://doi.org/10.1007/978-3-030-24864-2_14

in the life of mothers and grandmothers (Taubman – Ben-Ari, Ben Shlomo, & Findler, 2012), the potential for personal growth of heterosexual versus lesbian mothers (Shenkman, 2018), satisfaction in life among first-time fathers (Taubman – Ben-Ari, Skvirsky, Bar Shua, & Horowitz, 2017).

Development of the theory of positive psychology has also led to the expansion of therapeutic models for mothers and fathers transitioning to parenthood. This transition was previously probed principally via psychodynamics (Espasa, 2004), which places the emphasis on the manner in which unconscious content from the parent's past evokes anxiety, which in turn arouses the use of defence mechanisms and/or creates parental psychopathology. In contrast, new models focus on the present, seeking to promote growth in the wake of the stressful experience. Moreover, the emergence of the inter-subjective approach, also known as the "psychology of two people," led to the introduction of terms such as mutual relations between the therapist and the patient, as well as to concern for the manner in which arousal of suffering in the patient awakens suffering in the therapist (Aron, 1996).

In therapeutic terms, the existentialist approach draws on these principles and elaborates on them. It holds that a person exists at one and the same time in four existential dimensions (physical, psychological, social, and spiritual), which, although differentiated from each other, are also closely interconnected. Unlike therapists adopting other approaches, the existentialist therapist is not concerned with the development of the patient's personality profile or with an attempt to interpret events in the patient's life by means of an understanding of their mind. Instead, they examine which of the dimensions in the patient's life are stable and which are precarious and in need of support and strengthening.

Quantitative tools are generally used to examine the theoretical concepts deriving from the existentialist approach, such as meaning in life, a search for this meaning (Steger, Frazier, Oishi, & Kaler, 2006; see also Morse & Steger, Chap. 1 in this volume), and an awareness of mortality (Levasseur, McDermott, & Lafreniere, 2015; see also Solomon, Chap. 11 in this volume). This chapter presents a different approach: a convergence of diagnostic tools, therapy, and evaluation based on an understanding of existential psychodynamics as described by Yalom (1980). We begin by outlining the principles of existentialist therapy, and then explain how it deals with fundamental questions raised in the transition to parenthood. Finally, we describe an intervention model for new parents based on this approach, illustrating its principles by means of two clinical cases.

14.2 What Is Existential Psychotherapy?

Existential psychotherapy is a form of dynamic mental therapy that developed, like other approaches, as a by-product of Freud's (1914) psychodynamic theory. The principal difference between existentialist and Freudian therapy lies in the emphasis they place on the element of drive in the individual. The classic Freudian approach holds that a person's inborn drive clashes with the demands of the environment (initially the external, and subsequently the internal environment), arousing anxiety, with which the person copes through defence mechanisms that enable the drive to be expressed indirectly. In contrast, the existentialist approach maintains that the basic conflict is not between the inborn drive and the environment, but rather between the individual and existential givens (concerns and the individual's inherent traits), which are an integral part of their very existence in the world. An awareness of these concerns leads to anxiety, with which a person copes through defence mechanisms, some conventional, such as those described by Freud, Anna Freud, and Sullivan, and others unique, designed to cope specifically with existential fears (Yalom, 1980).

14.3 Ultimate Concerns

Yalom (1980) defines four ultimate concerns that lie at the core of the dynamic-existential conflict:

1. *Death*—Although we live in the present, we know he says, that one day we will cease to exist, creating a conflict between awareness of inevitable death and the desire to continue living. "It is not easy for individuals to live every moment being aware of death; nor can individuals live frozen in fear, so they develop methods to soften death's terror. We project ourselves into the future through our children, we grow rich and famous, ever larger; we develop compulsive protective rituals; or embrace an impregnable belief in an ultimate rescuer" (Yalom, 2008, p. 5). The transition to parenthood underscores this existential issue since the moment people become parents they realize that they are responsible for the life of a new generation. In other words, they are made aware of the fact that they are next in line to die.
2. *Freedom*—This refers to the lack of an organized external template that determines our actions, such as study, work, or relationships. That is to say, freedom connotes the absence of solid ground under our feet, giving rise to a conflict between the void and the yearning for terra firma. A key existential dynamic then, is the clash between our confrontation with groundlessness and our wish for ground and structure (Yalom, 1980, p. 9). The term "groundlessness" is used to describe the subjective experience felt when confronting existential freedom and the anxiety that may be generated when one encounters the reality of absolute self-responsibility in an existential sense. Yalom adds, "Viewed from the perspective self-creation, choice, and will, and action, freedom is psychologically complex and permeated with anxiety" (Yalom, 2002, p. 141). The total dependence of the infant and the parent's absolute self-responsibility from now on accentuates the loss of the freedom and spontaneity that previously characterized the parents' lives. From now on, their lives will be determined by the child who is utterly dependent on them.
3. *Existential isolation*—i.e., fundamental isolation from other people and from the world. "No matter how close each of us becomes to another, there remains a

final unbridgeable gap; each of us enters existence alone and must depart from it alone. The existential conflict is thus, the tension between our awareness of our absolute isolation and our wish to be part of a larger whole" (Yalom, 1980, p. 9). Childbirth is a powerful experience that calls attention to the existential isolation of new parents, who will never regain what they once had. This experience remains with them, constantly requiring them to trade their previous personal and social frames of reference for new ones that typify young parents.

4. *Meaninglessness*—If we are destined to die and, in the final analysis, we are alone in the world, what meaning is there to life? Is it possible under the given existential conditions to create meaning? Such questions generate a conflict between the search for meaning and the recognition that we live in a universe that has no meaning.

> An existential position holds that the world is contingent—that is, everything that is could as well have been otherwise; that human beings constitute themselves, their world, and their situation within that world; that there exists no "meaning," no grand design in the universe, no guidelines for living other than those the individual creates. The problem, then, in most rudimentary form is, How does a being who needs meaning find meaning in a universe that has no meaning? (Yalom, 1980, p. 423).

Yalom claims that, meaning in life is the outcome of an internal dialogue with the world. Many people mistakenly believe that the transition to parenthood, that is, the creation of a new human being, will fill their lives with meaning. In practice, however, what they feel is meaninglessness. In and of itself, creating life does not impart meaning. What does is the parent's ability to conduct an existential dialogue on the experience.

An additional difference between existential and Freudian dynamics lies in the question of how deeply the therapist delves in attempting to identify the patient's conflicts (Freud, 1914). Freud described the child as a being that develops through coping with psychosexual phases through which the psychic apparatus is constructed: id, ego, and superego. Each developmental stage is built on the achievements or fixations of previous stages. According to this approach, the therapist could be said to conduct an archaeological excavation in an attempt to reach down to the most ultimate conflicts. Since the existentialist dynamic does not uphold the developmental model, an in-depth probe into a basic concern does not necessarily investigate a person's past, but rather examines the relationship between the individual and the space around them. The past is important only insofar as it impacts daily existence and helps or hinders the grappling with existential concerns.

Existentialist theoreticians (Binswanger, 1963; van Deurzen, 1984; Yalom, 1980) relate to the manner in which the ultimate concerns in life, and in the clinic, are seen through four existential dimensions. Each dimension brings the person face to face with both their aspirations and their fears.

1. *The physical dimension*—i.e., the material world and the individual's attitude toward the constraints and challenges that this dimension poses. The existential aspiration in this dimension is survival: the achievement of existential security.

2. *The social dimension*—that is, the attitude toward others living side by side with the individual, and the public domain in which social norms, social conventions, and interpersonal dynamics impact behavior and worldview. The individual oscillates between the desire to be accepted and the fear of rejection and isolation. Their relationships with others always swing between those stemming from power (a healthy motive) and those deriving from the need to control others (an unhealthy motive).
3. *The psychological dimension*—or the individual's attitude toward themselves as delineated through internal reflection. A person fluctuates between a crystallized identity and self-confusion.
4. *The spiritual dimension*—i.e., the individual's attitude to the beliefs, concepts, values, and principles underlying their life. This dimension represents the individual's general world image, which largely determines the perception of the quality of the other dimensions and the meaning of life. A person vacillates between existential meaning and existential emptiness, the aspiration being to adopt an all-encompassing worldview that will help them understand a strange and alienated world.

Existentialist therapy relates to features in the particular individual's personality and environment, the way in which they influence their level of anxiety, and the defence mechanisms they employ to cope with existential concerns. While some of these defence mechanisms are traditional, such as suppression or denial, unique mechanisms can also be used to cope with existentialist experiences, ultimate rescuer defense is less effective than the belief in personal specialness.

For example, a defence mechanism that appears in response to the concern about the finality of life, or one defined as the person's belief in his specialness and his "protection from harm" (Yalom, 2008, p. 5). According to Yalom (1980), another of these unique mechanisms is the protection of the "ultimate rescuer" (p. 129). Here people depend on others being potential saviors, particularly because of their belief that they are controlled by external forces. Dependence on others leads to a feeling of powerlessness and low self-efficacy. In cases of meaninglessness or a sense of existential isolation, some people choose the defence of merging with a strong figure or another entity (group, goal, or project). As they are using others in order to feel less anxious, the relationships that develop are not genuine. A final common mechanism used against a sense of responsibility is to temporarily opt for loss of control. People may behave irresponsibly, even toward themselves, and may even develop compulsive behavior as a defence against the need to assume responsibility. Yalom claims that a full caring relationship while conducting therapy includes the following components: "transference, parataxic distortions, ulterior motives and goals—all must be swept away before an authentic relationship with another can prevail" (Yalom, 1980, p. 381).

14.4 Identification of Ultimate Concerns

A major question is how can the nature of ultimate concerns be uncovered? According to Yalom: "out of the depth of the relationship", the therapist "helps the patient to face isolation and to apprehend his solitary responsibility for his own life—that is the patient who has created his life predicament and that, alas, it is the patient and no one else, and who can alter it". (Yalom, 1980, p. 406).

The conditions for a successful therapeutic process are simple: isolation, quiet, time, and detachment from daily disturbances. If we can arrive at the root of our own being, we will be able to confront the existential facts of life. This process of deep inner contemplation is frequently accelerated by immediate experiences or "border situations," such as coming face to face with death, dealing with fateful and irreversible decisions, or the collapse of the basic psychic scheme of things that impart meaning.

14.5 Transition to Parenthood as an Existential Experience

The transition to parenthood can be perceived as a seminal experience. The decision to become a parent is generally a conscious one, but from the moment we make the transition to parenthood we have to cope with an irreversible reality that inherently contains, alongside the joy, a sense of loss—loss of one's former shape, loss of previous relationships, loss of free time, and so on. The transition to parenthood also entails a loss of former identities. For example, the new mother goes from being the "daughter of" or the "wife of" to being the "mother of." She now belongs to a group of mothers of babies that expands to additional groups as life progresses (Taubman – Ben-Ari et al., 2009). It is not surprising, therefore, that in "Hate in the Countertransference," Winnicott (1949) lists a total of 16 reasons why mothers feel hatred toward their babies, even to the point where they harbor thoughts of murder.

The past decades have seen recognition of the fact that while the transition to parenthood generally awakens feelings of satisfaction and joy, it can also be a source of stress (Keizer, Dykstra & Poortman, 2010). By its very nature, this life event is accompanied by profound changes in the parents' relationship with each other (Cowan & Cowan, 1992) as well as changes in the social (Claxton & Perry-Jenkins, 2008) and occupational domains (Hynes & Clarkberg, 2005). In the past, research focused on the way this stress can lead to mental suffering. In recent years, however, the understanding that stress can also lead to feelings of contentment, joy, and meaning in life (Taubman – Ben-Ari et al., 2012) has been gaining ground.

To the best of our knowledge, this understanding, based on empirical findings, has yet to be translated into an existentialist intervention model that reflects the questions evoked in men and women in the wake of the transition to parenthood. To fill this gap, we propose a cyclical model of psycho-existentialist attentiveness that comprises the following stages:

1. The therapist listens to the ultimate concerns raised by the client through their narrative.
2. The therapist allows the client's narrative to resonate profoundly in their mind in order to attain a deep psycho-existentialist understanding of the discourse.
3. The therapist constructs an intervention that is as appropriate as possible in view of the basic concerns reflected in the client's narrative.

14.6 Stages of the Therapist-Client Encounter

14.6.1 Stage 1: First Encounter—Listening to the Client's Ultimate Concerns

The client talks to the therapist about their emotional experience using free association, and the therapist allows the way the client narrates the experience of basic concerns to resonate in their mind. "The way the client narrates the experience" refers to all the different means of expression employed, including verbal and nonverbal, such as body language, facial expression, and intonation. In respect to the therapist, "allows…the experience…to resonate in their mind" refers to the primary process from the existentialist standpoint, as described by Winnicott (1956) in "Primary Maternal Preoccupation." This process takes place during the early stages of the therapeutic encounter, when the therapy has not yet evolved into something concrete and the therapist-client dyad has not yet been formed. It begins with the client contacting the therapist, continues with the first meeting with the therapist at the clinic door, and proceeds with the client sitting on the couch and narrating their experiences in their own unique way. It is important to remember that this initial stage is critical. When a therapist meets a client for the first time, they do not know which emotional layer has been damaged and are unfamiliar with its particular features. Unlike purely medical treatment, where a practitioner seeks to determine an optimal medical protocol by deciding which system is damaged, in the case of emotional injury, diagnosis must not only determine which system, or dimension, has been damaged, but also what existential defence strategy the client has used to avoid feeling the festering wound inside. Thus, the therapist must be prepared to open up all areas of their own symbolic and regressive emotional space in order to fully take in the client's experience before trying to diagnose it.

14.6.2 Stage 2: Allowing the Client's Regressive Area to Resonate Profoundly in the Mind in Order to Obtain a Deep Existentialist-Dynamic Understanding of the Discourse

The therapist needs to be patient and wait until they can identify which psycho-geographical dimensions in the client have been harmed (physical, social, psychological, spiritual). In the words of Bollas (1987), "I found that the effort to discover where I am, what I am, who I am, how I should function, and in which of the client's psycho-developmental periods I was living, took months, if not years. The ability to tolerate and value this necessary uncertainty defines one of our most important clinical duties toward our client" (p. 278). Here, Bollas is talking about countertransference revelations and stressing the need for therapists not just to identify which psycho-developmental dimension is involved, but to actually *spend time* there. Thus, the second stage is marked by two elements: identifying the dimension in which the damage has occurred and actually entering that dimension by enabling the client's basic concerns to resonate in the mind. This resonance is critical, as it allows the therapist to decide whether to orient the intervention toward the client's verbal-oedipal regions that would employ the traditional tools at their disposal, or to construct an intervention oriented toward the non-verbal regressive dimensions, and to initially access these dimensions inside themself.

14.6.3 Stage 3: Constructing a Therapeutic Intervention

At this stage, the therapist has worked out in which psycho-existential dimension they are with the client and can plan an appropriate intervention. This requires that the therapist connect with their own areas of basic concerns and develop an intervention by reflecting on them. In other words, we might think of the therapist and client as travellers journeying down an unmarked road together without necessarily "thinking" or "speaking." All they have to help them navigate the road is a primitive road map that uses psycho-biological signs. As they proceed, the client communicates and the therapist absorbs, utilizing the subjective tools at their disposal to plan the treatment. Like a mother caring for an infant in what Winnicott (1960) calls the stage of "absolute dependence," the therapist knows that the unmarked road is followed by an easier road where there are words and thoughts. But the unmarked road must be travelled first in order to reach it.

The transition from the pre-verbal to the verbal stage occurs when the therapist creatively works through thoughts that the client is unable to articulate and presents them to the client for the first time in their new guise. This can only happen after the therapist and client have spent a long time on the unmarked psychological road, and have gotten to know each other as they traverse this difficult terrain. Along the way, they approach the edges of the unfamiliar existential region, move back, move closer again, and move further away. They will only be able to talk about the difficulties of spending time in this region and the special tools they will need for the treatment to succeed after they have deciphered the contents of the region together. As they amass one sign after another, they start to put a name to the region that was previously "nameless and formless" (Winnicott, 1971). The therapist's creative translation allows clients to engage in dialogue with their basic concerns and the extreme zones they inhabit, and to feel the pain they cause without fleeing from it. They now know they are not alone in the torture chamber of their mind. This three-stage process is illustrated below by two clinical Vignettes.

14.7 Vignette 1: Alma

Alma (29) has been married for three years and is in the seventh month of her first pregnancy. She is a high school teacher. Her mother died a year ago following a prolonged battle with cancer. After a period of intense sadness over the loss, Alma decided she wanted a child. In the first months of her pregnancy she was elated, but on reaching her seventh month she started feeling sad again. She began to distance herself from her partner, David, and her friends, and requested early maternity leave from her teaching job in order to "gear up" for the event. It was at this stage that she came for therapy.

Alma enters the room, and, despite her large stomach, curls up into a fetal position on the sofa.

The therapist registers a sense of childhood distress due to the absence of containing and supportive parenting.

Alma relates in a monotone: "*My mother died a year ago. We were close. This pregnancy was supposed to fill me with meaning. In the beginning it did, but now it's nothing special. Only my body is full and ugly. I've never been so fat. I don't have the energy for David. I don't have the energy for friends. I don't have the energy for this baby that will be born soon.*"

The therapist absorbs the physical position in which Alma is sitting, her neediness, the void that has opened up with the death of her mother, and the talk of her full figure, and says: "*It sounds as though your mother filled you with a lot of strength. Now that she is gone, there is no one who can do what she did for you.*"

Alma: "*We were best friends. You can't compare it with my husband, David, or my friends.*"

Therapist: "*Your mother's absence appears to be extremely painful. You miss her presence, her support, her embrace, and her containment. Your mother responded to your existential needs the way David and your friends can never do.*"

Alma: "*I thought the baby would be the answer to those needs. I wanted so much to get pregnant. But I suddenly realized that when the baby is born I will be older, and in general I think about all my friends' children who were small and cute and now they're nothing special. What point is there if they grow up? We grow up and then we die.*"

The therapist identifies depression related to the inability to find a way to protect herself in the face of the cycle of life and its ultimate finality. She also senses Alma's vulnerability because of the inability of her friends to give her back what she lost. She says: "*Your mother's absence constitutes a reminder of our inevitable end and leads to the question: What is there to live for if in the end we all die?*"

Alma: "*True.*"

Therapist: "*I'm here to offer you support and to look after you in the journey we will take together, in the face of the awareness of the finality of life that has come into such sharp focus since your mother died. By taking this journey with me you will be able to progress to the next stage in your life — being a mother — and you be able to inject new meaning into your life.*"

Alma: "*Doesn't talking about this with me scare you?*"

The therapist interprets Alma's question as though she were saying: "Do you think you'll be up to the task? Isn't it too big for you?" She feels Alma is touching on her own basic concerns and says: "*It might be scary sometimes, but I think the things that fill my life with meaning allow me to look this fear in the eye and live with it.*"

Alma changes her position. Sitting upright she says: "*It's strange. Even though we're talking about death and the fear of death, I have a sense of relief.*"

Therapist: "*Awareness of what scares us allows us to make way for new things. In the coming months, there are many things that you will have to make way for. Together we will attempt to fertilize the ground that will enable all these things to grow.*"

14.7.1 Analysis of Vignette 1

Here, the therapist made use of the physical sensations and emotions conveyed by Alma to identify the imbalance between the various dimensions in her life and the basic concern that lay at the root of the conflict that brought her to therapy. As stated above, the transition to parenthood is itself an extreme state. In this case, it came on the heels of another extreme experience—the death of her mother—leading to a sharp inner awareness of death and the finality of life. Consequently, Alma interpreted even the new life she was creating through the experience of death prevailing inside her.

Through inner resonance of the existentialist concerns brought by the client, the therapist saw how the encounter with death led to an imbalance in several life dimensions. In the psychological dimension, Alma found it difficult to form her new identity as a mother and sensed confusion over her loss; in the social dimension, Alma wished to belong but found it hard to be part of the various relationships in her life (with her partner and friends) while she was still grieving over the tangible loss of contact with her mother. All this created an imbalance in the spiritual dimension, resulting in a sense of emptiness and meaninglessness. Based on her diagnosis, the therapist decided to emphasize the basic concern and the circumstances that aroused it. She provided space for the loss of the mother both through direct talk about the quality of the connection between her and Alma and through the verbal images she used, such as fertilizing and growing, which she registered via the patient's body positions. The support and embrace Alma received from the therapist, along with the therapist's ability to relate to her own basic concern regarding death and the finality of life, gave her the sense that there were two people in the room who harbored the same fears but had found different ways to cope with them. Thus, she began to perceive an initial sense of relief that enabled her to embark on the joint therapeutic journey.

14.8 Vignette 2: Ron

Ron (40) is married and the father of a three-month-old baby. He works in hi-tech. He arrived for consultation in a panic over the feelings that had overcome him since the birth of his daughter.

Ron: "*I got married relatively late. I had a lot of female partners and travelled all over the world. You could say I squeezed the most out of every opportunity life offered. I met my wife, who is 10 years younger than me, during one of my business trips abroad. We were together for three years before we got married. We both know how to give the other person his space, and in this sense our relationship is right for me. Soon after we got married, my wife got pregnant. Both of us wanted a child and we waited excitedly for the baby to come. But after she was born, something like two or three weeks later, I began to feel imprisoned. It was like everything revolved around feeding and changing diapers. My wife also changed. Now I feel that I made a mistake in bringing this girl into the world, and I'm really scared. I honestly feel like leaving home and flying off to India. I've come to you as a last resort. I don't know what to do.*"

The therapist discerns a profound experience of grieving and distress, making it difficult for Ron to make himself available for someone else's needs. It appears that for the first time in his life, he has to invest most of his emotional and physical resources in another (the baby). The therapist says: "*Instead of giving you a sense of stability, becoming a father has wrought havoc on you. Your inner sense of freedom to choose, to be your own master, has suffered a blow!*"

Ron: "*But why? I looked forward to this baby so much.*"

Therapist: "*You looked forward to being a father, but you didn't anticipate the sense of responsibility involved, the curtailing of personal freedom, the loss of mastery over your life. You've given yourself over entirely to seeing to someone else's needs.*"

Ron: "*Look, I bring home a good salary and the child doesn't lack for anything. I love her, but…maybe I really do need a break. There's a good reason I keep thinking about going to India. That's where I got my head together when I was young.*"

The therapist identifies an imbalance in the psychological dimension aroused by the fear of responsibility. She understands that Ron is coping with this fear by means of the defence mechanism of shirking responsibility (going to India), and says: "*The concern for your daughter's needs is very important, but it's also accompanied by losses, such as a demanding routine. And you have to adjust to a new life style that's different from what you were used to before. The situation fills you with so much fear that you're prepared to go all the way to India to escape.*" Thus, the therapist stages a direct confrontation with the basis of the new conflict in Ron's life: the conflict between the freedom to consider only his own needs, as he did before the baby, and the need to care for someone else.

Ron: "*To be honest, I tried to join an Internet forum for new fathers. But I got depressed by all the talk of things like getting up in the middle of the night, playing in the park, all sorts of things that just aren't me.*"

Here the therapist identifies the use of another defence mechanism, the attempt to belong. But it didn't work and didn't succeed in allaying Ron's concerns.

Therapist: "*This group is supposed to serve as a support system, but it just revealed the gaps between the new identity as a father that you have to forge and your true state. You're not there yet. You have to allow time and space for the pain of forgoing the life you once had and will never have again.*"

Ron: "*I don't know if I made the right decision in becoming a father.*"

Therapist: "*It's frightening to think that there are decisions we make in life that are irreversible and we have to bear responsibility for them.*"

Ron: "*Do I have any chance of coping with it?*"

Therapist: "*The very fact that you came here indicates that you want to try and take responsibility for your new situation. I suggest that the first thing we do is to try to understand what it means for you to accept responsibility and when you did it in the past.*" Further discussions with Ron considered the various choices he had made in his life and whether they involved accepting responsibility. In light of the existentialist approach, the focal point of these talks was the manner in which the previous experiences shed light on his current decision, rather than Ron's personality traits.

14.8.1 Analysis of Vignette 2

Ron came for therapy on finding that he had difficulty coping with his anxiety over the encounter with responsibility and the intense involvement with another person, as well as with profound grief over what would never be his again: the ability to think mainly of himself. He tried to escape in various ways from the burdensome responsibility that aroused existential anxiety, whether by attempting to belong to a group of other new fathers, or fantasizing about going to India. He was confused by the contradiction between the love he felt for his daughter and the fact that he chose to have a child on the one hand, and his regret at deciding to become a father and the need to give up almost all his personal freedom on the other.

The therapist understood that what Ron wished to flee from most of all was the sense of weighty responsibility that had descended upon him, and not his daughter, whom he loved. She also understood the upheaval caused by the fact that his decision to become a father was irreversible and entailed life-long responsibility. The conflict that Ron presented was confusing because it related to a new situation that was born of a conscious decision, while at the same time it seemed to describe the feelings of someone who has had things forced upon him and has been robbed of his freedom. The therapist understood that after having absolute control over his own time for forty years, the circumstances in which Ron now found himself could be frightening and even feel deterministic. Although he was clearly highly defensive in respect to the encounter with basic concerns, she felt that the fact that he came for therapy indicated that he wanted help in other subjective experiences, as well as in his first attempts at investing in others (the social dimension). Ron would seem to be at the start of a journey involving a search for new meaning that is much less narcissistic and more social in nature.

14.9 Concluding Discussion

The existentialist approach proposes a different way of looking at the various aspects of the inner reality that clients bring to the meeting with the therapist. It includes diagnosing the basic concerns the individual is confronting, and pinpointing the imbalance consequently created in the various dimensions in their life. As an extreme situation, the transition to parenthood in and of itself arouses basic concerns and creates an imbalance, since it is essentially a transition to a new routine and reality. Although this imbalance is generally temporary, in more severe cases it may require therapeutic intervention.

In this chapter we have proposed a therapeutic model based on the principles of the existentialist approach consisting of three stages: Listening to the client's narrative; allowing it to resonate profoundly in the mind in order to obtain a deep psycho-existential understanding of it; and constructing an intervention based on that regressive resonance to address the client's problem as specifically as possible. The clinical vignettes we have presented illustrate the use of the model, and show how the therapist can absorb the client's inner experience, on both the physical and emotional level, in order to diagnose their realm of conflict in the face of basic concerns, and subsequently construct a suitable intervention.

One of the interesting questions that arise in this context is why certain people are more successful than others in confronting basic concerns in the transition to parenthood. The answer may be found in recent empirical studies examining the personal growth of new parents. The findings suggest that in the face of extreme events, the factor that contributes most to a person's growth and development are their personal, personality, and environmental resources. Research reveals that those who possess a high level of such resources manage to survive the challenges that are part and parcel of stressful situations, but evidence a low level of growth. In contrast, those who embark on the journey of coping with stress with fewer resources experience greater pain, but undergo significant personal growth over time. This finding has been explained by the fact that people with fewer resources discover inherent strengths in themselves and in their environment of which they were previously unaware (Taubman – Ben-Ari et al., 2009).

In view of this understanding, this chapter can be said to highlight the role of the existentialist therapist in guiding clients with a low level of resources through the transition to parenthood. Using the model, we propose, the therapist can walk through the process hand-in-hand with the client at their own pace. In order to identify this pace, the therapist must first internalize the nature of the client's confrontation with the basic concerns in their life. This task may become increasingly complex in the coming years in light of the ongoing development of reproductive technologies. Such technologies are already posing new challenges for the existentialist clinic dealing with the transition to parenthood, among them: confronting basic concerns in pregnancies resulting from egg or sperm donations; same-sex parenthood; single parenthood, etc.

Finally, the transition to parenthood is discussed here as an extreme experience, but it is important to bear in mind that other extreme experiences may occur simultaneously. For example, the transition to grandparenthood, when a son or daughter gives birth to the first grandchild, also represents an upheaval. Awareness of these issues on the part of therapists working with first-time parents could open new channels in the clinic, as well as contribute to the process of growth and development of the client, and consequently of their whole family.

References

Aron, L. (1996). *A meeting of minds: Mutuality in psychoanalysis*. Hillsdale, NJ: The Analytic Press.

Binswanger, L. (1963). *Being-in-the-world* (J. Needleman, Trans.). New York: Basic Books.

Bollas, C. (1987). *The shadow of the object: Psychoanalysis of the unthought known* (pp. 200–236). New York: Columbia University Press.

Bonanno, G. A., Papa, A., Moskowitz, J. T., & Folkman, S. (2005). Resilience to loss in bereaved spouses, bereaved parents and bereaved gay men. *Journal of Personality and Social Psychology, 88*(5), 827–843.

Claxton, A., & Perry-Jenkins, M. (2008). No fun anymore: Leisure and marital quality across the transition to parenthood. *Journal of Marriage and Family, 70*(1), 28–43.

Cowan, C. P., & Cowan, P. G. (1992). *When partners become parents: The big life change for couples*. New York: Basic Books.

Espasa, F. P. (2004). Parent-infant psychotherapy, the transition to parenthood and parental narcissism: Implications for treatment. *Journal of Child Psychotherapy, 30*(2), 155–171.

Frankl, V. E. (1984). *Man's search for meaning: An introduction to logotherapy*. New York: Symon & Schuster.

Freud, S. (1914). *Remembering, repeating and working through*. The standard edition of the complete psychological works of Sigmund Freud (Vol. XII). London: Hogarth Press.

Hynes, K., & Clarkberg, M. (2005). Women's employment patterns during early parenthood: A group-based trajectory analysis. *Journal of Marriage and Family, 67*(1), 222–239.

Keizer, R., Dykstra, P. A., & Poortman, A. (2010). The transition to parenthood and well-being: The impact of partner status and work hour transitions. *Journal of Family Psychology, 24*(4), 429–438.

King, L. A., & Patterson, C. (2000). Reconstructing life goals after the birth of a child with Down syndrome: Finding happiness and growing. *International Journal of Rehabilitation and Health, 5*(1), 17–30.

Levasseur, O., McDermott, M. R., & Lafreniere, K. (2015). The multidimensional mortality awareness measure and model: Development and validation of a new self-report questionnaire and psychological framework. *Omega: Journal of Death and Dying, 70*(3), 317–341.
Sawyer, A., & Ayers, S. (2009). Post-traumatic growth in women after childbirth. *Psychology and Health, 24*(4), 457–471.
Seligman, M. E. P., & Csikszentmihalyi, M. (2000). Positive psychology: An introduction. *American Psychologist, 55*(1), 5–14.
Shenkman, G. (2018). The association between basic need satisfaction in relationship and personal growth among lesbian and heterosexual mothers. *Journal of Social & Personal Relationships, 35*(2), 246–262.
Steger, M., Frazier, P., Oishi, S., & Kaler, M. (2006). The meaning in life questionnaire: Assessing the presence of and search for meaning in life. *Journal of Counseling Psychology, 53*(1), 80–93.
Taubman – Ben-Ari, O., Ben Shlomo, S., & Findler, L. (2012). Personal growth and meaning in life among first-time mothers and grandmothers. *Journal of Happiness Studies, 13*(5), 801–820.
Taubman – Ben-Ari, O., Ben Shlomo, S., Sivan, E., & Dolizki, M. (2009). The transition to motherhood: A time for growth. *Journal of Social and Clinical Psychology, 28*(8), 943–970.
Taubman – Ben-Ari, O., Skvirsky, V., Bar Shua, E., & Horowitz, E. (2017). Satisfaction in life among fathers following fertility treatment. *Journal of Reproductive and Infant Psychology, 35*(4), 334–341.
Tedeschi, R. G., & Calhoun, L. G. (2004). Posttraumatic growth: Conceptual foundations and empirical evidence. *Psychological Inquiry, 15*(1), 1–19.
van Deurzen, E. (1984). Existential psychotherapy. In W. Dryden (Ed.), *Individual therapy in Britain*. London: Harper and Row.
Widows, M. R., Jacobsen, P. B., Booth-Jones, M., & Fields, K. K. (2005). Predictors of posttraumatic growth following bone marrow transplantation for cancer. *Health Psychology, 24*(3), 266–273.
Winnicott, D. W. (1949). Hate in the counter-transference. *The International Journal of Psychoanalysis, 30*, 69–74.
Winnicott, D. W. (1956). *Through pediatrics to psychoanalysis: Collected papers* (pp. 300–306). London: Karnac.
Winnicott, D. W. (1960). *The maturational processes and the facilitating environment* (pp. 37–56). London: Karnac.
Winnicott, D. W. (1971). *Playing and reality*. London: Routledge.
Yalom, I. D. (1980). *Existential psychotherapy*. New York: Basic Books.
Yalom, I. D. (2002). *The gift of therapy*. New York, NY: Harper Collins.
Yalom, I. D. (2008). *Staring at the sun*. San Francisco, CA: Jossey-Bass.

Chapter 15
Health Behavior, Health Promotion, and the Transition to Parenthood: Insights from Research in Health Psychology and Behavior Change

Martin S. Hagger and Kyra Hamilton

15.1 Introduction

The transition to parenthood represents a period of considerable change and stress, and may have adverse effects on psychological health as well as physical health (Bleidorn et al., 2016; Doss & Rhoades, 2017; Marshall, Simpson, & Rholes, 2015). Loss of sleep, increased workload, limited 'leisure' or 'down' time, restrictions on socializing with partner, and management of the balance between family, work, and social commitments may all have substantive impact on health outcomes for parents (Barimani, Vikström, Rosander, Forslund Frykedal, & Berlin, 2017). Although these demands may be mitigated later on, the initial disruptions that occur during early parenthood may lead to parents 'falling out' of health habits (Da Costa et al., 2017). In addition, parents have increased responsibilities to care for the health of their children (e.g., making sure their children eat health-promoting food, engage in physical activity, are protected from the sun) and, when their children are older,

Martin Hagger's contribution was supported by a Finnish Distinguished Professor Programme (FiDiPro) award from Business Finland.

M. S. Hagger (✉) · K. Hamilton
Health Psychology and Behavioral Medicine Research Group, Faculty of Health Sciences, School of Psychology and Speech Pathology, Curtin University, GPO Box U1987, Perth, WA 6845, Australia
e-mail: martin.hagger@curtin.edu.au

M. S. Hagger
School of Applied Psychology, Griffith University, Mt. Gravatt, QLD, Australia

Faculty of Sport and Health Sciences, University of Jyväskylä, Jyväskylä, Finland

K. Hamilton
Health and Psychology Innovations (HAPI) Lab, School of Applied Psychology, Griffith University, Mt. Gravatt, QLD, Australia
e-mail: kyra.hamilton@griffith.edu.au

O. Taubman – Ben-Ari (ed.), *Pathways and Barriers to Parenthood*,
https://doi.org/10.1007/978-3-030-24864-2_15

'socialize' them into taking up healthy habits (Hamilton, Daniels, White, Murray, & Walsh, 2011; Hamilton & White, 2011, 2012).

Strategies that enable parents to initiate and maintain health behaviors during the transition to parenthood may be important means to increase the physical and psychological health of parents (Hamilton, Cox, & White, 2012; Hamilton et al., 2011). Research into the self-regulation of health behavior (i.e., getting people to be better able to change behavior for themselves), can provide useful insight into techniques and strategies that can be used to promote better engagement in health behavior during the transition to parenthood and life as a parent in general. Researchers in the field of health psychology have applied theories of social cognition to identify the important factors that determine parents' participation in health behaviors (e.g., Hamilton, Cleary, White, & Hawkes, 2016; Hamilton, Hatzis, Kavanagh, & White, 2015; Hamilton, Kirkpatrick, Rebar, White, & Hagger, 2017). These factors include beliefs, attitudes, self-efficacy, perceived barriers, normative beliefs, and personality factors that relate to health behaviors and their lifestyle (McMillan & Conner, 2007). Based on these factors, specific techniques that may be useful in promoting self-regulation of health behavior in parents have been identified including goal setting, planning, skill building, and cue-monitoring (Hamilton & White, 2014). The effectiveness of these techniques has been shown in producing greater participation in health behaviors (e.g., physical activity, healthy eating, reduced alcohol consumption) and health outcomes including reduced stress and increased life satisfaction, psychological well-being, and quality of life (Kwasnicka, Dombrowski, White, & Sniehotta, 2016). The techniques can be utilized by practitioners interested in parent and child health in simple, low burden interventions and health messages that can promote better health behaviors in new parents. In this chapter, we (a) identify the key health issues facing adults transitioning to parenthood particularly with respect to their own health behaviors, and the need to engage in new health related behavior to maintain and promote the good health of their child; (b) review the social cognitive theories that have been applied to predict and understand health behavior in parents; and (c) identify theory-based behavior change strategies and interventions aimed at promoting behaviors that will lead to salient health outcomes of this population and their children.

15.2 Thinking Behaviorally: Promoting Health in the Transition to Parenthood

The arrival of a new born child presents considerable challenges to parents, whether that be parents transitioning into parenthood with the arrival of their first-born child or parents continuing the transition process with the arrival of additional children. During this life-stage, priorities and attention often shift from work, social, and other everyday commitments and activities to the role of caregiver, and parents are confronted with the need to find sufficient time and resources in what may be an already full agenda to care for their new child as well as care for other family members they may be responsible for (Rolle et al., 2017). This overwhelming sense of an 'ethic of care', which is especially felt by mothers (Hamilton & White, 2010c), makes it difficult, then, for parents to prioritize their own health needs over the needs of their parenting responsibilities. Taken together, the many challenges parents face during the years of establishing a young family and the shift in focus to the priority of the child and others may influence parents' interest and ability to be involved in personal health behaviors, and health behaviors previously engaged in prior to parenthood may become of lower priority and/or sacrificed to accommodate the new demands on their time (Hamilton & White, 2010c; Perales, del Pozo-Cruz, & del Pozo-Cruz, 2015). Such behavioral shifts may have also occurred prior to the birth of the child. For example, mothers will likely find that the physiological changes and demands of pregnancy make engaging in health behaviors more challenging and, as a result, may opt out of certain behaviors, often with the motive of reengaging with them postpartum (Merkx, Ausems, Bude, de Vries, & Nieuwenhuijze, 2017).

An important consideration that likely affects decisions to engage in behaviors is resource availability. Parenthood, especially in the early period of adjustment, is particularly demanding, and loss of sleep along with the demands of the new caregiving role and the need to adjust most components of the daily routine to care for the child may take a toll on energy and lead to increased perceptions of fatigue (Hamilton & White, 2010a, 2011). Parents may not feel like engaging in health behaviors that require considerable effort (e.g., exercise) and, thus, may opt to engage in habitual, easy-to-enact behaviors (e.g., television viewing) in order to free up time for rest or socializing. Furthermore, parents may want to take the time to share time with their partner or enjoy free time with their child, and may feel that their energy should be focused on these at the expense of health behaviors.

A number of behaviors important to promoting and maintaining good physical and mental health, and minimizing risk of chronic illness (e.g., regular physical activity), may decline in the transition to parenthood (Bellows-Riecken & Rhodes, 2008). Epidemiological research demonstrates that four key health behaviors, participating in regular physical activity, eating healthily, refraining from smoking, and keeping alcohol consumption within guideline levels is associated with an 11–14 year reduction in all-cause mortality (Ford, Zhao, Tsai, & Li, 2011). These behaviors should, therefore, be viewed as priorities for all adults including new parents. However, parenthood may present challenges to regular engagement in these behaviors. For example, time available for physical activity may be perceived as limited (Hamilton & White, 2011), and parents' attention to the dietary needs of the child may shift their focus from their own eating habits (Bassett-Gunter et al., 2013). In contrast, parenthood may present new opportunities to engage in health behaviors (Hamilton & White, 2010c). For example, pregnancy and the arrival of a new child may serve as a 'flashbulb' impetus for mothers and fathers, respectively, to quit smoking (Moan, Rise, & Andersen, 2005). Parents may find that catering for the new child also results in greater scrutiny of their own diet (Merkx et al., 2017), and presents a new reason to start exercising by taking their newborn for walks in a perambulator (Thompson, Vamos, & Daley, 2017).

In addition to challenges faced with engaging in behaviors to promote with own health, new parents also need to consider the adoption of behaviors that will ensure the good health of their child. These behaviors go beyond everyday caregiving behaviors aimed at maintaining current health, such as feeding, sleep, shelter, and general hygiene, but encompass behaviors that will ensure long term health and prevent illness in the future. These include single behaviors like immunization from communicable diseases such as tuberculosis, measles, mumps, and rubella (Bishop, Holden, Ogollah, Foster, & Team, 2016), extending breast feeding which has been linked to reduced obesity and metabolic syndrome in children (Ekelund et al., 2009), regular attendance to health clinics for checkups (Sawyer et al., 2016), protection from the sun (Hamilton, Kirkpatrick, Rebar, White, et al., 2017), introducing solid foods into the child's diet (Hamilton et al., 2011), eating fruit and vegetables and limiting discretionary choices (Spinks & Hamilton, 2016), limiting screen-time (Hamilton, Spinks, White, Kavanagh, & Walsh, 2016), improving physical activity (Hamilton & Schwarzer, 2017; Hamilton, Thomson, & White, 2013; Rhodes et al., 2016), and improving oral health (Van den Branden, Van den Broucke, Leroy, Declerck, & Hoppenbrouwers, 2013). In some cases, the behaviors will be prompted by usual care offered to parents after the birth of a child, as in the case of vaccination, while others require considerable deliberation and planning. Transitioning to parenthood, therefore, requires parents to identify these key behaviors and engage in sufficient planning to enact them.

15.3 Social Cognitive Theories and Health Behavior

Given the importance of parents' regular engagement in health-promoting behaviors, and their avoidance of health-compromising behaviors, to optimal personal health and the health of their child, initiatives, such as interventions, campaigns, and clinic-based advice from health professionals, aimed at to promoting health behaviors should be considered (Tully et al., 2017). Such initiatives need to be grounded in factors known to be related to the target health behavior, particularly factors are derived from social cognitive theory (Biddle, Hagger, Chatzisarantis, & Lippke, 2007). Identifying social cognitive correlates of parent health behaviors in the transition to parenthood may assist in the identification of the potentially manipulable factors that may form the targets for initiatives seeking to change behavior to promote better parent and child health (Hamilton et al., 2012; Hamilton & White, 2012). Application of theories of social cognition have been a prominent means adopted by health behavior researchers to identify antecedent factors that relate to health behavior and the processes involved.

Social cognitive theories are considered to have utility in health behavior prediction as they outline the factors relating to individuals decision-making in social contexts based on beliefs derived from previous experience and an evaluation of the outcomes and consequences of future social action (Biddle et al., 2007). Central to theories of social cognition is the assumption that individuals' behavior is eminently predictable provided the researcher has knowledge of all sets of social information, and co-occurring processes, on which individuals base their decisions. In addition, social cognitive theories assume that individuals are rational decision-makers and their decisions to act are determined by their processing of the available information on the course of action and its future outcomes (Bandura, 1986). When applying social cognitive theories to health behavior, therefore, the focus is on how individuals' beliefs about future participation in a health behavior of interest relates to their actual participation in the behavior.

A prominent approach adopted to predict and understand health behaviors across multiple contexts is the reasoned action approach, a social cognitive theory that arose from attitude-based theories and focus on the impact of belief-based judgements on future behavior (Fishbein & Ajzen, 2010). The prototypical form of the reasoned action approach is the theory of planned behavior (Ajzen, 1991). Central to the theory is the construct of intentions, a motivational construct which reflects an individual's judgement on how much they will plan and invest effort in pursuing a future behavior. For example, the stronger new parents' intention to participate in physical activity, the greater the likelihood that they will perform that behavior in future. The theory proposes that intentions are a function of three sets of belief-based constructs, attitudes, subjective norms, and perceived behavioral control. Attitudes reflect an individual's positive or negative judgement of the behavior, subjective norms reflects perceptions that the behavior is something salient others (e.g., partner/spouse, family, friends) want them to do, and perceived behavioral control reflects perceptions that the individual has the capacity to perform the behavior and to overcome barriers that may impede doing the behavior. In terms of process, intentions are proposed to *mediate* the effect of attitudes, subjective norms, and perceived behavioral control on behavior. This means that individuals with positive attitudes, subjective norms, and perceptions of control are more likely to align their future intentions with those beliefs and are, therefore, more likely to engage in the behavior in future.

Attitudes, subjective norms, and perceived behavioral control are belief-based constructs (Ajzen, 1991). According to the theory of planned behavior, these constructs serve as summary accounts of the sets of beliefs an individual holds about performing the behavior in future. One set of beliefs, summarized by the attitude construct, reflect the individual's beliefs about whether the behavior will result in certain outcomes (known as *behavioral beliefs*) and whether those outcomes are desirable or important to the individual (known as *outcome expectancies*). These beliefs, therefore, reflect whether an individual beliefs toward the behavior will lead to outcomes and how much that outcome is important to them. For example, a new parent might think that eating less added sugar might lead to less fluctuations in energy levels, an outcome they deem to be important. The identification of an expected outcome and a judgment of its importance is known as an expectancy-value model of attitudes. Similarly, an expectancy-value model of subjective norms comprises beliefs about salient referents (e.g., partner, friends; *normative beliefs*) and the extent to which one is likely to act in accordance with their views (*motivation to comply*). The same model applied to perceived behavioral control identifies beliefs about extent of control over the behavior (e.g., lack of time; *control beliefs*) and the strength or importance of that control (*perceived power*) to the individual. Together these sets of beliefs are proposed as direct measures of the attitude, subjective norms, and perceived behavioral control constructs and are said to be antecedent to these constructs. Behavioral, normative, and control beliefs toward a particular behavior are usually identified through open-ended belief elicitation from a sample of people from the target population. The beliefs provide potential target for intervention in persuasive communications aimed at changing health behavior.

The theory of planned behavior has been shown to be an important means to understand some key health behaviors in the transition to parenthood. The theory has been applied to predict and understand health behaviors during pregnancy such as physical activity (Hamilton, Fleig, Henderson, & Hagger, 2017; Rhodes et al., 2014b), smoking cessation (De Wilde et al., 2017), and healthy eating (Malek, Umberger, Makrides, & Zhou, 2017). For example, Rhodes et al. (2014b) examined the predictors of physical activity participation using the theory of planned behavior in mothers and fathers who were either expecting their first child, and those expecting their second child. They found that perceived behavioral control was much more important among mothers expecting their first child in particular. De Vivo, Hulbert, Mills, and Uphill (2016) meta-analysis of research studies applying the theory of planned behavior to predict physical activity participation during pregnancy supported theory hypotheses, but also noted a particularly strong effect for subjective norms on intentions, larger than the size of the effects for this construct usually found in studies in other populations. The authors speculated that this might indicate the importance of social support and normative information in forming intentions to physical activity during pregnancy, which is unsurprising given the likely additional needs associated with exercising when pregnant.

The theory has also been applied to parental behaviors to promote the health of their children including sun safety behavior (Hamilton, Kirkpatrick, Rebar, & Hagger, 2017; Hamilton, Kirkpatrick, Rebar, White, et al., 2017), breastfeeding (Lau et al., 2017), introducing to solids (Hamilton et al., 2011), eating fruit and vegetables and limiting discretionary choices (Spinks & Hamilton, 2016), limiting screen-time (Hamilton, Spinks, et al., 2016), improving physical activity (Hamilton & Schwarzer, 2017; Hamilton et al., 2013), improving oral health (Van den Branden et al., 2013). The research has generally lent support for the importance of all three components in predicting intentions, again with higher contributions of subjective norms relative to studies in other populations given the importance of social support and normative influences on child care. Research has also explored the role of specific beliefs in determining the key belief-based factors that relate to parental behaviors to promote child health (Hamilton, Cleary, et al., 2016; Hamilton et al., 2011; Hamilton et al., 2015; Hamilton, Kirkpatrick, Rebar, White, et al., 2017; Hamilton, Spinks, et al., 2016). In one example, Hamilton, Cleary et al. (2016) demonstrated the importance of behavioral beliefs (improve child mental well-being, decrease parental distress, promote healthy habits in child), normative beliefs (spouse/partner, friends), and control beliefs (inconvenience, lack of time) on parents' intentions and behavior to limit their young children's screen time viewing.

There has also been research on the theory-based predictors of the health behaviors of parents themselves using the theory of planned behavior (Cowie, White, & Hamilton, 2017; Hamilton et al., 2012; Hamilton & White, 2010b, 2012; Rhodes et al., 2014a). Unsurprisingly, a large proportion of the research has focused on predicting behaviors that have been shown to be correlated with chronic disease risk and associated conditions that predispose people to those risks (e.g., Hamilton & White, 2014; Moan et al., 2005; Rhodes et al., 2014a). A substantive body of research has focused on physical activity participation and healthy eating in mothers and fathers of new born children (Hamilton et al., 2012; Hamilton & White, 2010a, 2014). For example, research applying the theory of planned behaviors has demonstrated that control beliefs are particularly important predictors of physical activity participation in young mothers, and the effects of those beliefs tend to be higher in this population compared to young adults without children (Rhodes et al., 2014a). This study also identified some key barriers such as domestic duties and inclement weather as salient perceived barriers. Overall, research examining the salient behavioral and control beliefs from theory of planned behavior has suggested that interfering with other commitments, inconvenience, lack of time, and tiredness and fatigue, as prominent reasons for not participating in physical activity (Hamilton & White, 2010a, 2011).

The theory of planned behavior is not without limitations (Sniehotta, Presseau, & Araújo-Soares, 2014). One limitation is that it does not encompass all possible influences on health behavior and it has been criticized for shortfalls in its predictive capacity. Researchers have therefore augmented the theory with the aim of increasing its capability in predicting behavior. Research adopting augmented versions of the theory of planned behavior to predict the health behaviors of parents has demonstrated the importance of family norms (i.e., beliefs that a particular behavior is 'typical' and 'expected' within the individual's family) and moral norms (i.e., personal beliefs of moral obligation to perform or refuse to perform a certain behavior) and social support from key groups. For example, Hamilton and White (2012) demonstrated unique effects for family norms, friend support, and an 'active parent' identity on physical activity participation among both mothers and fathers in families with young children. These findings suggest that having an identity of being a physically active parent and general consideration of child care and, importantly, the extent of perceived support for child care, are important factors in decisions of parents to participate in health behaviors. Unsurprisingly, moral norms feature prominently in parents' decisions to engage in health-related behaviors which may have direct impact on the health of their children such as smoking (Moan et al., 2005). This is a unique health behavior as it has consequences for both the parent and the child, and given the importance of moral norms, the transition to parenthood may constitute an acute opportunity to intervene to change such behaviors. Where parents may have lacked motivation or rationale for quitting smoking to promote their own behaviors prior to parenthood, becoming a parent may present a unique opportunity to encourage parents to quit smoking. Interventions that promote parent identity along with quit smoking messages may have greater chances of success.

Additional components have also shown to have particular importance when it comes to behaviors in which new parents can participate to promote child health including role construction, moral norms, and anticipated regret. Researchers have identified these constructs as important determinants of health behaviors in behavioral contexts where individuals feel they have high social responsibility or there is strong social pressure to conform according to conventional values or norms. This is likely to be the case for new parents engaging in health behaviors to maintain the good health of their child. For example, role construction has been shown to independently predict parents' intentions for a range of child health behaviors (Hamilton, Kirkpatrick, Rebar, White, et al., 2017; Hamilton, Spinks, et al., 2016; Spinks & Hamilton, 2016). Role construction regarding parental involvement for childhood behavior is thought to be influenced by beliefs about desired child outcomes, responsibility for these outcomes, perceptions of important others, and parental behaviors related to those beliefs and expectations (Hoover-Dempsey & Sandler, 1997). In contrast to subjective norms in the theory of planned behavior, where the motivational orientation for action is derived out of significant others' approval (Ajzen, 1991), the motivational roots of role construction derives from parents' consideration of the relevant responsibilities for, and commitments toward, their child. This motivation arises from self and social affirmation of their role as a parent, which leads them to behave accordingly to fulfil these obligations and remain consistent with the standards attached to the role.

Anticipated regret is also a variable that has been introduced as a separate predictor within the theory of planned behavior. Parents' anticipation that they will regret not performing a behavior that they know might promote the health of their child is likely to have a strong influence on motivation. Recent studies have indicated that parental anticipated regret is a strong unique predictor of parents' intentions to engage in behaviors that promote child health such as breastfeeding (Shepherd, Walbey, & Lovell, 2017) and physical activity (Hamilton, Kirkpatrick, Rebar, White, et al., 2017). Together these results suggest that the decisions of parents of young children to engage in behaviors that promote the health of their child depends not just on their attitudes, subjective norms, and perceived behavioral control, but also on their beliefs related to their perceived moral and social obligations, and the extent to which they will regret not performing the behavior in the future.

A further limitation of the theory of planned behavior, and similar social cognitive theories, is the exclusive focus on reasoned, conscious processes (Ajzen, 2002; Hagger, 2017a). The theory assumes that engagement or desistence from a behavior is the result of a decision-making process involving conscious deliberation over the merits and detriments of the course of action. However, contemporary theoretical approaches in psychology recognize that many everyday behaviors are determined by automatic, non-conscious processes (Hagger, 2017a; Hagger & Chatzisarantis, 2014; Strack & Deutsch, 2004). Such behavioral enactment is fast, efficient, and derived from learned contingencies between action and conditions in the environment that cue up or determine the behavior. These actions may be akin to habits, which are developed over time through repeated performance of the behavior with consistent presence of cues or contexts that become inextricably linked to the action. The behavior is then enacted in a rapid, efficient way on presentation of these cues. This has given rise to 'dual process' models of behavior, in which behavior is a function of the deliberative and automatic pathways depending on factors such as experience with the behavior and the strength of the cues (Hagger & Chatzisarantis, 2014; Sheeran, Gollwitzer, & Bargh, 2013; St Quinton & Brunton, 2017).

Research examining the role of implicit processes in the context of the transition to parenthood have been relatively sparse. Hamilton, Kirkpatrick, Rebar, and Hagger's (2017) study on sun safety demonstrated the importance of habit as an independent predictor of parents' performance of sun protection behaviors for their child. The habit construct represents the 'automatic' nature of the behavior, and measures referred to the extent to which the behavior was done without thinking or conscious effort. The effects of habit were also independent of intentions, which is consistent with dual process approaches to the theory given that intentions represent the more reasoned, deliberative path to action. While there have been relatively few applications of dual process approach to predict health behaviors in new parents, they offer considerable potential in enabling researchers to gain a more complete understanding of the complex processes that determine health behaviors in this population.

15.4 Theory-Based Behavior-Change Interventions

Organizations and health professionals such as public health departments, clinicians, nurses, and parent groups with an interest in promoting child and parent health have aimed to develop effective behavior change interventions that are likely to encourage health promoting behaviors in new parents. There has been considerable focus on the content, design, and development features of health behavior interventions that will maximize their effectiveness (Abraham, 2012; Leventhal, Weinman, Leventhal, & Phillips, 2008; Michie, 2008). Many past and current health behavior change interventions have been developed on a relatively ad hoc basis focusing on a rudimentary and heuristic understanding of behavior. This has led to literature of behavioral interventions that are poorly described with inconclusive findings with respect to their effectiveness and efficiency. Recent innovations in the field of behavioral medicine and implementation science have aimed to gain a clearer understanding of the components of interventions that are effective in changing behavior across contexts, and to systematize the content of behavioral interventions and their descriptions. The focus is to develop common descriptions and an evidence base informed by behavioral theory that will provide practitioners with clear guidance on the content and design of interventions that are optimally effective in changing behavior. This knowledge means practitioners can then implement their behavior change interventions with a high degree of confidence that they will attain clinically-relevant outcomes in promoting health and reducing chronic disease risk.

The content and description of behavior change interventions has been greatly facilitated by the development of taxonomies of behavior change methods or techniques (Kok et al., 2016; Michie et al., 2011). These are organized lists with definitions of the unique, irreducible components of interventions that are effective in changing behavior. The purpose of the taxonomies is to isolate the individual methods that 'do the work' in changing behavior, and provide a common set of terms to describe those methods. The methods have frequently be labelled the 'active ingredients' of behavioral interventions. The methods are unique in that they cannot be further broken down into separate methods or techniques, and each may be used individually or in conjunction with other methods to evoke behavior change in the target population. A number of taxonomies have been proposed, and the general approach has been to identify and refine the number, definitions, and content of techniques through expert consensus. The taxonomies provide investigators and practitioners with the systematic tools necessary to accurately describe behavioral interventions and develop intervention content.

The development of effective behavior change interventions entails a number of important initial considerations relating to the behavioral problem including identifying the health problem and population in need of change (e.g., low levels of physical activity in parents of new born children) and the behavior that needs to change (e.g., promoting regular participation in physical activity) (Abraham, 2012). These initial considerations are important as they require clear specification of the population of interest and the specific behavior that needs to change. The latter considerations may seem obvious, but in many cases interventionists are seldom explicit in the population they wish to target and the specific behavior, or set of behaviors, they wish to change. It is also important to specify means to assess change and the criterion against which clinically-relevant success is defined. For example, progress in smoking cessation could be defined in terms of a reduction in the frequency of smoking, such as the number of cigarettes smoked, but a complete cessation of smoking for a given period of time may be considered the outcome with clinical significance.

Once the target problem, population, and behavior have been defined, the key components of the intervention need to be considered: identification of the key change mechanisms that are responsible for a change in the target behavior, and specification of the behavior change methods that will activate the change mechanisms to evoke behavior change (Abraham, 2012; Bartholomew Eldredge et al., 2016; Hagger, 2017b). These two components will determine the content of the intervention, the processes by which the intervention is expected to change behavior, and how its effectiveness is to be evaluated. The components entail a basic process model of intervention, which is derived from behavioral theories such as the social cognitive theories identified in the previous section and research on behavior change methods of behavioral interventions. The process model identifies the mechanism by which active intervention content changes behavior by changing internal factors derived from social cognitive theories of behavior, such as those reviewed in the previous section. The basic process model is illustrated in Fig. 15.1. In the model, methods adopted in interventions are depicted as predicting a psychological mediator which, in turn, relates to participation in the behavior. The psychological mediator, therefore, serves as an intermediary between the intervention and behavior engagement and, therefore, describes *how* the intervention works; through changing the social cognitive variables that are the antecedents of health behavioral participation. Identification of the relevant psychological mediator or multiple mediators of an intervention should begin with identifying the key theoretical constructs that have been

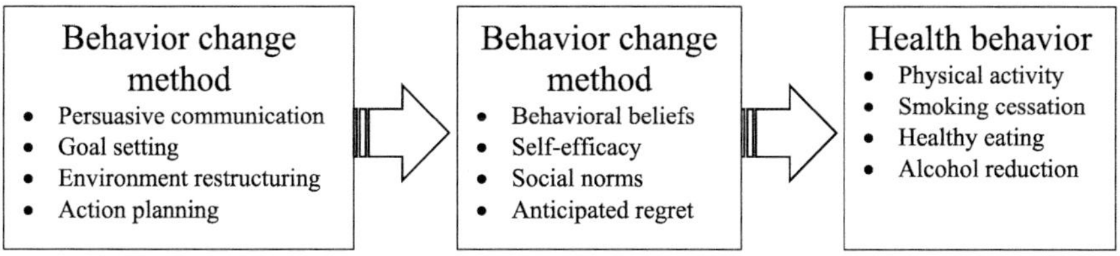

Fig. 15.1 Basic process model of the effects of behavior change methods from behavioral interventions on health behavior change mediated by social cognitive constructs

previously identified as antecedents of the behavior of interest in formative research. For example, parents' intentions to apply sunscreen to their child immediately prior to sun exposure may be related to their attitudes and perceptions of control. These should, therefore, be matched or 'mapped' on to the relevant behavior change methods (Abraham, 2012; Kok et al., 2016). This mapping process is an important step in the development of theory-based behavior change interventions because it provides an explicit link between the content of the intervention and the mechanism by which the content is expected to evoke a change in behavior.

Based on this systematic approach, the starting point for behavior change interventions to promote health behaviors in parents, and to promote parents adopting behaviors to promote the health of their children, should be the identification of the constructs that should be the targets of behavior change methods. Behavior change methods from taxonomies that are theoretically related to changing the target constructs can then be identified and form the content of future interventions. Although there are many behavior change methods—a recent taxonomy, for example, identified 93 unique methods—some methods are closely aligned with theoretical constructs, have a stronger evidence base for their effectiveness, and more widely used than others (Michie et al., 2013). For example, there are groups or clusters of change methods that relate to particular theoretical constructs. Abraham (2012) and others (Bartholomew Eldredge et al., 2016; Kok et al., 2016) have classified change methods according to the theoretical constructs they target. These include methods for changing personal beliefs (instrumental attitudes), risk perceptions, and feelings (affective attitudes), and normative beliefs (social norms), motivation, and self-efficacy. Methods to change personal beliefs, risk perceptions, and feelings generally rely on provision of information and persuasive communication regarding the behavior of interest, and the possible positive or negative outcomes. For example, positive attitudes toward a behavior can be enhanced by providing information on the benefits of doing the behavior and downplaying or discrediting beliefs about negative aspects or costs; and risk perceptions such as beliefs about susceptibility of an illness and linking it to a behavior such as promoting medication adherence through persuasive communications highlighting the health risks of not taking the medication. Social norms can be enhanced using methods such as providing examples of salient groups to which the individual belongs and what is normally done in those groups, or by providing group-level feedback on behavior. Self-efficacy can be promoted using methods that provide successful experience with the behavior, prompting goal setting, providing positive feedback of successful performance of the behavior, and motivation can be enhanced by setting personally-relevant goals and incentivizing performance of the behavior. Most of these methods is expected to enhance motivation, but certain forms of motivation, such as intrinsic motivation, can be enhanced using autonomy supportive techniques such as providing rationale, acknowledging conflict, and providing choice (Hagger & Chatzisarantis, 2015).

Behavioral interventions aimed at promoting health behavior in new parents have targeted change in behavioral beliefs and attitudes (e.g., Beardslee, Wright, Rothberg, Salt, & Versage, 1996; Massey, Decety, Wisner, & Wakschlag, 2017). The interventions are often based on social cognitive theories like the theory of planned behavior in which beliefs feature prominently as a predictor of behavior. The interventions aim to change attitudes and beliefs so that they are more positive or favorable toward a particular course of action, such as participating in physical activity or quitting smoking over a given time period and in a given context use persuasive communications that 'present a case' for the health behavior to the population of interest (Johnson, Wolf, & Maio, 2017). Importantly, the messages should serve to emphasize the positive, adaptive outcomes and advantages for performing the behavior, and allay the negative, maladaptive consequences regarding the behavior in accordance with the specific behavioral beliefs identified for that population. For example, research examining parents' beliefs on performing sun safety behaviors for their children cited "provide peace of mind", "lack of accessibility", and "having a rule in place" as important advantages of the behavior (Hamilton, Kirkpatrick, Rebar, White, et al., 2017). The content of the persuasive communication should, therefore, highlight that performing these behaviors will provide parents with peace of mind regarding the child's protection from the sun, and should emphasize the importance of having a rule about protective behaviors and being in the sun (e.g., "no hat, no sun") and make sure that access to sun safety precautions is always available (e.g., hat/bonnet, sunscreen, umbrellas). In another example, research examining parents' beliefs for their own physical activity behavior cited "improve my parenting practices" and "interfere with my other commitments" as important advantages and disadvantages, respectively of the behavior (Hamilton & White, 2011). Persuasive communication to improve parents' physical activity performance could, therefore, focus on health messages that portray parents as being more tolerant with their children after going for a brisk walk and that interfering with other commitments is not a necessary outcome of regular physical activity, such as providing parents with suggestions of how they can obtain required levels of physical activity that fit within their daily routines (e.g., engaging in more moderately active play with their children, doing house work more vigorously). In summary, health behavior interventions aimed at changing the attitudes and beliefs of new parents should be based on formative research on population- and behavior-specific beliefs matched with behavior change strategies that present the case for the behavior. These should be embedded in persuasive communications using the appropriate delivery method in contexts where new parents are likely to receive the messages.

A further behavior change method that likely impacts motivation through beliefs is goal setting. Theories of goal setting indicate that motivation to engage in a particular behavior can be promoted by emphasizing or highlighting outcomes or goals that are meaningful to the actor. Highlighting meaningful, attractive goals will likely stimulate positive beliefs with respect to engaging in the behavior in future. Research and theory on goal setting suggest that the features and content of goals are important to promoting motivation, and goals are more likely to be pursued if they are consistent with some key features. Promoting setting of appropriate goals that are interesting and engaging, realistic, optimally challenging, measurable, and timed, will likely lead individuals to align their sets of beliefs to be consistent with attaining the goal. For example, *Baby Steps* (Hamilton, Kavanagh, et al., 2016) is a modular, self-paced program designed to provide infant care and wellbeing information and tools relevant for mothers and fathers during late pregnancy until their infant is around 6 months of age. One specific element to the experimental condition, the *Wellbeing Program*, is that participants can choose tips to send to the *My Plans* tool, which functions as a goal-setting, problem-solving, and behavioral activation tool. Participants are encouraged to develop plans to incorporate the chosen tips into their life including setting a specific date and time when the plan will be attempted, or a regular frequency at which they will complete the plan. For example, a participant using the *Self Care* module could select the *Talk to someone about what's stressing you* tip, and choose to develop a plan to *Book an appointment with my General Practitioner* and to complete the plan on a self-selected date. Participants are able to monitor, review, and update their plans throughout their use of the program, and can mark plans as completed.

The promotion of change in self-efficacy is also a viable target for interventions aimed at promoting the health behaviors in parents. Self-efficacy, a construct reflecting individuals specific self-confidence in engaging in a particular behavior and closely aligned with perceived behavioral control (Bandura, 1986), can be promoted using a number of different behavior change methods including providing experiences of success, modeling the behavior, mental imagery, and self-monitoring. Self-efficacy is promoted through adaptive, positive experiences with behavior, consistent with the premise from social learning theory that individuals' confidence and motivation for behaviors is learned through experience and observation, which can be direct (e.g., experiencing success with the behavior) or indirect (e.g., watching others' successful participation). Behavior interventions can capitalize on this process by providing guidance on how to engage in the behavior successful through role models, providing feedback on successful performance, prompting individuals to visualize successful participation, and providing opportunities to monitor progress. These strategies promote greater motivation or intentions to participate in the behavior in the future by promoting greater confidence that future performances will be met with success. For example, interventions that have manipulated mastery experience (i.e., prompting successful behavior practice) and vicarious experience (i.e., observing a model performing the behavior) have been shown to produce high levels of self-efficacy, as has providing feedback on past or others' performance (Ashford, Edmunds, & French, 2010; Luszczynska & Schwarzer, 2003).

Given the proliferation of dual process theories and, in particular, the pervasive effects of non-conscious, automatic processes in determining health behavior for many behaviors and across multiple populations (Hagger, 2017a; Hagger, Trost,

Keech, Chan, & Hamilton, 2017; Strack & Deutsch, 2004), testing effects of interventions informed by automatic processes may have important implications for behavior change in health domains. When behaviors are determined by social cognitive factors like attitudes and self-efficacy, numerous strategies exist that have been shown to affect behavior change through change in these factors (e.g., attitude change through persuasive communication, self-efficacy change through goal setting). However, such strategies may not be effective when behavior is determined by cognitive processes. For example, new parents attempting to follow a healthy diet may fall back on their habitual eating patterns that have been well-learned, reinforced over time, and are easy to execute. It takes considerable cognitive effort to alter behavior patterns, and, in particular, suppress the well-learned behavioral patterns.

Behavioral scientists have therefore advocated environmental restructuring, cue-monitoring, and action planning as possible strategies to manage habitual behavior (Hagger et al., 2016; Verhoeven, Adriaanse, de Vet, Fennis, & de Ridder, 2014). Cue monitoring requires the individual to identify the potential cues or prompts that instigate an unwanted behavior and to increase vigilance for situations when the unwanted cue arises. For example, a father trying to quit smoking would identify the situations where he typically smokes and maintain vigilance when those cues arise. Diaries and other monitoring devices can assist in this regard. The goal is for the individual to be consciously aware of the cue and when it occurs rather than the cue appearing unnoticed, a scenario carries with it a high probability that the behavior will be enacted. Once the individual has identified the cue, strategies can be developed to manage them and create alternative courses of action. Environmental restructuring involves changing the environment to reduce or eliminate the potential for cues to initiate an unwanted behavior. Identifying the context or cue that initiates an unwanted behavior is an important first step. For example, for many new parents having unhealthy, 'junk' food available in the household serves as a cue to snacking and eating unhealthily. Ensuring that those foods are not available in the household and replacing them with healthier choices is a simple restructuring activity that removes the cue. Action planning involves developing a plan for an alternative course of action when the cue for the unwanted behavior is presented. Specifying an action plan requires an individual to specify an alternative course of action, when it will be enacted, where it will be performed, and how the individual will perform it. For example, a mother trying to cut down on her alcohol intake may have identified being offered another alcoholic drink by her friend when paying her a house visit or meeting her in a restaurant as a cue. Her action plan might specify refusing the drink in the social situation (when and where) by saying that she is trying to increase her fluid intake and will take a thirst quenching alternative (how). Research has suggested that specification of such plans may lead to the alternative being sufficiently accessible to bypass the well-learned unwanted cued-up by the situation when making decisions (Adriaanse, Gollwitzer, De Ridder, de Wit, & Kroese, 2011). Together these strategies can be implemented to assist parents break the routine afforded by their automatic, well-learned habitual behaviors in favor of healthier alternatives.

15.5 Summary and Conclusion

The transition to parenthood is an exciting new phase in the life of mothers and fathers. It also presents considerable challenges, particularly when it comes to behavioral health promotion and illness prevention. Parents have new responsibilities to engage in health behaviors that will promote the health of the new infant. They also find participating in behaviors that will promote their own health more challenging. We have reviewed research applying social cognitive theories to identify the factors relating to parental health behaviors to promote the health of their child and their own health. Research has identified attitudes, subjective norms, and perceived control and self-efficacy as important behavioral determinants. Research has also identified role construction, group norms, moral norms, and anticipated regret as key factors that motivate new parents to engage in behaviors that promote health in their child. Social factors, such as social support and normative information, are also of particular important to parents for their own behavior. We have also provided a review of how the formative research adopting social cognitive theories can inform behavior change interventions, and the relevant procedures necessary to develop those interventions. Specifically, we outlined the key stages in the process of intervention development including identification of the target behavior and population, the mechanisms that will likely lead to behavior change (e.g., the psychological factors involved), and the behavior change methods that target these mechanisms to bring about change in the behavior, and can be included in behavioral interventions. We have provided examples of the key strategies that might be used to promote health behaviors in new parents including persuasive communications, goal setting, environmental restructuring, cue-monitoring, and action planning. Although this is not a comprehensive overview of the kinds of strategies that may be used in behavior interventions in the transition to parenthood, it provides significant examples of the importance of utilizing evidence from behavioral science to design interventions that use methods that will be optimally effective in promoting the health behavior in parents and children during the transition to parenthood.

References

Abraham, C. (2012). Mapping change mechanisms onto behaviour change techniques: A systematic approach to promoting behaviour change through text. In C. Abraham & M. Kools (Eds.), *Writing health communication: An evidence based guide* (pp. 99–116). Thousand Oaks, CA: Sage.

Adriaanse, M. A., Gollwitzer, P. M., De Ridder, D. T. D., de Wit, J. B. F., & Kroese, F. M. (2011). Breaking habits with implementation intentions: A test of underlying processes. *Personality and Social Psychology Bulletin, 37*(4), 502–513.

Ajzen, I. (1991). The theory of planned behavior. *Organizational Behavior and Human Decision Processes, 50*(2), 179–211.

Ajzen, I. (2002). Residual effects of past on later behavior: Habituation and reasoned action perspectives. *Personality and Social Psychology Review, 6*(2), 107–122.

Ashford, S., Edmunds, J., & French, D. P. (2010). What is the best way to change self-efficacy to promote lifestyle and recreational physical activity? A systematic review with meta-analysis. *British Journal of Health Psychology, 15,* 265–288.

Bandura, A. (1986). *Social foundations of thought and action: A social-cognitive theory*. Englewood Cliffs, NJ: Prentice-Hall.

Barimani, M., Vikström, A., Rosander, M., Forslund Frykedal, K., & Berlin, A. (2017). Facilitating and inhibiting factors in transition to parenthood—Ways in which health professionals can support parents. *Scandinavian Journal of Caring Sciences, 31*(3), 537–546.

Bartholomew Eldredge, L. K., Markham, C. M., Ruiter, R. A. C., Fernández, M. E., Parcel, G. S., & Kok, G. (2016). *Planning health promotion programs: An intervention mapping approach* (4th ed.). San Francisco, CA: Jossey-Bass.

Bassett-Gunter, R. L., Levy-Milne, R., Naylor, P. J., Downs, D. S., Benoit, C., Warburton, D. E. R., et al. (2013). Oh baby! Motivation for healthy eating during parenthood transitions: A longitudinal examination with a theory of planned behavior perspective. *International Journal of Behavioral Nutrition and Physical Activity, 10,* 11.

Beardslee, W. R., Wright, E., Rothberg, P. C., Salt, P., & Versage, E. (1996). Response of families to two preventive intervention strategies: Long-term differences in behavior and attitude change. *Journal of the American Academy of Child and Adolescent Psychiatry, 35*(6), 774–782.

Bellows-Riecken, K. H., & Rhodes, R. E. (2008). A birth of inactivity? A review of physical activity and parenthood. *Preventive Medicine, 46,* 99–110.

Biddle, S. J. H., Hagger, M. S., Chatzisarantis, N. L. D., & Lippke, S. (2007). Theoretical frameworks in exercise psychology. In G. Tenenbaum & R. C. Eklund (Eds.), *Handbook of sport psychology* (3rd ed., pp. 537–559). New York, NY: Wiley.

Bishop, A., Holden, M. A., Ogollah, R. O., Foster, N. E., & Team, E. B. S. (2016). Current management of pregnancy-related low back pain: a national cross-sectional survey of UK physiotherapists. *Physiotherapy, 102*(1), 78–85.

Bleidorn, W., Buyukcan-Tetik, A., Schwaba, T., van Scheppingen, M. A., Denissen, J. J. A., & Finkenauer, C. (2016). Stability and change in self-esteem during the transition to parenthood. *Social Psychological and Personality Science, 7*(6), 560–569.

Cowie, E., White, K. M., & Hamilton, K. (2017). Physical activity and parents of very young children: The role of beliefs and social-cognitive factors. *British Journal of Health Psychology*. Advance Online Publication.

Da Costa, D., Zelkowitz, P., Letourneau, N., Howlett, A., Dennis, C.-L., Russell, B., et al. (2017). HealthyDads.ca: What do men want in a website designed to promote emotional wellness and healthy behaviors during the transition to parenthood? *Journal of Medical Internet Research, 19*(10), e325.

De Vivo, M., Hulbert, S., Mills, H., & Uphill, M. (2016). Examining exercise intention and behaviour during pregnancy using the theory of planned behaviour: A meta-analysis. *Journal of Reproductive and Infant Psychology, 34*(2), 122–138.

De Wilde, K., Maes, L., Boudrez, H., Tency, I., Temmerman, M., & Clays, E. (2017). Analysis of smoking cessation beliefs in pregnant smokers and ex-smokers using the Theory of Planned Behavior. *Journal of Public Health-Heidelberg, 25*(3), 267–274.

Doss, B. D., & Rhoades, G. K. (2017). The transition to parenthood: Impact on couples' romantic relationships. *Current Opinion in Psychology, 13,* 25–28.

Ekelund, U., Anderssen, S., Andersen, L. B., Riddoch, C. J., Sardinha, L. B., Luan, J., et al. (2009). Prevalence and correlates of the metabolic syndrome in a population-based sample of European youth. *American Journal of Clinical Nutrition, 89*(1), 90–96.

Fishbein, M., & Ajzen, I. (2010). *Predicting and changing behavior: The reasoned action approach*. New York, NY: Psychology Press.

Ford, E. S., Zhao, G. X., Tsai, J., & Li, C. Y. (2011). Low-risk lifestyle behaviors and all-cause mortality: Findings from the national health and nutrition examination survey III mortality study. *American Journal of Public Health, 101*(10), 1922–1929.

Hagger, M. S. (2017a). Health behaviour and the reflective-impulsive model. In R. Deutsch, B. Gawronski, & W. Hoffman (Eds.), *Reflective and impulsive determinants of human behavior* (pp. 157–172). New York: Routledge.

Hagger, M. S. (2017b). The role of attitudes in physical activity. In D. Albarracín & B. T. Johnson (Eds.), *Handbook of attitudes* (2nd ed., Vol. 2). New York, NY: Psychology Press.

Hagger, M. S., & Chatzisarantis, N. L. D. (2014). An integrated behavior-change model for physical activity. *Exercise and Sport Sciences Reviews, 42*(2), 62–69.

Hagger, M. S., & Chatzisarantis, N. L. D. (2015). Self-determination theory. In M. T. Conner & P. Norman (Eds.), *Predicting and changing health behaviour: Research and practice with social cognition models* (3rd ed., pp. 107–141). Maidenhead, UK: Open University Press.

Hagger, M. S., Luszczynska, A., de Wit, J., Benyamini, Y., Burkert, S., Chamberland, P.-E., et al. (2016). Implementation intention and planning interventions in health psychology: Recommendations from the Synergy expert group for research and practice. *Psychology & Health, 31*(7), 814–839.

Hagger, M. S., Trost, N., Keech, J., Chan, D. K. C., & Hamilton, K. (2017). Predicting sugar consumption: Application of an integrated dual-process, dual-phase model. *Appetite, 116,* 147–156.

Hamilton, K., Cleary, C., White, K. M., & Hawkes, A. (2016). Keeping kids sun safe: Exploring parents' beliefs about their young child's sun-protective behaviours. *Psycho-Oncology, 25,* 158–163.

Hamilton, K., Cox, S., & White, K. M. (2012). Testing a model of physical activity among mothers and fathers of young children: Integrating self-determined motivation, planning, and theory of planned behavior. *Journal of Sport and Exercise Psychology, 34*(1), 124–145.

Hamilton, K., Daniels, L., White, K. M., Murray, N., & Walsh, A. (2011). Predicting mothers' decisions to introduce complementary feeding at 6 months: An investigation using an extended Theory of Planned Behaviour. *Appetite, 56,* 674–681.

Hamilton, K., Fleig, L., Henderson, J., & Hagger, M. S. (2017). Being active in pregnancy: Theory-based predictors of physical activity among pregnant women. *Women & Health*. Advance Online Publication.

Hamilton, K., Hatzis, D., Kavanagh, D. J., & White, K. M. (2015). Exploring parents' beliefs about their young child's physical activity and screen time behaviours. *Journal of Child and Family Studies, 24*(9), 2638–2652.

Hamilton, K., Kavanagh, D., Connolly, J., Davis, L., Fisher, J., Halford, K., et al. (2016). Baby Steps—An online program promoting the wellbeing of new mothers and fathers: A study protocol. *JMIR Research Protocols, 5*(3), e140.

Hamilton, K., Kirkpatrick, A., Rebar, A., & Hagger, M. S. (2017). Child sun safety: Application of an integrated behavior change model. *Health Psychology, 36*(9), 916–926.

Hamilton, K., Kirkpatrick, A., Rebar, A., White, K. M., & Hagger, M. S. (2017). Protecting young children against skin cancer: Parental beliefs, roles, and regret. *Psycho-Oncology, 26*(12), 2135–2141.

Hamilton, K., & Schwarzer, R. (2017). Making plans to facilitate young children's physical activity: The role of psycho-social mediators and moderators. *Journal of Child and Family Studies*. Advance Online Publication.

Hamilton, K., Spinks, T., White, K. M., Kavanagh, D. J., & Walsh, A. M. (2016). A psychosocial analysis of parents' decisions for limiting their young child's screen time: An examination of attitudes, social norms and roles, and control perceptions. *British Journal of Health Psychology, 21*(2), 285–301.

Hamilton, K., Thomson, C. E., & White, K. M. (2013). Promoting active lifestyles in young children: Investigating mothers' decisions about their child's physical activity and screen time behaviours. *Maternal and Child Health Journal, 17*(5), 968–976.

Hamilton, K., & White, K. M. (2010a). Identifying parents' perceptions about physical activity: A qualitative exploration of salient behavioural, normative and control beliefs among mothers and fathers of young children. *Journal of Health Psychology, 15*(8), 1157–1169.

Hamilton, K., & White, K. M. (2010b). Parental physical activity: Exploring the role of social support. *American Journal of Health Behavior, 34*(5), 573–584.
Hamilton, K., & White, K. M. (2010c). Understanding parental physical activity: Meanings, habits, and social role influence. *Psychology of Sport and Exercise, 11,* 275–285.
Hamilton, K., & White, K. M. (2011). Identifying key belief-based targets for promoting regular physical activity among mothers and fathers with young children. *Journal of Medicine and Science in Sport, 14,* 135–142.
Hamilton, K., & White, K. M. (2012). Social influences and the physical activity intentions of parents of young-children families: An extended theory of planned behavior approach. *Journal of Family Issues, 33*(10), 1351–1372.
Hamilton, K., & White, K. M. (2014). Strategies for developing and delivering a parental physical activity intervention: Answers to the what and how. *Journal of Physical Activity & Health, 11,* 152–164.
Hoover-Dempsey, K. V., & Sandler, H. M. (1997). Why do parents become involved in their children's education? *Review of Educational Research, 67*(1), 3–42.
Johnson, B. T., Wolf, L., & Maio, G. (2017). Persuasive communication influences on attitudes. In B. T. Johnson & D. Albarracín (Eds.), *The handbook of attitudes*. New York, NY: Psychology Press.
Kok, G., Gottlieb, N. H., Peters, G.-J. Y., Mullen, P. D., Parcel, G. S., Ruiter, R. A. C., et al. (2016). A taxonomy of behavior change methods: An intervention mapping approach. *Health Psychology Review, 10*(3), 297–312.
Kwasnicka, D., Dombrowski, S. U., White, M., & Sniehotta, F. F. (2016). Theoretical explanations for maintenance of behaviour change: A systematic review of behaviour theories. *Health Psychology Review, 10*(3), 277–296.
Lau, Y., Htun, T. P., Lim, P. I., Ho-Lim, S. S. T., Chi, C., Tsai, C., et al. (2017). Breastfeeding attitude, health-related quality of life and maternal obesity among multi-ethnic pregnant women: A multi-group structural equation approach. *International Journal of Nursing Studies, 67,* 71–82.
Leventhal, H., Weinman, J., Leventhal, E. A., & Phillips, L. A. (2008). Health psychology: The search for pathways between behavior and health. *Annual Review of Psychology, 59,* 477–505.
Luszczynska, A., & Schwarzer, R. (2003). Planning and self-efficacy in the adoption and maintenance of breast self-examination: A longitudinal study on self-regulatory cognitions. *Psychology and Health, 18,* 93–108.
Malek, L., Umberger, W. J., Makrides, M., & Zhou, S. J. (2017). Predicting healthy eating intention and adherence to dietary recommendations during pregnancy in Australia using the Theory of Planned Behaviour. *Appetite, 116,* 431–441.
Marshall, E. M., Simpson, J. A., & Rholes, W. S. (2015). Personality, communication, and depressive symptoms across the transition to parenthood: A dyadic longitudinal investigation. *European Journal of Personality, 29*(2), 216–234.
Massey, S. H., Decety, J., Wisner, K. L., & Wakschlag, L. S. (2017). Specification of change mechanisms in pregnant smokers for malleable target identification: A novel approach to a tenacious public health problem. *Frontiers in Public Health, 5,* 12.
McMillan, B., & Conner, M. (2007). Health cognition assessment. In A. B. S. Ayers, C. McManus, S. Newman, K. Wallston, J. Weinman, & R. West (Eds.), *Cambridge handbook of psychology, health and medicine* (2nd ed., pp. 260–266). Cambridge, UK: Cambridge University Press.
Merkx, A., Ausems, M., Bude, L., de Vries, R., & Nieuwenhuijze, M. J. (2017). Factors affecting perceived change in physical activity in pregnancy. *Midwifery, 51,* 16–23.
Michie, S. (2008). What works and how? Designing more effective interventions needs answers to both questions. *Addiction, 103*(6), 886–887.
Michie, S., Ashford, S., Sniehotta, F. F., Dombrowski, S. U., Bishop, A., & French, D. P. (2011). A refined taxonomy of behaviour change techniques to help people change their physical activity and healthy eating behaviours: The CALO-RE taxonomy. *Psychology & Health, 26*(11), 1479–1498.
Michie, S., Richardson, M., Johnston, M., Abraham, C., Francis, J., Hardeman, W., et al. (2013). The behavior change technique taxonomy (v1) of 93 hierarchically clustered techniques: Building an

international consensus for the reporting of behavior change interventions. *Annals of Behavioral Medicine, 46*(1), 81–95.

Moan, I. S., Rise, J., & Andersen, M. (2005). Predicting parents' intentions not to smoke indoors in the presence of their children using an extended version of the theory of planned behaviour. *Psychology & Health, 20*(3), 353–371.

Perales, F., del Pozo-Cruz, J., & del Pozo-Cruz, B. (2015). Long-term dynamics in physical activity behaviour across the transition to parenthood. *International Journal of Public Health, 63*(3), 301–308.

Rhodes, R. E., Blanchard, C. M., Benoit, C., Levy-Milne, R., Naylor, P. J., Downs, D. S., et al. (2014a). Belief-level markers of physical activity among young adult couples: Comparisons across couples without children and new parents. *Psychology & Health, 29*(11), 1320–1340.

Rhodes, R. E., Blanchard, C. M., Benoit, C., Levy-Milne, R., Naylor, P. J., Downs, D. S., et al. (2014b). Social cognitive correlates of physical activity across 12 months in cohort samples of couples without children expecting their first child, and expecting their second child. *Health Psychology, 33*(8), 792–802.

Rhodes, R. E., Spence, J. C., Berry, T., Deshpande, S., Faulkner, G., Latimer-Cheung, A. E., et al. (2016). Understanding action control of parental support behavior for child physical activity. *Health Psychology, 35*(2), 131–140.

Rolle, L., Prino, L. E., Sechi, C., Vismara, L., Neri, E., Polizzi, C., et al. (2017). Parenting stress, mental health, dyadic adjustment: A structural equation model. *Frontiers in Psychology, 8,* 10.

Sawyer, M. G., Reece, C. E., Bowering, K., Jeffs, D., Sawyer, A. C. P., Peters, J. D., et al. (2016). Usage, adherence and attrition: how new mothers engage with a nurse-moderated web-based intervention to support maternal and infant health. A 9-month observational study. *Bmj Open, 6*(8), 11.

Sheeran, P., Gollwitzer, P. M., & Bargh, J. A. (2013). Nonconscious processes and health. *Health Psychology, 32*(5), 460–473.

Shepherd, L., Walbey, C., & Lovell, B. (2017). The role of social-cognitive and emotional factors on exclusive breastfeeding duration. *Journal of Human Lactation, 33*(3), 606–613.

Sniehotta, F. F., Presseau, J., & Araújo-Soares, V. (2014). Time to retire the theory of planned behaviour. *Health Psychology Review, 8*(1), 1–7.

Spinks, T., & Hamilton, K. (2016). Investigating mothers' decisions to give their 2–3 year old a nutritionally balanced diet. *Nutrition Education and Behavior, 48,* 250–257.

St Quinton, T., & Brunton, J. A. (2017). Implicit processes, self-regulation, and Interventions for behavior change. *Frontiers in Psychology, 8,* 346.

Strack, F., & Deutsch, R. (2004). Reflective and impulsive determinants of social behavior. *Personality and Social Psychology Review, 8,* 220–247.

Thompson, E. L., Vamos, C. A., & Daley, E. M. (2017). Physical activity during pregnancy and the role of theory in promoting positive behavior change: A systematic review. *Journal of Sport and Health Science, 6*(2), 198–206.

Tully, L. A., Piotrowska, P. J., Collins, D. A. J., Mairet, K. S., Black, N., Kimonis, E. R., et al. (2017). Optimising child outcomes from parenting interventions: Fathers' experiences, preferences and barriers to participation. *Bmc Public Health, 17,* 14.

Van den Branden, S., Van den Broucke, S., Leroy, R., Declerck, D., & Hoppenbrouwers, K. (2013). Measuring determinants of oral health behaviour in parents of preschool children. *Community Dental Health, 30*(1), 19–25.

Verhoeven, A. A. C., Adriaanse, M. A., de Vet, E., Fennis, B. M., & de Ridder, D. T. D. (2014). Identifying the 'if' for 'if-then' plans: Combining implementation intentions with cue-monitoring targeting unhealthy snacking behaviour. *Psychology & Health, 29*(12), 1476–1492.

Chapter 16
Blossoming and Growing in the Transition to Parenthood

Orit Taubman – Ben-Ari

16.1 Introduction

> Through the veil of fog and cloak of confusion, after three weeks of striving to talk motherhood, it's clear to me that being a mother is a complicated paradox: depression and confusion mixed with laughter and joy, satisfaction and amazement alongside frustration and disappointment, enchantment and gentleness along with anger and distress, devotion and compassion as well as fear and anxiety, weakness and helplessness together with pride and strength, a heartwarming smile and grit teeth. All of them live side by side in one soul, battling each other, clenching their fists, which pop open when a tiny hand clutches your fingers. (Women Talk Motherhood, Forum for New Mothers, http://www.medabrotimahut.co.il/2015/03)

The birth of a child, especially a first child, is considered a vulnerable period in parents' lives, a time when joy, fulfillment, and satisfaction exist side by side with distress, fears, and difficulty. Parenthood brings with it substantial challenges to personal identity, the organization of daily activity, and family structure and functioning (Arendell, 2000; Haga, Lynne, Slinning, & Kraft, 2012). This may explain why research suggests that both men and women experience a variety of affective disorders during pregnancy and the first year after childbirth (Cameron, Sedov, & Tomfohr-Madsen, 2016; Mann, Gilbody, & Adamson, 2010; Parfitt & Ayers, 2014). One of the negative implications of childbirth that has received the most attention is Post-Traumatic Stress Disorder (PTSD). A recent systematic review and meta-analysis of PTSD literature reported mean prevalence rates of 3.3% in community samples during pregnancy and a further 4% postpartum, mostly related to traumatic events during the birth (Yildiz, Ayers, & Phillips, 2017; see also Ayers and Sawyer, Chap. 12 in this volume). Prevalence is even higher in high risk samples, such as following a premature birth (e.g., Horsch et al., 2016).

O. Taubman – Ben-Ari (✉)
The Louis and Gabi Weisfeld School of Social Work, Bar Ilan University, Ramat Gan, Israel
e-mail: taubman@biu.ac.il

O. Taubman – Ben-Ari (ed.), *Pathways and Barriers to Parenthood*,
https://doi.org/10.1007/978-3-030-24864-2_16

Parental mental health in the child's early years is a significant public health concern due to the association between mental health problems and a variety of adverse outcomes for women, their partners, their relationships with their children, and the children's development, both in the short- and the long-run (Ayers, Bond, Bertullies, & Wijma, 2016; Kingston, Tough, & Whitfield, 2012; Shaw et al., 2009; Webb, Ayers, & Rosan, 2018). Consequently, considerable effort has been devoted to understanding and describing parental psychopathology (e.g., Yim, Tanner Stapleton, Guardino, Hahn-Holbrook, & Dunkel Schetter, 2015) and designing suitable interventions (e.g., Werner, Miller, Osborne, Kuzava, & Monk, 2015). Unfortunately, for decades, both researchers and practitioners focused on the costs of the transition to parenthood, and especially motherhood, endorsing a view of mental health as the absence of mental illness, rather than "a state of well-being in which every individual realizes his or her own potential, can cope with the normal stresses of life, can work productively and fruitfully, and is able to make a contribution to her or his community" (World Health Organization, 2004). As a result, psychopathology, however important it may be, is overrepresented in perinatal studies of parental mental health (Nishi & Usuda, 2017).

A change in the literature began to appear, however, with the introduction of Positive Psychology and its spotlight on positive aspects of threatening events, as well as on assets that enable certain individuals to cope effectively with difficult life events (e.g., Bassi et al., 2017). Growing interest in this approach has led to expanded research on psychological well-being (Ryff, 1989, 2014), subjective well-being (Diener, 1984, 2000), and positive outcomes such as happiness, satisfaction, and meaning in life (Steger, Frazier, Oishi, & Kaler, 2006), along with positive resources such as optimism (Carver & Scheier, 2001), hope (Snyder, 2002), resilience (Bonanno, Westphal, & Mancini, 2011), and social support (Schaefer & Moos, 1998).

Since its introduction in the 1990s, the concept of posttraumatic growth (PTG; Tedeschi & Calhoun, 1995) has attracted considerable attention. PTG was first defined as a positive psychological change experienced as the result of a struggle with highly challenging life circumstances. Although several scholars have developed tools designed to assess these changes, the posttraumatic growth inventory (PTGI; Tedeschi & Calhoun, 1996) remains the most widely used measure (Helgeson, Reynolds, & Tomich, 2006; Linley & Joseph, 2004). It comprises five factors: **Relating to Others**, referring to positive changes in interpersonal relationships, such as increased compassion, openness, or a greater sense of closeness; **New Possibilities**, experienced as the development of new paths or opportunities in life; **Personal Strength**, relating to higher self-reliance or a greater sense of personal strength; **Spiritual Change**, i.e., a better understanding of personal spirituality or stronger religious faith; and **Appreciation of Life**, or greater appreciation of the value of life. PTG is not a direct result of the trauma, but of the struggle in the aftermath of the trauma as the individual attempts to cope with their shattered assumptions about the world. These include a sense of meaning in life, belief in a fair world, an understanding of why individuals think and act the way they do, the nature of one's relationships with others, recognition of one's abilities, strengths, weaknesses, and expectations for the future, spiritual or religious beliefs, and perceptions of one's own worth as an individual (Cann et al., 2010).

Importantly, posttraumatic growth can coexist with the distress aroused by the stressful event (Calhoun & Tedeschi, 2013). Moreover, a person can experience growth in some dimensions but not in others, and not all individuals who undergo trauma experience posttraumatic growth (Beck & Watson, 2016).

Although initially developed to assess posttraumatic growth following severe trauma, such as natural disasters, life-threatening illness, or the death of a loved one (Tedeschi & Calhoun, 2004), over time research has provided considerable evidence of the PTGI's suitability for measuring the response to stress-evoking events that are less traumatic, such as romantic breakups, university studies, and as most relevant to the current discussion, developmental life events and transitions, including the transition to parenthood (Taubman – Ben-Ari, Findler, & Sharon, 2011), grandparenthood (Taubman – Ben-Ari, Ben Shlomo, & Findler, 2014), and a child's entry to first grade (Ben Shlomo & Taubman – Ben-Ari , 2017). These findings have brought about an essential change: the replacement of the term "posttraumatic growth" with "personal growth," enabling us to relate to the same phenomenon in situations that are stressful but not traumatic.

16.2 Establishing the Validity of Personal Growth Among Parents

In the process of a large scale set of studies to explore the experience of personal growth among parents (Taubman – Ben-Ari et al., 2011), we found ourselves struggling to defend the idea that personal growth actually exists in the wake of normative events, and that it is indeed experienced by parents. We therefore interviewed different groups of parents, and then more systematically, asked mothers to describe how their lives had changed since giving birth. We (Taubman – Ben-Ari et al., 2011) then conducted three studies employing three different procedures and three independent samples to examine the applicability of the PTGI to this population.

In the first study, new mothers were asked to respond to an open-ended question regarding changes in their lives following the birth of their first child. Their responses were content analyzed, and the resulting themes were compared to the PTGI dimensions. Four of the dimensions were reflected in the mothers' reports, the only exception being increased spirituality and religious faith. Hence, the PTGI appeared to provide fairly good coverage of the themes raised by the participants regarding positive changes in the wake of the transition to motherhood, suggesting its validity for use with new mothers. However, as we wished to establish the validity of the PTGI in the whole population, Study 2 compared sub-groups of mothers: new and more experienced mothers whose children were aged 4; mothers who delivered pre- and full-term babies; and mothers of twins and singletons. The participants in this more diverse sample were again asked to describe changes in their life since the birth of the child or children, and again, the themes that emerged from content analysis were compared to the five dimensions of the PTGI. In this sample, too, themes corresponding to the same four PTGI dimensions appeared in all sub-groups of mothers shortly after delivery, as well as in the reports of mothers of 4-year-olds.

Encouraged by these results, we went a step further and decided not to rely solely on self-reports. In Study 3, mothers were asked to complete the PTGI, and their mothers were asked to report on their daughters' growth. By comparing the results, we examined the convergent validity of the PTGI, a procedure previously employed in studies of trauma survivors (Shakespeare-Finch & Enders, 2008; Weiss, 2002). Moreover, by using an external source to corroborate the self-report, we believed we could achieve a more objective assessment of growth and overcome the limitations of a possible social desirability bias. What we found was that the reports of the mothers and their own mothers were significantly correlated, so that the higher the growth experienced by the mother, the greater growth reported for them by the grandmother. Not only did this study again validate the PTGI dimensions for mothers, but the procedure also provided at least an initial answer to the interesting question of whether the experience of growth in the transition to motherhood was only a personal sense, or whether it might be perceived and acknowledged by other people in the mother's environment as well.

Similar findings were obtained in a phenomenological study of 15 English-speaking women from around the world who perceived their childbirth as traumatic (Beck & Watson, 2016). Four themes indicating posttraumatic growth emerged from this study, and closely resembled the five dimensions of the PTGI.

Evidence also comes from a Canadian study on fathers of late pre-term babies (Benzies & Magill-Evans, 2015) in which 8 months postpartum, participants described fatherhood as an opportunity for growth through personal change (higher responsibility, maturity, more hopefulness, and patience) and their perception of life (expectations about the future). Furthermore, they described the transition to fatherhood as better than they had expected and reported that it had made a huge difference in their lives.

In studies assessing the prevalence of the experience of growth among mothers, between one-third and one-half of the women reported at least a moderate level of growth (Sawyer & Ayers, 2009; Sawyer, Ayers, Young, Bradley, & Smith 2012; Sawyer, Nakić Radoš, Ayers, & Burn, 2015; see also Ayers and Sawyer, Chap. 12 in this volume). As these samples were not clinical and had no specific or unique characteristics, they highlight the fact that even completely normative life events may give rise to the experience of personal growth. Moreover, they are consistent with the contention that it is the subjective experience of the event, rather than the event itself, which impels the development of growth (Linley & Joseph, 2004).

16.3 The Association Between Stress and Personal Growth Among Parents

One of the trademarks of personal growth is that it occurs in the aftermath of stress, so that a certain degree of distress is a prerequisite for growth. Two contradictory hypotheses have been derived from this principle. The first is that highly stressful events, or a higher perception of stress, would be related to more growth because such events are more likely to challenge fundamental assumptions and therefore afford a greater potential for growth (Park, 1998; Stanton, Bower, & Low, 2006). The second is that distress and growth are independent constructs that can coexist and are not necessarily correlated (Tedeschi & Calhoun, 1995, 2004).

Numerous studies of parents have tested the first hypothesis, relating either to the experience of labor itself or to particularly stressful situations, such as parenthood following fertility treatments, giving birth prematurely, or having twins (e.g., Spielman & Taubman – Ben-Ari, 2009; Taubman – Ben-Ari, Findler, & Kuint, 2010; Taubman – Ben-Ari, Skvirsky, Bar Shua, & Horowitz, 2018). In some cases, the second hypothesis has been invoked as an explanation when no correlations were found (e.g., Sawyer et al., 2012). To date, however, the literature remains inconclusive and inconsistent.

One of the first studies, conducted in the UK (Sawyer & Ayers, 2009), found no significant association between PTSD symptoms and growth following childbirth among women up to 36 months after labor. However, a further study by the same group (Sawyer et al., 2012) found that the only birth event that predicted growth among women 8 weeks after childbirth was type of delivery, with women who had undergone a caesarean section (elective or emergency) displaying higher levels of growth than those who had had a normal vaginal delivery. This finding is consistent with the view that more severe events stimulate greater growth (Park, 1998; Stanton et al., 2006). Obviously, an obstetric procedure such as a caesarean section may contribute to the stressfulness of the experience and increase the traumatic nature of the event (Olde, van der Hart, Kleber, & van Son, 2006).

Nevertheless, the same study indicated that growth was unrelated to PTSD symptomatology in the wake of childbirth, consistent with the view that distress and growth can coexist (Tedeschi & Calhoun, 1995, 2004). The main predictor of the growth of new mothers was posttraumatic stress symptoms reported during pregnancy in response to a recent stressful event. Thus, for more vulnerable women, childbirth was more likely to be perceived as a crisis, leading to higher growth after the delivery (Sawyer et al., 2012).

In yet another study that compared UK and Croatian women, depression or posttraumatic stress symptoms among UK mothers were again unrelated to growth (Sawyer et al., 2015). However, these results were not replicated in the Croatian sample, where higher levels of posttraumatic symptoms predicted higher reported growth. The authors suggest that Croatian women might have experienced posttraumatic reactions to the war they had experienced as children, which affected their well-being (Frančišković et al., 2007), and this greater level of distress precipitated growth (Sawyer et al., 2015).

A study conducted in Japan among women during pregnancy and four weeks after childbirth (Nishi & Usuda, 2017) found that women who gave birth for the first time (which the authors consider a more challenging and meaningful experience then having additional children) reported higher PTG a month after childbirth. Similarly, in a series of Israeli studies we found that giving birth to premature baby/ies (presumably a more stressful event than full-term birth) was systematically related to reports of higher personal growth. For example, in a study comparing both primiparous and multiparous mothers of premature twins to mothers with either full-term twins or single babies one year after childbirth (Taubman – Ben-Ari et al., 2010), mothers of premature twins experienced greater personal growth than the other groups. These results were replicated in a later study that added a group of mothers of premature singletons, where mothers of preterms (either single babies or twins) experienced higher personal growth than mothers of full-terms (Noy, Taubman – Ben-Ari, & Kuint, 2015).

Both mothers and fathers of premature babies also reported greater personal growth than parents of full-term babies when examined one month, six months, and two years after the birth of their first child (Porat-Zyman, Taubman – Ben-Ari, & Spielman, 2017; Spielman & Taubman – Ben-Ari, 2009; Taubman – Ben-Ari & Spielman, 2014). Importantly, only among mothers were the more intimidating objective features of the infant's condition related to sense of growth. Thus, the lower the infant's week of gestation, birthweight, and Apgar scores, the more growth the mother reported (Spielman & Taubman – Ben-Ari, 2009). Even 4 years postpartum, premature birth still contributed significantly and positively to personal growth (Taubman – Ben-Ari, Skvirsky, Strauss, & Morag, in press). In an attempt to delve deeper into the dynamic behind this finding, it was found that premature birth was associated with an increase in mental health over time, which, in turn was positively related to higher personal growth four years later (Porat-Zyman, Taubman – Ben-Ari, Kuint, & Morag, in press).

Finally, a study comparing single mothers by choice with mothers in a couple relationship up to two years following the birth of their first child found that single mothers reported greater personal growth than those in a couple relationship (Chasson & Taubman – Ben-Ari, 2019). As being a single mother, even by choice, may engender a greater sense of burden and accountability (Hertz, 2006), and may evoke criticism for the decision to raise a child without a father (Bock, 2000), it can be seen as a more stressful circumstance. Thus, again, greater stress was found to be related to a higher level of personal growth.

Two exceptions to these seemingly systematic findings concern events similarly expected to be highly stressful: undergoing fertility treatment, and giving birth to twins. However, no differences in personal growth were found between parents who conceived following fertility treatments and those who conceived spontaneously (Noy et al., 2015; Porat-Zyman et al., 2017; Taubman – Ben-Ari & Spielman, 2014; Taubman – Ben-Ari et al., 2018), and no differences in growth were evidenced in studies comparing mothers of twins and singletons (Noy et al., 2015; Taubman – Ben-Ari et al., 2010). It may be that although fertility treatments indeed arouses higher levels of stress during treatment and pregnancy (Burns, 2007; Gameiro, Moura-Ramos, Canavarro, & Soares, 2010), it does not have long-term effect on personal growth after parenthood is achieved (Hjelmstedt, Widstrom, Wramsby, & Collins, 2004). In the case of twins, although parenting twins is more demanding (e.g., Olivennes, Golombok, Ramogida, & Rust, 2005), the birth of twins has become more normative, and may no longer undermine existing conceptions (Noy et al., 2015).

Stressful circumstances are conceptualized as a sort of objective characteristic of different events. However, there may be a gap between what is considered a stressful life event and what is perceived as stressful by the individual. Theoretical models argue that subjective appraisals of stress are more important than the objective characteristics of the event or the objective indicators of stress in determining growth (Linley & Joseph, 2004; Tedeschi & Calhoun, 2004).

Several studies on the transition to parenthood have sought to specifically measure stress, rather than merely conjecturing as to which circumstances are more stressful. For example, one study of new fathers (up to 18 months following the birth) examined parenting stress and personal growth, and found a positive association between them (Taubman – Ben-Ari et al., 2018).

Another study compared mothers of preterms whose babies were medically determined to be at low risk with those whose infants were judged to be at moderate-high risk (Rozen, Taubman – Ben-Ari, Strauss, & Morag, 2018). Although mothers in the moderate-high risk group were expected to report more growth than those in the low risk group, this prediction was confirmed only on the PTGI dimension of Spirituality. This finding should be considered with caution, however, as the PTGI is a bit limited in relation to spirituality, and the concept of spirituality is particularly sensitive to cultural variability (Tedeschi, Cann, Taku, Senol-Durak, & Calhoun, 2017).

Rozen et al. also measured the level of perceived stress. Whereas no linear connection was found, a curvilinear effect (an inverse U shape curve) emerged between perceived stress shortly after the birth and personal growth at infant age of two months (corrected for prematurity), showing that women reporting moderate levels of stress experienced higher growth on four dimensions. In other words, the more the level of stress diverged from the mid-point (whether higher or lower), the less growth was reported. It is important to note that no difference was found in the mother's perceived, subjective, stress between the two groups, which were divided according to the objective, medically-defined risk to their infants. Although this may sound counterintuitive, as one might expect harsher circumstances to necessarily be more stress-arousing, it is consistent with the results of a meta-analysis showing that, in contrast to the common assumption, mothers of pre- and full-terms report only slight differences in perceived stress (Schappin, Wijnroks, Uniken Venema, & Jongmans, 2013). These differences may be even smaller when all the mothers in the sample gave birth prematurely, as was the case in this study. This finding is extremely significant, as it provides evidence that subjective stress is the product of a large number of variables, and does not derive directly from the objective severity of the event.

Consistent with the basic premise of the theory of personal growth, the curvilinear associations that emerged in the study by Rozen et al. (2018) indicate that perceived stress is more important than objective stress in generating growth (Barr, 2011; Linley & Joseph, 2004; Tedeschi & Calhoun, 2004). Furthermore, they lend credence to the contention that it is moderate levels of stress that are a significant predictor of growth, as reported by recent studies examining the curvilinear associations between perceived stress and posttraumatic stress in the context of personal growth following other traumatic events (Coroiu, Körner, Burke, Meterissian, & Sabiston, 2016; McLean et al., 2013; Shakespeare-Finch & Lurie-Beck, 2014; Tsai, El-Gabalawy, Sledge, Southwick, & Pietrzak, 2015). A low level of stress may not be sufficient to trigger the meaningful change that leads to growth. On the other hand, a high level of stress may require such a large investment of mental and cognitive resources to regulate emotions and process the event that it leaves no room for the experience of growth (Rozen et al., 2018). In other words, mothers with high levels of stress may be struggling with PTSD symptoms or other forms of distress, and this struggle impedes the association between stress and personal growth. If this is the case, it provides support for the hypothesis that distress and personal growth are not correlated, but adds the caveat that this is true only beyond a certain degree of distress (or below a certain degree).

Furthermore, whereas most studies have examined the total growth score, Rozen et al. (2018) examined all five growth dimensions individually, and found that the birth of preterms generated personal growth on the dimensions of New Possibilities, Personal Strength, Relations with Others, and marginally, Appreciation of Life. In comparison, among bereaved Japanese young adults, curvilinear associations were found only on the dimensions of Relating to Others and the combined factor of Spirituality and Appreciation of Life (Taku, Tedeschi, & Cann, 2015). Thus, as the authors suggest, the likelihood of experiencing growth in each PTG domain, as well as its connection with stress, is conceivably affected by the nature of the event, and therefore growth may not be evidenced on all dimensions.

This contention is supported by the fact that Rozen et al.'s (2018) study was essentially different from all the other studies we conducted on mothers of preterms. Our previous studies compared the response to the birth of preterms and full terms, whereas this study compared the response of mothers of preterms on two levels of risk. Thus, it is reasonable to assume that the discrepancy between the findings derives from the nature of the event being investigated. In other words, when the normative life event of full-term birth is compared with the stress-related event of premature delivery, the mothers of preterms report more growth (Noy et al., 2015; Taubman – Ben-Ari & Spielman, 2014; Taubman – Ben-Ari et al., 2010). However, when the event in both groups induces enough stress to generate significant growth, the differences between them become less discernible.

16.4 Changes in Personal Growth Over Time

One issue that has received insufficient attention is how personal growth changes over time. The vast majority of studies have been cross-sectional in nature, so that little is known about both the longitudinal course and the long-term predictors of PTG. Among the few longitudinal studies that have been conducted following events such as breast cancer, most have relied on sample means, have followed participants for 3–6 months, and report stable mean levels of PTG (e.g., Silva, Crespo, & Canavarro, 2012). Longer-term longitudinal studies (mostly around 18–24 months) have identified increasing PTG 18 months after a diagnosis of breast cancer, followed by a levelling off (Danhauer et al., 2013). Other studies have examined the trajectories of PTG among women with breast cancer and military veterans over a 2-year period, and found multiple trajectories (e.g., Danhauer et al., 2015; Tsai, Sippel, Mota, Southwick, & Pietrzak, 2016), including no change, increase over time, and decrease over time.

In the first study to examine personal growth in two phases of the transition to motherhood, pregnancy and shortly after the birth of the first child (Taubman – Ben-Ari, Ben Shlomo, Sivan, & Dolizki, 2009), mothers reported higher growth two months after childbirth than during pregnancy. Further studies corroborated this finding among mothers and fathers (Porat-Zyman et al., 2017; Taubman – Ben-Ari & Spielman, 2014), showing that personal growth is a continuous and developing experience, with the level of growth two years after the birth higher than that measured one month after delivery. Similarly, among fathers up to 18 months following the birth of their first baby, personal growth was found to be greater the older the infant (Taubman – Ben-Ari et al., 2018), and the personal growth of mothers four years following childbirth was higher than three years earlier, with growth at one year being the most predictive variable of growth at four years (Taubman – Ben-Ari et al., in press).

16.5 Intrapersonal and Interpersonal Contributors to Personal Growth

Most studies examining personal growth in the transition to parenthood focus around one major question: What variables contribute to this experience. The variables that have received the greatest attention fall into three groups: demographic; intrapersonal (including personality, cognitive appraisals and coping styles); and interpersonal.

Starting with demographics, studies consistently show that mothers report higher growth than fathers (Porat-Zyman et al., 2017; Spielman & Taubman – Ben-Ari, 2009; Taubman – Ben-Ari & Spielman, 2014; Taubman – Ben-Ari et al., 2014). This is in line with the results of a meta-analysis of general PTG studies, which indicates a small to moderate **gender** difference (Vishnevsky, Cann, Calhoun, Tedeschi, & Demakis, 2010). The transition to parenthood inevitably has a stronger impact on mothers than fathers, including the physiological changes of pregnancy, birth, and nursing, and often a greater need to give up independence and former way of life (Nicolson, 1999). These larger life changes may be associated with a more powerful sense of personal growth. Moreover, it is obvious that in sociological, psychological, and cultural terms, parenting is a highly gendered experience. Consequently, men and women enact parenthood from different starting points, their experiences and trajectories diverge in many ways over time, and the meaning of fathering is distinct from that of mothering (Palkovitz, Trask, & Adamsons, 2014).

Another relevant demographic variable is parent's **age**. Younger age is associated with higher personal growth among mothers (Sawyer & Ayers, 2009; Sawyer et al., 2012, 2015; Taubman – Ben-Ari et al., 2010; Taubman – Ben-Ari, Ben Shlomo, & Findler, 2012), in line with general PTG studies indicating that younger individuals tend to report greater levels of growth than older individuals (see the meta-analysis by Shakespeare-Finch & Lurie-Beck, 2014). Tedeschi and Calhoun (2004) suggest that younger people might be more open to learning and changing, whereas older people might be less amenable to change. It is also possible that being a younger mother presents particular challenges, which may increase the opportunity for growth (Taubman – Ben-Ari et al., 2012).

In addition, a lower level of **education** has been related to higher personal growth (Noy et al., 2015; Rozen et al., 2018; Taubman – Ben-Ari et al., 2010). Finally, some studies have found an association between lower **economic status** and higher growth among both mothers and fathers (Rozen et al., 2018; Taubman – Ben-Ari et al., 2018), while in others, higher growth was related to better economic status among mothers (Chasson & Taubman – Ben-Ari, 2019; Noy et al., 2015).

In the case of intrapersonal characteristics, a large set of variables has been examined. Studies show that greater **optimism** was associated with greater growth among new fathers up to 18 months following the birth of their first child (Taubman – Ben-Ari et al., 2018), and that four years following childbirth, it contributed positively to personal growth among mothers (Taubman – Ben-Ari et al., in press). In addition, Japanese women reporting greater **resilience** during pregnancy displayed higher PTG a month after childbirth (Nishi & Usuda, 2017).

Another characteristic that has been the subject of several studies is the individual's attachment orientation. **Anxious attachment** contributed significantly to personal growth among parents of full- and pre-terms both 1 month postpartum (Porat-Zyman et al., 2017; Spielman & Taubman – Ben-Ari, 2009), and two years after the birth of their first child (Taubman – Ben-Ari & Spielman, 2014). In the latter study, however, **avoidant attachment** also contributed significantly to the growth of fathers. In contrast, another study of first-time mothers during pregnancy and following childbirth did not indicate a significant association between anxious attachment and personal growth (Taubman – Ben-Ari et al., 2009), and among mothers of preterms, lower attachment anxiety was related to a higher experience of personal growth on the dimensions of Spirituality and Personal Strength (Rozen et al., 2018).

In addition, both more **positive** and more **negative emotions** were associated with greater growth among first-time fathers (Taubman – Ben-Ari et al., 2018). Higher **self-esteem** was also associated with higher personal growth among first-time mothers of

1-month-old pre- and full-term babies (Spielman & Taubman – Ben-Ari, 2009), and self-esteem one year postpartum correlated positively with personal growth 4 years later (Taubman – Ben-Ari et al, in press). However, in another study, the lower a first-time mother's or father's self-esteem up to two years following childbirth, the higher his or her assessment of personal growth (Taubman – Ben-Ari et al., 2014), and other studies did not indicate any significant association between self-esteem and personal growth during the transition to motherhood (Rozen et al., 2018; Taubman – Ben-Ari & Spielman, 2014; Taubman – Ben-Ari et al., 2009, 2012). Such inconsistencies are characteristic of the PTG literature concerning associations of growth with self-esteem and other characteristics of adaptive mental health (Zoellner & Maercker, 2006).

Furthermore, in a longitudinal study of women during pregnancy and shortly after childbirth, higher **appraisal of challenge** of either pregnancy or motherhood contributed to higher personal growth at both points in time (Taubman – Ben-Ari et al., 2009). Similarly, a cross-sectional study of first-time mothers found that lower threat appraisal and higher challenge appraisal of motherhood contributed to greater growth (Taubman – Ben-Ari et al., 2012). These findings were corroborated in a study of both mothers and fathers and their own parents, which showed not only that the higher a parent's assessment of challenge, the higher personal growth they reported, but also that the higher one generation's assessment of challenge, the higher the other's personal growth, suggesting that a positive appreciation of the situation by both parents and grandparents might promote a sense of growth in the two generations at this important time in their life (Taubman – Ben-Ari et al., 2014).

Coping strategies also appear to play a part in parents' growth. In two samples of UK women 1 month to 36 months following childbirth, as well as in an Israeli sample of women shortly after childbirth, greater use of problem solving and guidance and support seeking strategies, termed active approach coping in the UK (Sawyer & Ayers, 2009; Sawyer et al., 2015), and problem-focused and support seeking coping in Israel (Taubman – Ben-Ari et al., 2009), were significantly associated with higher levels of personal growth. On the other hand, greater use of avoidance coping (e.g., denial) was positively related to growth in a Croatian sample (Sawyer et al., 2015).

It seems that in order to experience growth, a combination of personal resources and personality traits is required. An individual needs a positive life orientation, reflected in optimism, resilience, positive emotions, challenge appraisal, and perhaps a problem-focused approach to coping. At the same time, however, some degree of vulnerability is needed as well, as both negative emotions and anxious attachment orientation have also been related to personal growth. It is possible that in times of turmoil, such as during the stressful transition to parenthood, anxiously attached individuals feel more threatened (see also Mikulincer and Shaver, Chap. 18 in this volume), and these tendencies, along with the presence of a baby who is totally dependent on them, may cause them to feel overwhelmed and experience various negative emotions. This in turn may lead to strong efforts to obtain comfort and support from their attachment figures. Their ability to "survive" the experience may result in enhanced self-confidence, a heightened sense of trust, and a fuller understanding of the meaning of life and the value of family (Cadell, Regehr, & Hemsworth, 2003), which may be interpreted as growth (Taubman – Ben-Ari, 2012). If a parent sinks in despair and negatively ruminates about their difficulties, the option to experience growth will not be available to them. They have to embrace some kind of positive view of life to be able to go through the hardship and emerge a somewhat different person. And just as there is an optimal middle point for stress to affect personal growth, there seems to be some middle range for intrapersonal resources. Someone who is highly resilient and secure might not experience growth, as they do not feel they have learned anything new about themselves; those who are highly insecure and pessimistic may not be able to handle stress-evoking situations and be overwhelmed with despair or depression, and thus will not have the opportunity to sense growth. Only those who synergize both feelings of stress and a positive, more open, outlook, may be in a position to experience a sense of thriving, changing, and gaining from the transition to parenthood.

In addition, the inconsistencies in the findings for intrapersonal characteristics suggest the need to look more carefully into the various dimensions of personal growth. The common use of a total growth score may hide differences that relate to specific aspects of growth. Moreover, the fact that some studies produced different results for mothers and fathers may hint at disparate gender dynamics in the experience of personal growth. Both these possibilities should be explored in the future.

Beyond the personal traits that one brings to every situation, a major factor that appears in the general PTG literature (Tedeschi & Calhoun, 2004) is perceived **social support**. Similar to measures of stress, perceived support is thought to be a better indicator of whether someone's needs are being met than actual support (Lyons, 1991). The significance of this variable is confirmed in a meta-analysis of 46 studies reporting a moderate positive relationship between social support and growth following a range of stressful events (Prati & Pietrantoni, 2009). The presence of supportive others may promote self-disclosure, stimulate cognitive processing, and offer new perspectives, all of which can assist people in finding positive meaning in the situation with which they are coping.

In our own series of studies concerning the transition to parenthood, we related primarily to two support figures, the spouse and the parents' own parents (i.e., the grandparents), particularly their mothers, examining the associations between growth and the quality of these relationships and the perceived emotional and instrumental support they provide. We found quite consistently that a better relationship with the spouse and higher perceived support from this individual were positively related to personal growth. A better marital relationship was associated with higher growth during pregnancy among first time pregnant women (Taubman – Ben-Ari et al., 2009); better marital adaptation immediately after the birth was associated with higher growth one year after delivery among mothers of preterms (Taubman – Ben-Ari et al., 2010); and mothers who had a more positive perception of the parenting aspect of their marriage reported more personal growth a year postpartum (Noy et al., 2015).

Along the same lines, higher levels of personal growth were found among mothers who perceived more support from their own mothers (Noy et al., 2015; Taubman –

Ben-Ari et al., 2010). Up to two years after childbirth, higher frequency of meetings between first-time mothers and their own mothers was related to higher personal growth (Taubman – Ben-Ari et al., 2012), and among mothers of preterms, higher perceived maternal grandmother's emotional support was associated with greater personal growth on all five PTGI dimensions (Rozen et al., 2018). These findings are in line with the notion that people regard their mothers as one of the closest person to them throughout their lives (Antonucci, Akiyama, & Takahashi, 2004), and highlights the role of the grandmother in facilitating the personal growth of a mother, both in general and in the unique circumstances of a first or preterm baby. It is interesting to note that objective, medically-defined, risk levels moderated this association, so that for the growth dimensions of New Possibilities, Personal Strength, and Relationship with Others, the more mothers in a low risk group perceived maternal support, the higher the growth they reported, whereas maternal support was not associated with personal growth among mothers in a moderate-high risk group (Rozen et al., 2018).

Similarly, in our study of single mothers by choice, the association between perceived support and personal growth was moderated by group affiliation (being a single mother or in a relationship), so that among mothers in a couple relationship, there was a positive association between the support provided by the family and personal growth, but no significant association emerged between the two variables among single mothers by choice. In contrast, a positive association was found between the support provided by a significant other and personal growth among single mothers by choice, but not among mothers in a couple relationship (Chasson & Taubman – Ben-Ari, 2019). Thus, whereas family support appears to enhance the experience of growth among women in a relationship, the growth of women who have chosen to have a child on their own is not dependent on the support of their family. However, given the absence of a spouse or life partner, support from a different significant figure in their life is likely to strongly impact their ability to cope with their new role as mother, and consequently their experience of personal growth.

Additional evidence of the importance of social support comes from a study that compared women in lesbian-mother families with women in heterosexual families (Shenkman, 2018). It was found that the association between basic need satisfaction in the relationship (defined as the support the individual gets from the other person in the relationship for their sense of autonomy, competence, and relatedness; La Guardia, Ryan, Couchman, & Deci, 2000) and mother's personal growth in a range of years following childbirth was significant only for lesbian-mothers. The author suggests that for lesbians, becoming a mother often involves coping with and overcoming additional difficulties (e.g., undergoing fertility treatments, dealing with homophobia, etc.). In view of these added burdens, support in the form of satisfying basic needs may be more strongly associated with the positive construction of personal growth among biological lesbian mothers than among their heterosexual cohorts.

16.6 The Big Picture: What We Have Learned and What Is Left to Discover

The accumulated knowledge regarding growth following childbirth clearly indicates that personal growth is a relevant concept not only in respect to traumatic events, but also in the context of this normative life event. The literature reveals the relationship of parents' personal growth with stress, and with a host of demographic, intrapersonal, and interpersonal variables, as well as its dynamics over time. Moreover, it shows the importance of the individual's perception of the situation over the seemingly objective reality, and highlights the need for a positive outlook combined with a degree of vulnerability as prerequisites for the experience of personal growth.

Research into personal growth in parenthood is less than 10 years old. Although we have already gained significant knowledge, certain questions still remain unanswered. They include the specific contexts that enable personal growth, as well as the dynamics that encourage growth among some individuals and not others. The mere existence of the experience of personal growth in the transition to parenthood has been tested and validated in numerous studies, and has been found to be stronger in more demanding, threatening, and stress-related circumstances, such as giving birth to premature babies, following a cesarean section, or being a single mom. However, other events considered stressful, e.g., fertility treatment or having twins, have not yielded higher reports of personal growth over time. Thus, further research is needed for us to gain a more nuanced understanding of the development of personal growth among parents.

In regard to its dynamics, personal growth is one potential consequence of the cognitive effort to redefine basic beliefs and to rebuild the assumptive world (Calhoun & Tedeschi, 2006; Janoff-Bulman, 1992, 2006). The theory of personal growth postulates that between the initial challenge to core beliefs and the subsequent experience of growth, the individual needs to engage in appropriate cognitive work (Cann et al., 2010). It is therefore presumed that a significant factor in the path from cognitive threat to the assumptive world to growth is the degree to which the person engages in repeated thinking about the event. Repeated thought, or rumination, may lead to the accommodation of the assumptive world to the changed reality or to the assimilation of the event into the existing cognitive structures (Janoff-Bulman, 1992, 2006). Further research is needed to explore such processes as related specifically to parenthood.

In addition, studies of further resources that might help explain the rather sensitive mechanisms of growth are warranted. Among the variables worth examining in the context of parenthood are measurable constructs drawn from the field of trauma, such as questioning of the individual's basic belief system, intrusive rumination aroused by the event, and deliberate rumination meant to help process the event (Taku, Cann, Tedeschi, & Calhoun, 2015), or more basic personality characteristics, such as flexibility, which means the ability to shift between two patterns of response (e.g., focusing on the traumatic event in order to process it vs. detaching oneself from the event; Bonanno, Pat-Horenczyk, & Noll, 2011).

The PTG literature also relates to the question of how central the individual views the traumatic event to their life narrative, identity, and attribution of new experiences, demonstrating associations between event centrality and PTG, in-de-pen-dent of distress symptoms (Blix, Birkeland, Hansen, & Heir, 2015; Groleau, Calhoun, Cann, & Tedeschi, 2013). Although it may be assumed that the transition to parenthood is a central event in a person's life and identity, and may thus lead to personal growth, studies have yet to examine the specific nature of this connection. Research exploring, for example, theories of motivation (e.g., the motivation to become a parent, see also Solomon, Chap. 11 in this volume) and meaning (i.e., parenthood as a source of meaning, see also Steger and Morse, Chap. 1 in this volume) might help us better understand individual differences in the experience of personal growth.

Moreover, although studies indicate that growth is a process that evolves over time, continuing to develop during the first years after childbirth (Porat-Zyman et al., 2017; Taubman – Ben-Ari & Spielman, 2014), further research using a more comprehensive longitudinal design is required to gain a more thorough understanding of its potential multiple trajectories. In addition, men should be more represented in studies, both in examinations of their particular experience and in dyadic designs that relate to the couple's response to the transition to parenthood. Another population conspicuously absent from the literature are new families.

The cultural similarities found in the various studies indicate the universality of the phenomenon of parents' personal growth and its robustness across cultures. Nevertheless, certain differences have emerged, signifying the need to delve deeper to understand the cultural meanings associated with childbirth, parenthood and the experience of growth, the significance of the various dimensions of growth in different social contexts, and how much different societies are willing to acknowledge the stress generated by childbirth and personal growth as a legitimate outcome of this normative life event.

Furthermore, having recognized the existence of personal growth as a response to the transition to parenthood, we can now proceed to questions such as "What is the benefit of growth?" or "What does it predict?" In other words, growth can be used as an independent, moderating, or mediating variable, facilitating the examination of its trajectory over time as well as its association with other constructs, such as mental health or search for meaning.

Finally, in contrast to most events studied in the PTG literature, childbirth is usually planned, and even when it is not, it comes on the wake of a lengthy period of preparation. A better understanding of growth will therefore enable professionals to intervene and assist individuals or couples who struggle for meaning or the reconstruction of their core beliefs, helping them to overcome intrusive rumination and learn to replace it with deliberate self-awareness, positive reframing, and other techniques. Such interventions can ultimately enable more people to achieve life satisfaction, and offer them the opportunity to experience personal growth.

> Because of you, I reach the far edges of life, the good and the bad. Because of you I have begun to really live . I didn't even know that I wasn't actually living before. You're still so

tiny and fragile and utterly dependent on us, and yet, you have already taught me so much about myself, about you, about your father, about our family, about our friends, and about the whole world. It's amazing how much we adults can learn from one small child. (Women Talk Motherhood, Forum for New Mothers, http://www.medabrotimahut.co.il/2010/09)

References

Antonucci, T., Akiyama, H., & Takahashi, K. (2004). Attachment and close relationships across the life span. *Attachment & Human Development, 6*(4), 353–370.

Arendell, T. (2000). Conceiving and investigating motherhood: The decade's scholarship. *Journal of Marriage and the Family, 62*(4), 1192–1207.

Ayers, S., Bond, R., Bertullies, S., & Wijma, K. (2016). The aetiology of post-traumatic stress following childbirth: A meta-analysis and theoretical framework. *Psychological Medicine, 46*(6), 1121–1134.

Barr, P. (2011). Posttraumatic growth in parents of infants hospitalized in a neonatal intensive care unit. *Journal of Loss and Trauma, 16*(2), 117–134.

Bassi, M., Delle Fave, A., Cetin, I., Melchiorri, E., Pozzo, M., Vescovelli, F., & Ruini, C. (2017). Psychological well-being and depression from pregnancy to postpartum among primiparous and multiparous women. *Journal of Reproductive and Infant Psychology, 35*(2), 183–195.

Beck, C. T., & Watson, S. (2016). Posttraumatic growth after birth trauma: "I was broken, now I am unbreakable." *American Journal of Maternal Child Nursing, 41*(5), 264–271.

Ben Shlomo, S., & Taubman – Ben-Ari, O. (2017). Child adjustment to first grade as perceived by the parents: The role of parents' personal growth. *Stress and Health, 33*(2), 102–110.

Benzies, K. M., & Magill-Evans, J. (2015). Through the eyes of a new dad: Experiences of first-time fathers of late preterm infants. *Infant Mental Health Journal, 36*(1), 78–87.

Blix, I., Birkeland, M. S., Hansen, M. B., & Heir, T. (2015). Posttraumatic growth and centrality of event: A longitudinal study in the aftermath of the 2011 Oslo bombing. *Psychological Trauma: Theory, Research, Practice, and Policy, 7*(1), 18–23.

Bock, J. D. (2000). Doing the right thing? Single mothers by choice and the struggle for legitimacy. *Gender and Society, 14*(1), 62–86.

Bonanno, G. A., Pat-Horenczyk, R., & Noll, J. (2011a). Coping flexibility and trauma: The Perceived Ability to Cope with Trauma (PACT) scale. *Psychological Trauma: Theory, Research, Practice, and Policy, 3*(2), 117–129.

Bonanno, G. A., Westphal, M., & Mancini, A. D. (2011b). Resilience to loss and potential trauma. *Annual Review of Clinical Psychology, 7*, 511–535.

Burns, L. H. (2007). Psychiatric aspects of infertility and infertility treatments. *Psychiatric Clinics of North America, 30*(4), 689–716.

Cadell, S., Regehr, C., & Hemsworth, D. (2003). Factors contributing to post-traumatic growth: A proposed structural equation model. *American Journal of Orthopsychiatry, 73*(3), 279–287.

Calhoun, L. G., & Tedeschi, R. G. (2006). *Handbook of posttraumatic growth: Research and practice*. Mahwah, NJ: Lawrence Erlbaum.

Calhoun, L. G., & Tedeschi, R. G. (2013). *Posttraumatic growth in clinical practice*. New York: Routledge.

Cameron, E. E., Sedov, I. D., & Tomfohr-Madsen, L. M. (2016). Prevalence of paternal depression in pregnancy and the postpartum: An updated meta-analysis. *Journal of Affective Disorders, 206*, 189–203.

Cann, A., Calhoun, L.G., Tedeschi, R.G., Kilmer, R.P., Gil-Rivas, V., Vishnevsky, T., & Danhauer, S.C. (2010). The Core Beliefs Inventory: A brief measure of disruption in the assumptive world. *Anxiety, Stress, and Coping, 23*(1), 19–34.

Carver, C., & Scheier, M. (2001). Optimism, pessimism, and self-regulation. In E. Chang (Ed.), *Optimism and pessimism: Implications for theory, research, and practice* (pp. 31–55). Washington, DC: American Psychological Association.
Chasson, M., & Taubman-Ben-Ari, O. (2019). Single mothers by choice in the transition to motherhood. *Under Review.*
Coroiu, A., Körner, A., Burke, S., Meterissian, S., & Sabiston, C. M. (2016). Stress and posttraumatic growth among survivors of breast cancer: A test of curvilinear effects. *International Journal of Stress Management, 23*(1), 84–97.
Danhauer, S. C., Case, L. D., Tedeschi, R., Russell, G., Vishnvesky, T., & Triplett, K. (2013). Predictors of posttraumatic growth in women with breast cancer. *Psycho-Oncology, 22*(12), 2673–2683.
Danhauer, S. C., Russell, G., Case, L. D., Sohl, S. J., Tedeschi, R. G., Addington, E. L. ... Avis, N. E. (2015). Trajectories of posttraumatic growth and associated characteristics in women with breast cancer. *Annals of Behavioral Medicine, 49*(5), 650–659.
Diener, E. (1984). Subjective well-being. *Psychological Bulletin, 95*(3), 542–575.
Diener, E. (2000). Subjective well-being: The science of happiness and a proposal for a national index. *American Psychologist, 55*(1), 34–43.
Frančišković, T., Stevanović, A., Jelušić, I., Roganović, B., Klarić, M., & Grković, J. (2007). Secondary traumatization of wives of war veterans with posttraumatic stress disorder. *Croatian Medical Journal, 48*(2), 177–184.
Gameiro, S., Moura-Ramos, M., Canavarro, M. C., & Soares, I. (2010). Psychosocial adjustment during the transition to parenthood of Portuguese couples who conceived spontaneously or through assisted reproductive technologies. *Research in Nursing & Health, 33*(3), 207–220.
Groleau, J. M., Calhoun, L. G., Cann, A., & Tedeschi, R. G. (2013). The role of centrality of events in posttraumatic distress and posttraumatic growth. *Psychological Trauma: Theory, Research, Practice, and Policy, 5*(5), 477–483.
Haga, S. M., Lynne, A., Slinning, K., & Kraft, P. (2012). A qualitative study of depressive symptoms and well-being among first-time mothers. *Scandinavian Journal of Caring Sciences, 26*(3), 458–466.
Helgeson, V. S., Reynolds, K. A., & Tomich, P. L. (2006). A meta-analytic review of benefit finding and growth. *Journal of Consulting and Clinical Psychology, 74*(5), 797–816.
Hertz, R. (2006). *Single by chance, mothers by choice: How women are choosing parenthood without marriage and creating the new American family*. New York: Oxford University Press.
Hjelmstedt, A., Widström, A. M., Wramsby, H., & Collins, A. (2004). Emotional adaptation following successful in vitro fertilization. *Fertility and Sterility, 81*(5), 1254–1264.
Horsch, A., Tolsa, J. F., Gilbert, L., du Chêne, L. J., Müller-Nix, C., & Graz, M. B. (2016). Improving maternal mental health following preterm birth using an expressive writing intervention: A randomized controlled trial. *Child Psychiatry and Human Development, 47*(5), 780–791.
Janoff-Bulman, R. (1992). *Shattered assumptions*. New York: The Free Press.
Janoff-Bulman, R. (2006). Schema-change perspectives on posttraumatic growth. In L. G. Calhoun & R. G. Tedeschi (Eds.), *Handbook of posttraumatic growth: Research and practice* (pp. 81–99). Mahwah, NJ: Lawrence Erlbaum.
Kingston, D., Tough, S., & Whitfield, H. (2012). Prenatal and postpartum maternal psychological distress and infant development: A systematic review. *Child Psychiatry and Human Development, 43*(5), 683–714.
La Guardia, J. G., Ryan, R. M., Couchman, C. E., & Deci, E. L. (2000). Within-person variation in security of attachment: A self-determination theory perspective on attachment, need fulfillment, and well-being. *Journal of Personality and Social Psychology, 79*(3), 367–384.
Linley, P. A., & Joseph, S. (2004). Positive change following trauma and adversity: A review. *Journal of Traumatic Stress, 17*(1), 11–21.
Lyons, J. A. (1991). Strategies for assessing the potential for positive adjustment following trauma. *Journal of Traumatic Stress, 4*(1), 93–111.
Mann, R., Gilbody, S., & Adamson, J. (2010). Prevalence and incidence of postnatal depression: What can systematic reviews tell us? *Archives of Women's Mental Health, 13*(4), 295–305.

McLean, C. P., Handa, S., Dickstein, B. D., Benson, T. A., Baker, M. T., Isler, W. C. … Litz, B. T. (2013). Posttraumatic growth and posttraumatic stress among military medical personnel. *Psychological Trauma: Theory, Research, Practice, and Policy, 5*(1), 62–68.

Nicolson, P. (1999). Loss, happiness and postpartum depression: The ultimate paradox. *Canadian Psychology, 40*(2), 162–178.

Nishi, D., & Usuda, K. (2017). Psychological growth after childbirth: An exploratory prospective study. *Journal of Psychosomatic Obstetrics & Gynecology, 38*(2), 87–93.

Noy, A., Taubman – Ben-Ari, O., & Kuint, J. (2015). Well-being and personal growth in mothers of full-term and pre-term singletons and twins. *Stress & Health, 31*(5), 365–372.

Olde, E., van der Hart, O., Kleber, R., & van Son, M. (2006). Posttraumatic stress following childbirth: A review. *Clinical Psychology Review, 26*(1), 1–16.

Olivennes, F., Golombok, S., Ramogida, C., & Rust, J. (2005). Behavioral and cognitive development as well as family functioning of twins conceived by assisted reproduction: Findings from a large population study. *Fertility and Sterility, 84*(3), 725–733.

Palkovitz, R., Trask, B. S., & Adamsons, K. (2014). Essential differences in the meaning and processes of mothering and fathering: Family systems, feminist and qualitative perspectives. *Journal of Family Theory & Review, 6*(4), 406–420.

Parfitt, Y., & Ayers, S. (2014). Transition to parenthood and mental health in first-time parents. *Infant Mental Health Journal, 35*(3), 263–273.

Park, C. L. (1998). Implication of posttraumatic growth for individuals. In R. G. Tedeschi, C. L. Park, & L. G. Calhoun (Eds.), *Posttraumatic growth: Positive change in the aftermath of crisis* (pp. 153–177). Mahwah, NJ: Lawrence Erlbaum Associates.

Porat-Zyman, G., Taubman – Ben-Ari, O., Kuint, J., & Morag, I. (in press). Personal growth four years after premature childbirth: The role of change in maternal mental health. *Journal of Happiness Studies*.

Porat-Zyman, G., Taubman – Ben-Ari, O., & Spielman, V. (2017). Dyadic transition to parenthood: A longitudinal assessment of personal growth among parents of pre- and full-term infants. *Stress & Health, 33*(1), 24–34.

Prati, G., & Pietrantoni, L. (2009). Optimism, social support, and coping strategies as factors contributing to posttraumatic growth: A meta-analysis. *Journal of Loss and Trauma, 14*(5), 364–388.

Rozen, G., Taubman – Ben-Ari, O., Strauss, T., & Morag, I. (2018). Personal growth of mothers of preterms: Objective severity of the event, subjective stress, personal resources, and maternal emotional support. *Journal of Happiness Studies, 19*(7), 2167–2186.

Ryff, C. D. (1989). Happiness is everything, or is it? Explorations on the meaning of psychological wellbeing. *Journal of Personality and Social Psychology, 57*(6), 1069–1081.

Ryff, C. D. (2014). Psychological well-being revisited: Advances in the science and practice of Eudaimonia. *Psychotherapy and Psychosomatics, 83*(1), 10–28.

Sawyer, A., & Ayers, S. (2009). Post-traumatic growth in women after childbirth. *Psychology & Health, 24*(4), 457–471.

Sawyer, A., Ayers, S., Young, D., Bradley, R., & Smith, H. (2012). Posttraumatic growth after childbirth: A prospective study. *Psychology & Health, 27*(3), 362–377.

Sawyer, A., Nakić Radoš, S., Ayers, S., & Burn, E. (2015). Personal growth in UK and Croatian women following childbirth: A preliminary study. *Journal of Reproductive and Infant Psychology, 33*(3), 294–307.

Schaefer, J., & Moos, R. (1998). The context for posttraumatic growth: Life crises, individual and social resources, and coping. In R. Tedeschi, C. Park, & L. Calhoun (Eds.), *Posttraumatic growth: Positive changes in the aftermath of crisis* (pp. 99–126). Mahwah, NJ: Erlbaum.

Schappin, R., Wijnroks, L., Uniken Venema, M. M. A. T., & Jongmans, M. J. (2013). Rethinking stress in parents of preterm infants: A meta-analysis. *PLoS ONE, 8*(2), e54992.

Shakespeare-Finch, J., & Enders, T. (2008). Corroborating evidence of posttraumatic growth. *Journal of Traumatic Stress, 21*(4), 421–424.

Shakespeare-Finch, J., & Lurie-Beck, J. (2014). A meta-analytic clarification of the relationship between posttraumatic growth and symptoms of posttraumatic distress disorder. *Journal of Anxiety Disorders, 28*(2), 223–229.

Shaw, R. J., Bernard, R. S., Deblois, T., Ikuta, L. M., Ginzburg, K., & Koopman, C. (2009). The relationship between acute stress disorder and posttraumatic stress disorder in the neonatal intensive care unit. *Psychosomatics, 50*(2), 131–137.

Shenkman, G. (2018). The association between basic need satisfaction in relationship and personal growth among lesbian and heterosexual mothers. *Journal of Social and Personal Relationships, 35*(2), 246–262.

Silva, S., Crespo, C., & Canavarro, M. C. (2012). Pathways for psychological adjustment in breast cancer: A longitudinal study on coping strategies and posttraumatic growth. *Psychology & Health, 27*(11), 1323–1341.

Snyder, C. R. (2002). Hope theory: Rainbows in the mind. *Psychological Inquiry, 13*(4), 249–275.

Spielman, V., & Taubman – Ben-Ari, O. (2009). Parental self-efficacy and stress-related growth in the transition to parenthood: A comparison between parents of pre- and full-term babies. *Health and Social Work, 34*(3), 201–212.

Stanton, A., Bower, J., & Low, C. (2006). Posttraumatic growth after cancer. In L. G. Calhoun & R. G. Tedeschi (Eds.), *Handbook of posttraumatic growth: Research and practice* (pp. 138–175). Mahwah, NJ: Erlbaum Associates.

Steger, M. F., Frazier, P., Oishi, S., & Kaler, M. (2006). The meaning in life questionnaire: Assessing the presence of and search for meaning in life. *Journal of Counseling Psychology, 53*(1), 80–93.

Taku, K., Cann, A., Tedeschi, R. G., & Calhoun, L. G. (2015). Core beliefs shaken by an earthquake correlate with posttraumatic growth. *Psychological Trauma: Theory, Research, Practice, and Policy, 7*(6), 563–569.

Taku, K., Tedeschi, R. G., & Cann, A. (2015). Relationships of posttraumatic growth and stress responses in bereaved young adults. *Journal of Loss and Trauma, 20*(1), 56–71.

Taubman – Ben-Ari, O. (2012). Becoming and developing: Personal growth in the wake of parenthood and grandparenthood. In P. R. Shaver & M. Mikulincer (Eds.), *Meaning, mortality, and choice: The social psychology of existential concerns* (pp. 163–181). Washington DC: APA.

Taubman – Ben-Ari, O., Ben Shlomo, S., & Findler, L. (2012). Personal growth and meaning in life among first-time mothers and grandmothers. *Journal of Happiness Studies, 13*(5), 801–820.

Taubman – Ben-Ari, O., Ben Shlomo, S., & Findler, L. (2014). First-time parents' and grandparents' perceptions of personal growth: A dyadic approach. *Journal of Family Social Work, 17*(3), 229–250.

Taubman – Ben-Ari, O., Ben Shlomo, S., Sivan, E., & Dolizki, M. (2009). The transition to motherhood: A time for growth. *Journal of Social and Clinical Psychology, 28*(8), 943–970.

Taubman – Ben-Ari, O., Findler, L., & Kuint, J. (2010). Personal growth in the wake of stress: The case of mothers of preterm twins. *The Journal of Psychology, 144*(2), 185–204.

Taubman – Ben-Ari, O., Findler, L., & Sharon, N. (2011). Personal growth in mothers: Examination of the suitability of the Posttraumatic Growth Inventory as a measurement tool. *Women and Health, 51*(6), 604–622.

Taubman – Ben-Ari, O., Skvirsky, V., Bar Shua, E., & Horowitz, E. (2018). Personal growth of new fathers following assisted reproductive technology or spontaneous pregnancy. *Parenting: Science and Practice, 18*(3), 190–199.

Taubman – Ben-Ari, O., Skvirsky, V., Strauss, T., & Morag, I. (in press). Pre-term delivery, optimism and initial personal growth as predictors of mothers' long-term personal growth. *Journal of Reproductive and Infant Psychology.*

Taubman – Ben-Ari, O., & Spielman, V. (2014). Personal growth following the first child's birth: A comparison of parents of pre- and full-term babies. *Social Work Research, 38*(2), 91–106.

Tedeschi, R. G., & Calhoun, L. G. (1995). *Trauma and transformation: Growing in the aftermath of suffering.* Thousand Oaks, CA: Sage.

Tedeschi, R. G., & Calhoun, L. G. (1996). The posttraumatic growth inventory: Measuring the positive legacy of trauma. *Journal of Traumatic Stress, 9*(3), 455–471.

Tedeschi, R. G., & Calhoun, L. G. (2004). Posttraumatic growth: Conceptual foundations and empirical evidence. *Psychological Inquiry, 15*(1), 1–18.

Tedeschi, R. G., Cann, A., Taku, K., Senol-Durak, E., & Calhoun, L. G. (2017). The posttraumatic growth inventory: A revision integrating existential and spiritual change. *Journal of Traumatic Stress, 30*(1), 11–18.

Tsai, J., El-Gabalawy, R., Sledge, W. H., Southwick, S. M., & Pietrzak, R. H. (2015). Post-traumatic growth among veterans in the USA: Results from the National Health and Resilience in Veterans Study. *Psychological Medicine, 45*(1), 165–179.

Tsai, J., Sippel, L. M., Mota, N., Southwick, S. M., & Pietrzak, R. H. (2016). Longitudinal course of posttraumatic growth among U.S. military veterans: Results from the National Health and Resilience in Veterans Study. *Depression and Anxiety, 33*(1), 9–18.

Vishnevsky, T., Cann, A., Calhoun, L. G., Tedeschi, R. G., & Demakis, G. J. (2010). Gender differences in self-reported posttraumatic growth: A meta-analysis. *Psychology of Women Quarterly, 34*(1), 110–120.

Webb, R., Ayers, S., & Rosan, C. (2018). A systematic review of measures of mental health and emotional wellbeing in parents of children aged 0–5. *Journal of Affective Disorders, 225*, 608–617.

Weiss, T. (2002). Posttraumatic growth in women with breast cancer and their husbands: An intersubjective validation study. *Journal of Psychosocial Oncology, 20*(2), 65–80.

Werner, E., Miller, M., Osborne, L. M., Kuzava, S., & Monk, C. (2015). Preventing postpartum depression: Review and recommendations. *Archives of Women's Mental Health, 18*(1), 41–60.

World Health Organization. (2004). *Promoting mental health: Concepts, emerging evidence, practice (Summary report)*. Geneva: WHO.

Yildiz, P. D., Ayers, S., & Phillips, L. (2017). The prevalence of posttraumatic stress disorder in pregnancy and after birth: A systematic review and meta-analysis. *Journal of Affective Disorders, 208*, 634–645.

Yim, I. S., Tanner Stapleton, L. R., Guardino, C. M., Hahn-Holbrook, J., & Dunkel Schetter, C. (2015). Biological and psychological predictors of postpartum depression: Systematic review and call for integration. *Annual Review of Clinical Psychology, 11*, 99–137.

Zoellner, T., & Maercker, A. (2006). Posttraumatic growth in clinical psychology—A critical review and introduction of a two component model. *Clinical Psychology Review, 26*(5), 626–653.

Chapter 17
Attachment and the Transition to Parenthood

W. Steven Rholes and Ramona L. Paetzold

17.1 Introduction to Attachment Theory and Attachment Styles

The existence of an instinctive motive to form bonds of affection with particular individuals and to turn to those individuals to relieve distress is the essence of attachment theory. The most important function of attachment bonds is to protect infants and children from danger. Infants and children that seek out attachment figures when frightened have a survival advantage over those who do not.

The way in which the motive to seek safety from attachment figures manifests depends on a variety of environmental circumstances, chief among them the way that attachment figures react to efforts by infants and children to obtain support from them to relieve distress. Caring and supportive responses encourage the emergence of generalized expectations of supportive and protective attachment figures, and uncaring and unsupportive reactions do the opposite. The responses of attachment figures also help build mental models of the child's sense of self as loved and worthy of love or unloved and unworthy, and of attachment figures as loving and willing to provide support and comfort or unresponsive and rejecting of the child's bids for support (Bowlby, 1973, 1979).

W. S. Rholes (✉)
Department of Psychology, MS 4235, Texas A & M University, College Station, TX 77843-4235, USA
e-mail: s-rholes@tamu.edu

R. L. Paetzold
Department of Management, MS 4221, Texas A & M University, College Station, TX 77843-4221, USA
e-mail: rpaetzold@mays.tamu.edu

O. Taubman – Ben-Ari (ed.), *Pathways and Barriers to Parenthood*,
https://doi.org/10.1007/978-3-030-24864-2_17

Bowlby's (1979) initial research and theorizing concerned children's attachment to caregivers. However, he wrote that what holds for children holds for adults. In childhood, attachments start as bonds to particular others. However, as children's experiences with attachment figures broadens, generalized expectations for and understandings of attachment figures develop. These generalizations lead to routine perceptions of and patterns of behavior with attachment figures. Bowlby called these routines "working models."

The content of working models includes episodic memories of experiences with various attachment figures. It also typically include "rules" stored in semantic memory that guide behaviors with attachment figures. These rules may take the form of if/then propositions. For example, if I approach my father when I am afraid, he will respond favorably to this attempt to calm myself, or if my mother is angry, she will hurt me physically if I do not stay away from her. Working models may also include injunctions imposed by attachment figures that children are not to challenge the descriptions or explanations of events provided by attachment figures, even when such descriptions and explanations contradict children's experiences. For example, a mother may insist that a child's father is not dead but has just moved away, even after the child saw the father's deceased body. Or, a father may insist that problems within the family are the fault of the child, even when it might seem to the child that the father's alcoholism is the real cause. Or finally, a mother may insist that she loves her child and acts in his or her best interests when it is apparent to the child that she does not, or at least when the child suspects that she does not. Even as adults in psychotherapy, some people have difficulty re-examining the distorted realities of their lives promulgated by their attachment figures.

The work on attachment theory started by Bowlby (1973) has been continued by a generation of investigators in developmental, clinical, personality, and social psychology. The remainder of this chapter will address attachment relationships among adults, adults' working models, and their models of the self and the other each studied from the perspective of personality and social psychology. Mario Mikulincer and Phillip Shaver figure prominently in work done within this tradition due to their theory building and voluminous empirical research (see Mikulincer and Shaver, Chap. 18 in this volume).

Shaver and colleagues developed what has become the gold standard of self-report measures of attachment styles, the Experiences in Close Relationships scale (ECR; Brennan, Clark, & Shaver, 1998). The ECR assesses two dimensions of attachment, called attachment anxiety and attachment avoidance, which are relatively orthogonal. The ECR comports well with Bowlby's (1973) observations about attachment anxiety and compulsive self-reliance (now called avoidance). Mikulincer and Shaver (2016) write primarily about these two broad trends in or styles of affect, cognition, and behavior that guide interactions with attachment figures. In other words, they write primarily about personalities with avoidant or anxious tendencies, not about specific relationships involving avoidance or anxiety. In this way their work differs from much of Bowlby's (1973). Avoidance and anxiety are measured on continuous dimensions, but in this chapter we will discuss them using categorical terms to avoid the awkwardness of continually writing more avoidant or less anxious, etc.

Some of the most important characteristics of the behavior of avoidant people include lack of investment in and commitment to close relationships. Avoidant people are not comfortable examining and analyzing their relationships and the influence important relationships have had on their lives. Avoidant people do not want to, and typically do not, provide much help or support to relationship partners. Perhaps because of their distaste for caregiving, avoidant individuals also tend to be less interested in becoming a parent (Jones, Cassidy, & Shaver, 2015). Finally, avoidant adults do not rely on their close relationships for their sense of well-being. Other things, such as work, hobbies, travel, and the sense that they are free to do what they want to do tend to be more important. "Unencumbered" might be a good word to describe the life that avoidant people prize.

One of the most important qualities of the behavior of anxious adults is a proclivity for jealousy in romantic relationships. Jealousy seems to result from a fear that partners are not committed to them and may leave them. Anxious people want partners to be supportive, but they tend to think that they receive less support than they deserve. They also tend to under-perceive the amount of support than is actually provided (Collins & Feeney, 2004). Anxious people are less satisfied with their relationships than non-anxious people. Anxious people report low self-esteem, and they are highly vulnerable to psychopathological symptoms and disorders (Mikulincer & Shaver, 2016). Finally, unlike avoidant people, anxious people's satisfaction or dissatisfaction with their relationships is central to their sense of well-being. "Devoted" might be the best word to explain what anxious people want in relationship partners.

17.2 Parents' Well-Being: How Do Anxious and Avoidant Parents Fare During the Transition to Parenthood?

My colleague, Jeff Simpson, and I have conducted two studies of the transition to parenthood. The first began about 6 weeks before the birth of the parents' first child and ended about 7.5 months later (Rholes, Simpson, Campbell, & Grich, 2001; Simpson, Rholes, Campbell, Tran, & Wilson, 2003; Simpson, Rholes, Campbell, & Wilson, 2003). Our goal was to study parents' well-being during the transition, and our primary indicator of well-being was marital satisfaction. The second study also focused on well-being. It included marital satisfaction as a measure of well-being, but in addition it included depressive symptoms and feelings of closeness or distance with their child (Fillo, Simpson, Rholes, & Kohn, 2015; Kohn et al., 2012; Rholes et al., 2011; Wilson, Rholes, Simpson, & Tran, 2007). Couples completed questionnaires separately every 6 months, beginning approximately 6 weeks before the birth of their child and ending on their child's second birthday.

Attachment anxiety: Wilson et al. (2007) investigated women's responses to labor and delivery with questionnaires presented approximately two weeks after the birth of their infants. Feelings of closeness to their newborns and feelings of jealousy were our primary concern here. We expected anxious women to feel that they were not close to their babies, particularly when they felt jealous of their baby (i.e., felt that they were in competition with the baby for their partners' attention and affection). We found support for this hypothesis. Anxious women felt more jealousy than non-anxious women, and more jealous women in general felt less close to their infants. When jealousy was controlled for, however, anxious women felt closer to their infants than women who were not anxious. Jealousy, thus, seems to drive a wedge between anxious women and their babies.

Rholes et al. (2001) investigated perceptions of support available from romantic partners and its relationship to well-being. The support questionnaire asked about respondents' belief that support would be forthcoming from partners when needed. It did not assess support actually received. The hypothesis tested was that perceived support would predict marital satisfaction most strongly among anxious women. (Men's and women's data were analyzed separately in this study in part because the sexes did not always respond to the same questionnaires. For example, men were not asked to rate the support provided to them by their partners.) Consistent with the hypothesis, anxious women became more dissatisfied with their marriages over time when they thought their partners were not supportive. Anxious women who perceived their partners to be supportive, however, were as satisfied with their marriages as non-anxious women who also perceived their partners to be supportive. Non-anxious women were satisfied with their marriages no matter how much or how little support they perceived. These results confirm attachment theory's prediction that lack of support from partners undermines relationship satisfaction for some, but not all, people. To anxious people, a low level of support is destructive presumably because it confirms the negative view of attachment figures built into their working models. If a partner's lack of support further reinforces the view that no attachment figure will ever fully commit to them, it also reinforces the view, and fear, that they are essentially alone in the world. And, this could lead them be lonely, to believe that their lives lack meaning, to derive less purpose and satisfaction from rearing their children, to feel hopeless and depressed, and perhaps even to commit suicide. More encouragingly, this study's findings also show that anxious women who perceive their partners to be supportive can be as happy with their marriages as women who are not anxious. This reinforces attachment theory's view that relationships and attachment styles, not peoples' constitutional make-up, are the primary determinants of attachment-related behaviors and emotions.

Unfortunately, anxious people often fail to garner the level of support that they think they need. Collins and Feeney (2004) found that anxious people tend to perceive less support from their partners than is given. Romantic partners were video taped as they discussed a problem in their relationship. Partners then rated the support they thought they received from their partners and objective observers rated each partner's supportiveness. The researchers compared the two ratings of support and found that anxious partners' ratings were lower than the observers' ratings. Apparently, perceptual biases arising from negative views of romantic partners and expectations of non-support from attachment figures prevent anxious partners from seeing all of the support that their partners provide.

The problems that anxious people have with support are not due to perceptual biases exclusively. Rholes et al. (2001) found that the male partners of anxious women reported declining levels of support given to them during the transition regardless of the male partners' attachment styles. Disturbingly, men also attributed negative personality characteristics to their anxious partners. They viewed them as comparatively immature, needy, emotionally weak, and unstable, and these attributions fully mediated declines in support provided to anxious partners. Their partners' dependence and the amount of reassurance anxious women sought may have been judged by men to be excessive and may, thus, have caused a rift in the relationship.

Rholes et al. (2001) also found that among women, the correlations between attachment styles and relationship variables like the amount of support perceived or husbands' marital satisfaction were stronger at the time 2 testing session, when parents had been exposed to the stress of the transition for about 6 months, than they were in the comparatively less stressful pre-natal period. This finding is consistent with previous research that also shows that the apparent impact of attachment styles is greater during stressful conditions (Simpson, Rholes, & Nelligan, 1992). Attachment theory maintains that the attachment system varies in its activation and that it is more highly activated during stressful times (Bowlby, 1973). This means that the transition is a time when attachment styles should be more influential that they are at other times, and this highlights the importance of studying attachment styles during the transition period.

The findings for marital satisfaction in our second 2-year longitudinal study of the transition (Kohn et al., 2012) largely replicated those of Rholes et al. (2001). Men and women both reported lower levels of satisfaction if their partners were anxious. Women and men who were not anxious reported higher levels of marital satisfaction regardless of perceptions of support provided by their partners. Anxious women who perceived lower support reported less satisfaction than anxious women who perceived higher levels of support, and finally, anxious men were less satisfied with their marriages even when their partners offered higher levels of support.

The design of this study allowed us to look at the effects of partners on actors' marital satisfaction. Men were particularly dissatisfied with their marriages under two combined conditions: when their partners were anxious and when their anxious partners perceived them to be unsupportive. Men partnered with *non*-anxious women that perceived them to be unsupportive were relatively satisfied with their marriages. Anxious women who perceived their partners to be unsupportive may have engaged in a form of "toxic" behaviors that undermined their partners' satisfaction. When male partners perceived their female partners to be unsupportive, their marital satisfaction was unaffected regardless of their attachment style.

Rholes et al. (2011) investigated well-being as indicated by depressive symptoms. This study examined time since the birth of the child and respondents' gender as moderating factors. When anxious people perceived lower levels of support, women reported high depressive symptom levels at the beginning of the transition that remained high at least until her child was two years old. Men reported somewhat lower levels of depressive symptoms at the beginning of the transition, but their symptom levels increased over time and became as high as women's by the end of the study. When anxious people perceived higher support, their depression levels were relatively low, and they declined slightly over time. Men and women who were non-anxious reported lower symptom levels at the beginning of the study, which declined slightly over time. Like marital satisfaction, problems with depression tend to be the most problematic in people who are anxious and perceive less support available from their partners.

Avoidant Attachment. The association between depressive symptoms and avoidance was moderated by avoidant participants' feelings that their infant was interfering with their romantic relationship (Rholes et al., 2011). New parents who were avoidant and thought their infant was interfering by competing with them for the other parent's attention and affection showed higher levels of depressive symptoms. Perceptions that their baby was interfering with their outside activities (mostly leisure) was associated with more depressive symptoms among avoidant people as well. The findings regarding interference with the marital relationship may seem out of character for avoidant people. Relationships are multifaceted and serve multiple purposes and presumably different purposes for different kinds of people. Although seeking intimacy with partners is not high on the list of avoidant peoples' desires, having companionship with someone, having fun with someone, and related factors may be of great importance to them and that may be what they miss when their children seem to them to be interfering in their relationships.

Kohn et al. (2012) examined actor and partner effects on marital satisfaction in our 2-year study. They first found that marital satisfaction declined in general across the transition. Avoidance was associated with marital satisfaction, but the association depended on perceived family demands and work/family conflict. Avoidant actors were less satisfied with their marriages when they thought that the demands placed on them by family life were excessive and when they experienced higher levels of conflict between their family life and their work life. In both situations they can be described as "encumbered" when they want to be "unencumbered." One element of family demands that could be instrumental in lowering marital satisfaction is the demand to be involved in childcare. As Bowlby (1979) wrote, pressure to provide care to another is terrifying to avoidant people. Fillo et al. (2015) investigated marital satisfaction among avoidant people and the amount of infant care they provided in our 2-year study. Avoidant men who believed they were making higher contributions to childcare were among the people least satisfied with either their marriages or perhaps with the state of being married. They may yearn to be single again under these conditions. Moreover, their dissatisfaction grew over time. By the end of our investigation, when children were two years old, avoidant men that viewed themselves to be involved in higher levels of childcare were two standard deviations lower on marital satisfaction than non-avoidant men who also perceived themselves to be doing a lot of childcare. In general, avoidance had more impact on relationship satisfaction for men than women, perhaps because women are more strongly socialized into the parent role.

17.3 The Transition to Parenthood as an Opportunity for Personal Growth

What does personal growth mean in attachment theory? It is somewhat different from personal growth as it is discussed in humanistic psychology by authors like Maslow and Rogers. Growth from the perspective of attachment theory could mean ridding yourself of defenses that distort your understanding of the important events in your life that are related to the attachment system. It could mean being able to more accurately understand the people with whom you form romantic relationships, free of bias and defense. It could mean overcoming doubts about one's self-worth. All of these changes, however, come down to one thing: changing insecure attachment styles into secure ones. How this might happen is not entirely clear, and it seems likely to involve multiple processes. Bowlby (1980, pp. 230–231) presented one hypothesis regarding change in attachment styles. He hypothesized as follows: "there is certain information … that we find difficult to process. One example is information that is incompatible with our [working models]. In general, when new information clashes with established models…an old model may be replaced by a new one." Bowlby went on to describe this kind of change as slow and arduous because established models have for so long played a role in guiding behavior and organizing our thoughts about relationships.

We have conducted one study on the growth of security (or the decline of avoidance and/or anxiety) that was guided by Bowlby's (1973) hypothesis. Simpson, Rholes, Campbell, and Wilson (2003) examined change in attachment style occurring over a period of approximately 7.5 months, beginning approximately 6 weeks before the birth of parents' babies and ending when the babies were about 6 months old. These authors reasoned that the transition to parenthood might encourage change because it exposes parents to new information that may contradict assumptions built into their working models. This may lead them to reflect on their relationships, opening the way for change. The new information that may contradict established models can come from different sources. For example, one's behavior may change during the transition in ways that are inconsistent with an existing model, or one's relationship partner may behave in ways that clash with expectations contained in one's working model. Emotional responses to the infant (enjoyment, love, even awe) may also be a source of information that is incompatible with one's working model.

Simpson, Rholes, Campbell, and Wilson (2003) examined information that might come into one's awareness that changes the working model. They first analyzed change as a function of levels of perceived partner support as assessed at the prenatal testing session (6 weeks before the birth of the children). The authors reasoned that supportive partners of anxious people clash with their expectations of having a lack of support in their lives. Supportive partners, therefore, may cause anxious individuals to become less anxious. The results showed prospectively that perceptions of higher levels of partner support were associated with decreased levels of anxiety among women at the second testing session about 6 months after the birth of their infants. We did not ask men how supportive they found their partners to be.

Changes in avoidance also supported Bowlby's hypothesis. Providing support to partners is inconsistent with the avoidant working model and with a "terror" of becoming someone's caretaker, but men who perceived that they were providing higher levels of support to their partners at the pre-natal period were less avoidant at the 6-months testing session. We did not ask women how much support they gave to their male partners. Seeking support should also be inconsistent with the working models of avoidant people. An important goal of avoidant individuals is to keep the attachment system deactivated. To do so, avoidant people come to value independence, autonomy, and self-reliance, and they try to live guided by these values. They do not want others to depend on them and they do not want to become dependent on other people (Brennan et al., 1998). Support seeking, therefore, should be inconsistent with their working models. Women who reported more support seeking in the pre-natal test session were less avoidant at the 6-month testing session than they were before. To summarize, seeking support and feeling that support is available were each associated longitudinally with women becoming more secure, and giving support to their partners was associated longitudinally with men becoming more secure.

Would a study that attempted to replicate Simpson, Rholes, Campbell, and Wilson (2003) get the same results if it was conducted at a time other than the transition? In theory, it should. We can encounter information that is inconsistent with working models in a wide variety of settings, but how motivated are we at any given time to reconcile discrepant information? The transition period may be more conducive to change than other times. Greater interdependence of outcomes during the transition may make the good and bad aspects of relationships more salient. The attachment system should be more highly activated during the transition due to higher levels of stress (Mikulincer & Shaver, 2016). This could increase the cognitive availability of working models, making inconsistencies more noticeable and likely to produce change. The effects of the transition versus other periods on the likelihood of change is ultimately an unresolved empirical question. We bring it up to remind ourselves that the transition has a strong impact on new parents and in many ways is a unique experience.

17.4 New Directions in the Study of Attachment and the Transition to Parenthood

One way to extend research on the transition period would be to locate new behaviors that appear during the transition as a function of attachment style. To do this, one probably should scour the writings of Bowlby (1973, 1979). Another equally important way would be to use the theory to try to locate additional variables that moderate the effects of attachment styles during the transition. Additional factors that satisfy or aggravate the needs of people with insecure styles would probably be the most likely candidates. Finally, another way to move the field forward would be to ask whether there are new developments in attachment theory that might be relevant to the transition period. We want to conclude this chapter by reporting on a recent development in attachment theory, the introduction of the self-reported disorganized attachment style in adults.

The disorganized attachment style is quite different from avoidant and anxious styles. Avoidance and anxiety are organized methods of coping with the realities of getting attachment needs met when attachment figures do not play their caretaker role optimally. Anxious people cling, demand attention, and exaggerate the level of their distress, all to make what they see as an inattentive, uninvolved attachment figure respond to them. Avoidant people interact with attachment figures from a distance. As they see it, getting too close to attachment figures can antagonize them and lead them to further withdraw and further reject their needs for protection and comfort. Their interactions with attachment figures are an attempt to avoid neediness in an effort to keep the attachment figure as responsive as possible and to get their attachment needs met, at least minimally.

Disorganized behavior is different in that it does not appear to be a coherent coping strategy. It is the absence of a coherent strategy for getting attachment needs met when individuals are distressed. A principal cause of disorganized relationships is repeatedly experiencing a fear of attachment figures. When infants and children are repeatedly frightened by their attachment figure's behavior, disorganized relationships are expected to develop. Frightening behavior can come in many, sometimes subtle, forms. For instance, caregivers may seem to the child to be frightened of something that he or she does not see or understand. This can make the child afraid of the caregiver. Another fear-inducing behavior is absorption into dissociated states when interacting with the child. Overtly threatening behaviors, of course, also encourage disorganization as does sexualized treatment of the infant or child by the attachment figure (Lyons-Ruth & Jacobvitz, 2016).

Being fearful of an attachment figure creates a paradoxical state in which the attachment figure is both the cause and the solution to fear. Infants and children, when frightened, are "pushed" by the innate attachment system to turn to the caregiver for protection and relief of fear. Children's experiences with their attachment figures, however, may direct them to stay away. This "fright without solution" situation is one of the key psychological causes of disorganized attachments. For a discussion of other types of attachment figure behavior that can encourage disorganized attachments, see Lyons-Ruth and Jacobvitz (2016). At a more distal level of analysis, disorganization has been associated with long and repeated separations from attachment figures, severely inadequate care given to infants in orphanages, and physical or sexual abuse by caregivers (Bowlby, 1979; Lyons-Ruth & Jacobvitz, 2016).

Although most of the research on disorganization has involved infants and older children, the concept of disorganization in adults has a long history among developmental attachment researchers. They measure disorganization in connection with traumatic experiences. The Adult Attachment Interview (Main, Kaplan, & Cassidy, 1985) inquires about two kinds of trauma, child abuse and the death of someone close. Interviewees are classified as "unresolved/disorganized" depending on the way in which they talk about trauma. Deep absorption during questions about trauma, making statements about traumatic experiences that logically cannot be true, or losing touch with the context of the interview are examples of the behavior that characterizes interviewees placed in the unresolved/disorganized category. The concept of disorganization arrived at through pathways other than failure to resolve these two traumatic experiences does not exist among developmental researchers.

Paetzold, Rholes, and Kohn (2015) recently introduced a self-report measure of disorganization within adult romantic relationships. They view disorganization as including three major themes: confusion about romantic relationships, overt fear of romantic partners, and the idea that attachment figures are untrustworthy and trusting them can be dangerous. Efforts to validate the scale thus far have sought to determine whether the correlates of adult disorganization measured by this scale match the correlates of disorganization as assessed in infancy and childhood. Disorganization is considered the most insecure form of attachment. Therefore, developmentalists have focused on the relationship between disorganization and clinical variables.

Disorders found among adults with a childhood history of a disorganized relationship with an attachment figure prominently include dissociation and borderline personality, among others. Longitudinal studies of these disorders assess disorganization in infancy or later childhood and link it with adults' and older children's behavior and personality problems. Some key findings of these longitudinal studies are that infant and childhood disorganization are predictors of adult dissociation and borderline personality (Liotti, 1992; Ogawa, Sroufe, Weinfield, Carlson, & Egeland, 1997). Another finding is that early measures of disorganization predict later externalizing behavior (behavior that is angry, oppositional, aggressive, etc.) in older children (Fearon, Bakermans-Kranenburg, van Ijzendoorn, Lapsley, & Roisman, 2010; Groh, Roisman, van Ijzendoorn, Bakermans-Kranenburg, & Fearon, 2012).

Do adults who self-report disorganization behave in similar ways and have similar problems in adulthood? Are they more angry and aggressive in their relationships and more likely to report symptoms of dissociative and borderline disorders? Rholes, Paetzold, and Kohn (2016) found that women and men who scored high on the disorganization scale reported being more angry and aggressive toward their romantic partners. This study also showed that adult disorganization partially mediated the effects of child abuse on anger and aggression in relationships in adulthood. Paetzold, Rholes, and Andrus (2017) found that adults assessed as disorganized have dissociative tendencies, just like adults who were assessed as having disorganized relationships in infancy and childhood. They also found that disorganization and two forms of victimization, child abuse and current abuse by romantic partners, interacted to predict dissociation. The relationship between abuse and dissociation was more strongly positive when victims were more disorganized. Finally, in Paetzold et al. (2015) more disorganized adults had more symptoms of both depression and anxiety. This is significant because disorganized children also are vulnerable to depression (Groh et al., 2012).

How might disorganization in terms of relationships affect the transition to parenthood? The characteristics of disorganization in romantic relationships could easily affect spousal relationships during the transition in adverse ways. It could also affect the relationship with the newborn child. Because adults who are disorganized report more anger and aggression toward their partners at times other than the transition, the stress associated with the transition to parenthood could exacerbate such behavior, making the transition a particularly difficult time, perhaps especially for new mothers. Avoidance and anxiety have been linked to abusive behavior; a combination of avoidance and anxiety seems most likely to be associated with abuse (Mikulincer & Shaver, 2016). The connection between disorganization and abusive behavior is unstudied, but we do know that more disorganized adults report more often that they have behaved violently during a conflict with their partner (Rholes et al., 2016). Abusive behavior during the transition would, of course, have devastating effects. Thus, violence and aggression during the transition is a topic that strongly invites study.

The dissociative tendencies of adults with disorganized attachment styles may also prove to be important. Dissociative tendencies were mentioned above as an example of ways in which attachment figures incite fear in infants and young children, and fear is one of the factors involved in children developing disorganized relationships with attachment figures. The increased stress encountered during the transition could make dissociative tendencies more prevalent in the behavior of disorganized mothers and fathers. New, yet unpublished research by the authors of this chapter has found that the impact of disorganization on dissociation increases when adults have or have had problematic relationships with attachment figures as children or adults. Events within the transition may play the same role, increasing the strength of the connection between disorganization and dissociation. The connection between disorganization and symptoms of borderline personality are particularly troubling, as the romantic relationships of borderline people are often deeply disturbed. We are only beginning to scratch the surface of the problems associated with disorganization. Within a few years, the ways in which disorganization affects individuals during the transition should be better understood. In our opinion introducing disorganization into the study of the transition could be particularly fruitful for research.

To bring this chapter to an end, how can we summarize the findings that we have now in just one word? For anxious people going through the transition, the word would be Security. For avoidant individuals going through the transition the word would be Freedom.

References

Bowlby, J. (1973). *Attachment and loss. Vol 2. Separation, anxiety and anger*. New York, NY: Basic Books.

Bowlby, J. (1979). *The making and breaking of affectional bonds*. London: Travistock.

Bowlby, J. (1980). *Attachment and loss: Vol. 3. Loss, sadness and depression*. New York, NY: Basic Books.

Brennan, K. A., Clark, C. L., & Shaver, P. R. (1998). Self-report measurement of adult romantic attachment: An integrative overview. In J. A. Simpson & W. S. Rholes (Eds.), *Attachment theory and close relationships*. New York, NY: Guilford Press.

Collins, N. L., & Feeney, B. C. (2004). Working models of attachment shape perceptions of social support: Evidence from experimental and observational studies. *Journal of Personality and Social Psychology, 87*(3), 363–383.

Fearon, R. M. P., Bakermans-Kranenburg, M. J., Van Ijzendoorn, M. H., Lapsey, A., & Roisman, G. I. (2010). The significance of insecure attachment and disorganization in the development of children's externalizing behavior: A meta-analytic study. *Child Development, 81*(2), 435–456.

Fillo, J., Simpson, J. A., Rholes, W. S., & Kohn, J. L. (2015). Dads doing diapers: Individual and relational outcomes associated with the division of childcare across the transition to parenthood. *Journal of Personality and Social Psychology, 108*(2), 298–316.

Groh, A. M., Roisman, G. I., Van Ijzendoorn, M. H., Bakermans-Kranenburg, M. J., & Fearon, R. P. (2012). The significance of insecure and disorganized attachment for children's internalizing symptoms: A meta-analytic study. *Child Development, 83*(2), 591–610.

Jones, J. D., Cassidy, J., & Shaver, P. R. (2015). Adult attachment styles and parenting. In J. A. Simpson & W. S. Rholes (Eds.), *Attachment theory and research: New direction and emerging themes* (pp. 234–260). New York, NY: Guilford Press.

Kohn, J. L., Rholes, W. S., Simpson, J. A., Martin, A. M., Tran, S., & Wilson, C. L. (2012). Changes in marital satisfaction across the transition to parenthood: The role of adult attachment orientations. *Personality and Social Psychology Bulletin, 38*(11), 1506–1522.

Liotti, G. (1992). Disorganized/disoriented attachment in the etiology of the dissociative disorders. *Dissociation: Progress in the Dissociative Disorders, 5*(4), 196–204.

Lyons-Ruth, K., & Jacobvitz, D. (2016). Attachment disorganization from infancy to adulthood: Neurobiological correlates, parenting contexts, and pathways to disorder. In J. Cassidy & P. R. Shaver (Eds.), *Handbook of attachment: Theory, research, and clinical applications* (3rd ed., pp. 667–695). New York, NY: Guilford Press.

Main, M., Kaplan, N., & Cassidy, J. (1985). Security in infancy, childhood, and adulthood: A move to the level of representation. *Monographs of the Society for Research in Child Development, 50*(1–2), 66–104.

Mikulincer, M., & Shaver, P. R. (2016). *Attachment in adulthood: Structure dynamics and change* (2nd ed.). New York: Gilford Press.

Ogawa, J. R., Sroufe, L. A., Weinfeld, N. S., Carlson, E. A., & Egeland, B. (1997). Development and the fragmented self: Longitudinal study of dissociative symptomatology in nonclinical sample. *Development and Psychopathology, 9*(4), 855–879.

Paetzold, R. L., Rholes, W. S., & Andrus, J. L. (2017). A Bayesian analysis of the link between adult disorganized attachment and dissociative symptoms. *Personality and Individual Differences, 107*, 17–22.

Paetzold, R. L., Rholes, W. S., & Kohn, J. L. (2015). Disorganized attachment in adulthood: Theory, measurement, and implications of romantic relationships. *Review of General Psychology, 19*(2), 146–156.

Rholes, W. S., Paetzold, R. P., & Kohn, J. L. (2016). Disorganized attachment mediates the link from early trauma to externalizing behavior in adult relationships. *Personality and Individual Differences, 90*, 61–65.

Rholes, W. S., Simpson, J. A., Campbell, L., & Grich, J. (2001). Adult attachment and the transition to parenthood. *Journal of Personality and Social Psychology, 81*(3), 421–435.

Rholes, W. S., Simpson, J. A., Kohn, J. L., Wilson, C. L., Martin, A. M., III, Tran, S., et al. (2011). Attachment orientations and depression: A longitudinal study of new parents. *Journal of Personality and Social Psychology, 100*(4), 567–586.

Simpson, J. A., Rholes, W. S., Campbell, L., Tran, S., & Wilson, C. L. (2003a). Adult attachment, the transition to parenthood, and depressive symptoms. *Journal of Personality and Social Psychology, 84*(6), 1172–1187.

Simpson, J. A., Rholes, W. S., Campbell, L., & Wilson, C. L. (2003b). Changes in attachment orientations across the transition to parenthood. *Journal of Experimental Social Psychology, 39*(4), 317–331.

Simpson, J. A., Rholes, W. S., & Nelligan, J. (1992). Support seeking and support giving within couples in an anxiety provoking situation: The role of attachment styles. *Journal of Personality and Social Psychology, 62*(3), 434–446.

Wilson, C. L., Rholes, W. S., Simpson, J. A., & Tran, S. (2007). Labor, delivery, and early parenthood: An attachment theory perspective. *Personality and Social Psychology Bulletin, 33*(4), 505–518.

Chapter 18
Attachment, Caregiving, and Parenting

Mario Mikulincer and Phillip R. Shaver

18.1 Introduction

In his exposition of attachment theory, Bowlby (1973, 1980, 1982, 1988) emphasized the importance of positive interactions with caring and protective others (*attachment figures*) in times of need and the resulting sense of security (confidence that one is competent and lovable and that others will be supportive when needed) for emotion regulation, psychological well-being, and prosocial behavior. This sense of security allows a person to cope constructively with stressful events, maintain self-esteem and emotional stability, engage in satisfactory and harmonious interpersonal relations, and be empathic and compassionate toward needy and vulnerable others who seek care and attention (see Mikulincer & Shaver, 2016, for a review).

Originally, attachment theory (Bowlby, 1982) was formulated to explain infant-parent emotional bonding and the functioning of the *attachment behavioral system* (the system that governs people's—especially young children's—search for proximity to attachment figures in times of need) during infancy and early childhood. However, based on Bowlby's (1979, p. 129) claim that attachment needs and behaviors are active "from the cradle to the grave," adult attachment researchers have examined individual variations in attachment-system functioning within couple and family relationships. Specifically, they have shown that these individual differences underlie the quality of both couple relationships and parenting (see Jones, Cassidy, & Shaver, 2015; Mikulincer & Shaver, 2018, for reviews). In the case of parenting, the observed attachment-related variations are thought to reflect the underlying effects of attachment-system dynamics on the functioning of what Bowlby (1982) called the

M. Mikulincer (✉)
School of Psychology, Interdisciplinary Center (IDC) Herzliya, 46150 Herzliya, Israel
e-mail: Mario@idc.ac.il

P. R. Shaver
Department of Psychology, University of California, One Shields Avenue, Davis, CA 95616-8686, USA
e-mail: prshaver@ucdavis.edu

O. Taubman – Ben-Ari (ed.), *Pathways and Barriers to Parenthood*,
https://doi.org/10.1007/978-3-030-24864-2_18

"caregiving behavioral system"—an innate behavioral system in parents and other caregivers that responds to the needs of dependent others, especially (but not limited to) children. Our goal in this chapter is to summarize what we have learned about the link between the attachment and caregiving systems and understand how attachment security and insecurities shape parenting-related cognitions, feelings, and behavior.

We begin the chapter by explaining the behavioral system construct and showing how individual differences in a person's attachment system affect the functioning of the caregiving system. We then review adult attachment studies that show how individual differences in attachment security and insecurities explain variations in parenting-related desires and attitudes among childless adults, parenting-related expectations during pregnancy, emotional reactions during the transition to parenthood, and parent's cognitive, emotional, and behavioral reactions during interactions with their children during infancy, childhood, and adolescence.

18.2 A Behavioral Systems Perspective on Attachment and Caregiving

In explaining human behavior, Bowlby (1982) borrowed from ethology the concept of *behavioral system*, a species-universal neural program that organizes an individual's behavior in ways that increase the likelihood of survival and reproductive success. Each behavioral system is organized around a particular goal (e.g., attaining a sense of safety and security, providing support to a needy other) and includes a set of interchangeable, functionally equivalent behaviors that constitute the *primary strategy* of the system for attaining its goal (e.g., proximity seeking, empathically understanding another person's needs). These behaviors are automatically activated by stimuli or situations that make a particular goal salient (e.g., a signal of danger) and terminated by other stimuli or outcomes that signal attainment of the desired goal.

Bowlby (1973) believed that although behavioral systems are innate, experience shapes their parameters and strategies in various ways, resulting in systematic individual differences. According to Bowlby, the residues of such experiences are stored in the form of mental representations, or *working models of self and others,* that guide future attempts to attain a behavioral system's goal. With repeated use, these models become automatic and are important sources of within-person continuity in behavioral system functioning throughout development.

18.2.1 The Attachment Behavioral System

According to Bowlby (1982), the biological function of the attachment system is to protect a person from danger by assuring that he or she maintains proximity to loving and supportive attachment figures. The proximal goal of the system is to restore and strengthen the inner sense of attachment security, which normally terminates the system's activation. The goal of attaining security is made salient by perceived threats and dangers, which drive people to seek actual or symbolic proximity to attachment figures. During infancy, proximity seeking involves nonverbal expressions of need, such as crying and pleading, and locomotor behaviors (crawling, toddling) aimed at reestablishing and maintaining proximity to a caregiver (Ainsworth, 1991). In adulthood, this attachment strategy also includes many other means of establishing contact (e.g., talking directly to or phoning an attachment figure) as well as activating soothing mental representations of attachment figures (e.g., Mikulincer, Gillath, & Shaver, 2002).

The consolidation of a solid sense of attachment security following repeated positive interactions with supportive attachment figures in times of need promotes general faith in other people's good will; a sense of being loved, esteemed, understood, and accepted by relationship partners; and optimistic beliefs about one's ability to handle challenges, frustration, and distress. Bowlby (1988) considered attachment security to be a mainstay of mental health and social adjustment throughout life. A host of cross-sectional and longitudinal studies strongly support this view (see Mikulincer & Shaver, 2016, for reviews).

However, when attachment figures are not reliably available, responsive, and supportive, a sense of attachment security is not attained, negative working models are constructed, worries about self-protection and lovability are heightened, and strategies of affect regulation (which Cassidy & Kobak, 1988, called *secondary attachment strategies*) other than appropriate proximity seeking are adopted. Attachment theorists (e.g., Cassidy & Kobak, 1988; Mikulincer & Shaver, 2016) emphasize two such secondary strategies: *hyperactivation* and *deactivation* of the attachment system. Hyperactivation is manifested in energetic attempts to gain greater proximity, support, and protection, combined with a lack of confidence that it will be provided. Deactivation of the system involves inhibition of proximity-seeking tendencies, denial of attachment needs, maintenance of emotional and cognitive distance from others, and compulsive reliance on oneself as the only reliable source of comfort and protection.

When studying these secondary strategies during adolescence and adulthood, attachment researchers have focused mainly on a person's *attachment orientation*—a chronic pattern of relational cognitions and behaviors that results from a particular history of attachment experiences (Fraley & Shaver, 2000). These orientations can be conceptualized as regions in a continuous two-dimensional space (e.g., Brennan, Clark, & Shaver, 1998). One dimension, attachment-related *avoidance*, reflects the extent to which a person distrusts others' good will and relies on deactivating strategies for coping with threats and attachment insecurities. The other dimension, attachment *anxiety*, reflects the degree to which a person worries that relationship partners will be unavailable or unhelpful in times of need and relies on hyperactivating strategies. People who score low on both insecurity dimensions are said to be secure with respect to attachment or securely attached.

Although a person's attachment orientation is fairly stable over the life span (see Cassidy & Shaver, 2016, for updated reviews), one should note that it is actually the most dominant mental representation within a complex network of representations that includes other less dominant episodic, context-specific, and relationship-anchored memories and schemas (Collins & Read, 1994). Therefore, current experiences and contextual cues can cause less dominant attachment-related representations to become temporarily salient and lead a person to react and behave in ways that fit the currently salient representations. Many studies have experimentally primed security representations (*security priming*) and have found that even people with insecure attachment patterns react and behave in a more secure manner under the influence of such stimuli (e.g., Mikulincer & Shaver, 2001). In these experiments, presentation of pictures suggesting attachment-figure availability (e.g., a Picasso drawing of a mother cradling an infant in her arms); presentation of the names of actual people designated by participants as security-enhancing attachment figures; guided imagery concerning the availability and supportiveness of an attachment figure; visualization of the faces of security-enhancing attachment figures; and viewing the photograph of an attachment figure have all been found to increase participants' positive affect, self-esteem, optimism, empathy, prosocial behavior, and resilience, and to reduce negative attitudes toward outgroups (See Mikulincer & Shaver, 2016, for a review of these findings.)

18.2.2 The Caregiving Behavioral System

According to Bowlby (1982), human beings are born with a capacity to provide protection and support to others who are either chronically dependent or temporarily in need. Bowlby (1982) claimed that these behaviors are organized by a *caregiving behavioral system* that emerged over the long course of evolution because it improved the inclusive fitness of humans by augmenting the likelihood that children, siblings, and tribe members with whom a person shared genes would survive to reproductive age and succeed in producing and rearing offspring (Hamilton, 1964). Although the caregiving system presumably evolved primarily to increase the viability of an individual's own offspring and close relatives, it may also have been more generally adapted to respond to the needs of other tribe members, and it can be extended through socialization to include genuine concern for anyone in need (Wilson, 2014).

According to Bowlby (1982), the goal of the caregiving system is to reduce other people's suffering, protect them from harm, and foster their growth and development. That is, the caregiving system is designed to serve two major functions: (1) meeting another person's needs for protection in times of danger or distress (which Bowlby, 1982, called "providing a safe haven") and (2) supporting others' exploration, autonomy, and growth when exploration is safe and desirable (Bowlby, 1982, called this function "providing a secure base for exploration"). From this perspective, the goal of a care seeker's attachment system (to maintain a safe haven and secure base) is also the aim of his or her care provider's caregiving system. When a caregiver's behavioral system is activated by another person who needs help, the primary strategy of the system is to perceive the needy individual's problem accurately and provide effective aid. According to Collins, Guichard, Ford, and Feeney (2006), effective caregiving is characterized by two core qualities: sensitivity (being attuned to, and accurately interpreting, another person's signals of need) and responsiveness (validating the other person's needs, perceptions, and feelings; respecting his or her beliefs and values; and providing useful support).

Although Bowlby (1982) assumed that everyone is born with the potential to become an effective care provider, effective functioning of the caregiving system depends on several factors. Effective caregiving can be impaired by feelings, beliefs, and concerns that dampen or conflict with motivation to help or with the traits of sensitivity and responsiveness. It can also be impaired by deficits in social skills, fatigue, and problems in emotion regulation that cause a caregiver to feel overwhelmed by a needy other's pain or to wish to distance oneself physically, emotionally, or cognitively from the person's problems and distress (e.g., Cassidy, Stern, Mikulincer, Martin, & Shaver, 2018; Collins et al., 2006).

Following this reasoning, we (Shaver, Mikulincer, & Shemesh-Iron, 2010) proposed that if a person's caregiving system develops under favorable social circumstances, then compassion, empathy, sensitivity, and responsiveness become common reactions to other people's needs. However, if the caregiving system does not develop under favorable circumstances, because of an absence of parental modeling, training, and support, or because of interactions with parents that engender insecurities and worries, a person is likely to be less sensitive and less responsive with respect to other people's needs and suffering (see Shaver, Mikulincer, Gross, Stern, & Cassidy, 2016, for an extensive review).

18.2.3 Interplay of the Attachment and Caregiving Systems

Bowlby (1982) noticed that activation of the attachment system can interfere with the operation of the caregiving system, because potential caregivers may feel that obtaining safety and care for themselves is more urgent than providing care to others. At such times, people are likely to be so focused on their own vulnerability and need for protection that they lack the mental resources needed to attend sensitively to others' needs and respond effectively to them (Gilbert, 2014). Only when a sense of attachment security is restored can a potential caregiver perceive others to be not only potential sources of protection and support, but also worthy human beings who themselves need and deserve sympathy and support.

Reasoning along these lines, attachment theorists (e.g., Collins et al., 2006; Kunce & Shaver, 1994) hypothesized that attachment security provides an important foundation for effective caregiving. Moreover, a person who is more secure with respect to attachment is likely to have experienced and benefited earlier in life from effective care provided by responsive attachment figures. This means that secure adults have mental representations of compassionate and generous caregivers when they themselves occupy the caregiving role. Moreover, secure individuals' comfort with intimacy and interdependence allow them to respond favorably when another person is in need of support. In addition, secure people's positive working models of others make it easier for them to perceive others as deserving sympathy and support, whereas their positive self-representations allow them to feel confident that they can deal with others' needs or distress without being overwhelmed by them.

In contrast, attachment insecurities are likely to interfere with responsive care provision (e.g., Collins et al., 2006). Attachment anxiety leads people to focus on their own distress and unmet attachment needs, which may draw mental resources away from attending accurately to others' needs. Moreover, strong desire for closeness, support, and love related to attachment anxiety may taint caregiving motives with egoistic desires for acceptance and grateful approval, which can impair effective helping. The lack of comfort with closeness and negative working models of others that is associated with avoidant attachment may also interfere with the provision of sensitive and responsive care. People scoring high on attachment-related avoidance may back away rather than get involved with a needy and vulnerable person, preferring to detach themselves emotionally, cognitively, and physically.

In the remainder of this chapter, we review studies that test these theoretical ideas about the interplay of attachment and caregiving motives and processes within the context of parenting. We particularly focus on studies that have measured individual differences in adult attachment orientations and then have assessed parenting-related cognitions, feelings, and behaviors.

18.3 Evidence Concerning Attachment-Related Variations in Parental Caregiving

Many researchers have assessed parents' attachment orientations and examined their effects on mental representations of parenting, emotional reactions to the transition to parenthood, physiological responses to parenting-related stimuli, and parental caregiving behavior. Most such studies have focused on mothers' responses and have relied mainly on the Adult Attachment Interview (AAI, George, Kaplan, & Main, 1996) to assess adult attachment patterns. Nevertheless, the major findings have been replicated in studies that have focused on fathers or have used self-report attachment scales (for a review, see Jones et al., 2015).

18.3.1 Mental Representations of Parental Caregiving

According to attachment theory, adults preparing for parenthood and those who have already become parents develop mental representations of themselves as caregivers and of the parent-child relationship (Mikulincer & Shaver, 2016). Attachment insecurities can negatively bias these mental representations and raise worries and doubts about oneself as a parent and the quality of the relationship one will form with one's children.

Studies conducted among childless adults have found that attachment-related avoidance is consistently associated with less desire to have children (e.g., Rholes, Simpson, & Friedman, 2006; Wilson, Rholes, Simpson, & Tran, 2007). In addition, less secure non-parents have been found to be less positive when judging their ability to relate to children, imagining interactions with their own future child, and evaluating their closeness to that child (e.g., Rholes, Simpson, Blakely, Lanigan, & Allen, 1997; Scharf & Mayseless, 2011). Studies also indicate that more attachment-anxious people have more unrealistic, and perfectionist views of their imagined performance as parents (e.g., Snell, Overbey, & Brewer, 2005).

Conceptually similar results have been obtained in studies of adults who were already parents. Using either the AAI or self-report attachment scales, these studies reveal that less secure parents experienced less joy and pleasure during interactions with their children (e.g., Berlin et al., 2011; Rholes et al., 2006) and feel less close to them (e.g., Rholes, Simpson, & Blakely, 1995; Wilson et al., 2007). Several studies have also found that less secure people report heightened parenting-related distress (e.g., Fonseca, Nazaré, & Canavarro, 2013; Lionetti, Pastore, & Barone, 2015).

Less secure parents also scored lower on scales measuring parental satisfaction (e.g., La Valley & Guerrero, 2012; Rholes et al., 2006), and they appraised themselves as less able to cope with the demands and challenges of pregnancy, childbirth, and parenthood (e.g., Berant, Mikulincer, & Florian, 2001; Trillingsgaard, Elklit, Shevlin, & Maimburg, 2011). In addition, insecure mothers had more worries and anxieties about separation from their children (e.g., Taubman – Ben-Ari & Katz-Ben-Ami, 2008; Vasquez, Durik, & Hyde, 2002). Insecure parents also described themselves as less competent in accomplishing parenting tasks (e.g., Howard, 2010; Kohlhoff & Barnett, 2013), perceived greater costs in becoming a parent (e.g., Taubman – Ben-Ari, Ben Shlomo, Sivan, & Dolizki, 2009), and reported less competence in handling their children's distress (e.g., DeOliveira, Moran, & Pederson, 2005).

18.3.2 Emotional Reactions to the Transition to Parenthood

Having a baby is typically a joyful but stressful experience, but it can have different and even opposite psychological repercussions for some parents. For many parents, the transition to parenthood is a growth-inducing experience that increases their happiness and emotional well-being and heightens their sense of meaning in life. For other people, however, this transition can heighten personal and relational doubts and worries, erode relationship satisfaction, and increase the risk for depression (a form of distress that clinicians call *postpartum depression*). Research has consistently found that parents' attachment orientations influence individual variations in reactions to this transition (see Rholes & Paetzold, Chap. 17 in this volume). For example, insecure attachment (assessed during pregnancy or soon after delivery, using either the AAI or self-report scales) has been found to predict higher levels of postnatal depression over periods ranging from 6 months to 2 years (e.g., Iles, Slade, & Spiby, 2011; Rholes et al., 2011; Simpson, Rholes, Campbell, Tran, & Wilson, 2003). In addition, more anxious women and their male partners tend to perceive lower levels of spousal support and experience sharper declines in marital satisfaction, which in turn exacerbate depressive reactions (e.g., Kohn et al., 2012; Rholes, Simpson, Campbell, & Grich, 2001; Rholes et al., 2011). Interestingly, more avoidant men who believe their baby is interfering with their career or personal life or who feel that they are doing too much childcare also report sharper declines in marital satisfaction (e.g., Fillo, Simpson, Rholes, & Kohn, 2015; Kohn et al., 2012).

Attachment studies have also identified relational factors that mitigate the detrimental effects of attachment insecurities during the transition to parenthood. There is evidence, for example, that anxiously attached women do not show heightened postpartum depression when they perceive more support and care from their husbands (e.g., Rholes et al., 2011; Simpson et al., 2003) or when husbands themselves report more effective support of their wives during pregnancy (e.g., Conde, Figueiredo, & Bifulco, 2011). Thus, it seems that husbands' emotional support mitigates anxious wives' worries and concerns and thereby protects them from postpartum depression.

18.3.3 Parenting-Related Physiological Responses

Another line of research focuses on adults' brain responses to parenting-related stimuli (e.g., a picture of an infant's face, an infant's facial or vocal emotional expression) and examines how these responses are moderated by attachment orientations. For example, Riem, Bakermans-Kranenburg, van IJzendoorn, Out, and Rombouts (2012) found that attachment insecurities were associated with heightened amygdala activation (using functional Magnetic Resonance Imaging—fMRI) during exposure to infant crying in a sample of nulliparous women. In another fMRI study, Strathearn, Fonagy, Amico, and Montague (2009) found that less secure first-time mothers exhibited less activation in dopaminergic reward regions of the brain, such as the ventral striatum, in response to pictures of their own infant's emotional expressions. Taking together, these findings imply that insecure mothers' brains react to infant emotional expressions with heightened fear-related avoidance responses (amygdala hyperactivation) and inhibition of approach responses (ventral striatum deactivation), which in turn may prevent sensitivity and responsiveness to an infant's distress.

There is also evidence that autonomic responses to an infant's emotional expressions tend to be affected by attachment orientations (e.g., Ablow, Marks, Feldman, & Huffman, 2013; Schoenmaker et al., 2015; Spangler, Maier, Geserick, & von Wahlert, 2010). For example, Spangler et al. (2010) assessed first-time parents' mimicking responses (facial muscle activity) and eyelid reflexes (using a startle paradigm) to infant photographs depicting positive, neutral, and negative emotions. More secure parents showed more mimic responses to an infant's variations in emotional expressions—a sign of empathic, approach responses. In addition, avoidant parents showed heightened startle response to infants' expressions of negative emotions, implying an autonomic stress response to infants' signals of distress.

In exploring the hormonal basis of parental caregiving, Edelstein, Stanton, Henderson, and Sanders (2010) found that avoidant attachment was negatively associated with estradiol levels—a hormone that seems to sustain parenting behavior. In a subsequent study, Edelstein, Kean, and Chopik (2012) examined estradiol variations in response to a movie depicting an intimate parent-child interaction. Whereas women scoring low on avoidant attachment reacted to the parent-child clip with increased estradiol levels, those scoring high on avoidance did not.

18.3.4 Parental Caregiving Behavior

In one of the first studies of attachment-related predictors of maternal sensitivity, Haft and Slade (1989) administered the AAI to mothers of 9- to 23-month-old infants and videotaped interactions between them and their children, later coding the tapes for a mother's noticing of and attunement to her child's positive and negative emotions. As compared with insecure mothers, secure mothers were more consistent in reacting to their baby's emotions and needs. Anxious mothers attuned inconsistently to both positive and negative emotions, whereas avoidant mothers seemed to ignore negative emotions.

Following this pioneering study, dozens of studies have consistently documented attachment-related variations (using the AAI) in mother's sensitivity and responsiveness to their infants during videotaped free-play sessions and unstructured observations of everyday mothering behavior at home (e.g., Bernier & Matte-Gagné, 2011; Shlafer, Raby, Lawler, Hesemeyer, & Roisman, 2014). Specifically, insecure mothers are less attentive and responsive to their infant's needs than secure mothers, and are more distressed and intrusive when interacting with their infant. Some of these studies found attachment-related differences in parental behavior even when the AAI was administered before the child's birth, thus precluding an alternative explanation in terms of effects of children's temperament on mothers' attachment orientations.

In a recent diary study, Lang, Schoppe-Sullivan, Kotila, and Kamp Dush (2013) found that the link between attachment insecurities (assessed with a self-report scale) and parental behavior is more complex and depends on the nature of the assessed activities. For example, more anxious parents reported less engagement in exploration-focused activities with their infant (activities that stimulate and build the infant's knowledge). In addition, more anxious fathers (but not mothers) reported less engagement in proximity-focused activities (activities that involve physical or emotional connection with the infant).

Similar attachment-related variations have been reported in studies that have assessed the quality of support mothers provide to their preschool children during challenging cognitive tasks (e.g., Crowell, Warner, Davis, Marraccini, & Dearing, 2010; Whipple, Bernier, & Mageau, 2011). Specifically, secure mothers were rated by independent judges as warmer and more supportive than insecure mothers. In addition, whereas avoidant mothers were less sensitive and more controlling and task-focused (e.g., Crowell & Feldman, 1989; Whipple et al., 2011), anxious mothers gave confusing instructions (e.g., Crowell & Feldman, 1989), were distressed and intrusive when trying to help their children (e.g., Bosquet & Egeland, 2001), and provided less autonomy support (Whipple et al., 2011).

Additional studies assessed actual mothers' behavior during joint activities (e.g., playing, drawing, reading a book) with their preschool or school-aged children (e.g., Biringen et al., 2000; Busch, Cowan, & Cowan, 2008; Verschueren, Dossche, Marcoen, Mahieu, & Bakermans-Kranenburg, 2006). As expected, secure mothers displayed more warmth, responsiveness, and supportiveness than insecure mothers. They also tended to engage in more synchronous give-and-take interactions with their children, provided better task organization and structure, and had fewer difficult interactions with their children.

There is also evidence that insecure parents' non-optimal parenting behaviors are manifested during interactions with their adolescent offspring (e.g., García-Ruiz, Rodrigo, Hernández-Cabrera, & Máiquez, 2013; Jones, Brett, Ehrlich, Lejuez, & Cassidy, 2014; Jones & Cassidy, 2014). For example, Jones and Cassidy (2014) found that a mother's avoidance (assessed with a self-report scale) was related to less supportive behavior during a conflict management discussion with her adolescent offspring (as rated by observers). In addition, mother's avoidance was related to more hostile behavior toward the adolescent offspring and to the adolescent's less positive perceptions of the mother, which in turn tended to interfere with support provision and use of support during the conflict-laden discussion.

Beyond interfering with sensitive and responsive caregiving, attachment insecurities also impair the coordination of parenting by mothers and fathers (co-parenting). Talbot, Baker, and McHale (2009) asked couples transitioning to parenthood to complete the AAI and to participate in an assessment of co-parenting conflict and cohesion at 3 months postpartum. Maternal insecure attachment predicted higher levels of co-parental conflict, whereas paternal insecure attachment predicted lower co-parental cohesion. Similar findings were reported by Bouchard (2014) and Sheftall, Schoppe-Sullivan, and Futris (2010) who relied on self-report measures of attachment orientations.

18.4 Concluding Comments

Attachment theory and research provide good leads for fostering "good-enough" parenting and enjoying the transition to parenthood and interactions with growing children. Research clearly indicates that the functioning of the attachment behavioral system affects the workings of the caregiving system, making it likely that heightening attachment security will yield benefits in the realm of sensitive and responsive caregiving, which in turn will be manifested in positive and growth-oriented parenting cognitions, feelings, and behaviors. Research on attachment and caregiving suggests several ways to encourage this move toward attachment security and growth-oriented parenting. One is to care for children in ways that enhance their sense of security, which, besides having many benefits for the children themselves, makes it much more likely that they will be good parents in later years. Another way to heighten a person's sense of security is to have him or her regularly recall times when beneficial support was provided, or to imagine similar situations, perhaps even ones depicted in religious stories or inspiring works of art. Once a person has benefited from another's care, or deliberately imagined and emulated the kinds of care and concern for others exhibited by supportive parents, Jesus, the Buddha, or Gandhi, merely calling these exemplars to mind seems to have security-enhancing effects, as does exposure to pictures and drawings of examples of loving kindness. We suspect that many of these procedures foster sensitive and responsive caregiving in two ways, by enhancing a person's sense of security and by providing models of good caregiving.

References

Ablow, J. C., Marks, A. K., Feldman, S., & Huffman, L. C. (2013). Associations between first-time expectant women's representations of attachment and their physiological reactivity to infant cry. *Child Development, 84*(4), 1373–1391.

Ainsworth, M. D. S. (1991). Attachment and other affectional bonds across the life cycle. In C. M. Parkes, J. Stevenson-Hinde, & P. Marris (Eds.), *Attachment across the life cycle* (pp. 33–51). New York: Routledge.

Berant, E., Mikulincer, M., & Florian, V. (2001). Attachment style and mental health: A 1-year follow-up study of mothers of infants with congenital heart disease. *Personality and Social Psychology Bulletin, 27*(8), 956–968.

Berlin, L. J., Whiteside-Mansell, L., Roggman, L. A., Green, B. L., Robinson, J., & Spieker, S. (2011). Testing maternal depression and attachment style as moderators of early head start's effects on parenting. *Attachment & Human Development, 13*(1), 49–67.

Bernier, A., & Matte-Gagné, C. (2011). More bridges: Investigating the relevance of self-report and interview measures of adult attachment for marital and caregiving relationships. *International Journal of Behavioral Development, 35*(4), 307–316.

Biringen, Z., Brown, D., Donaldson, L., Green, S., Krcmarik, S., & Lovas, G. (2000). Adult attachment interview: Linkages with dimensions of emotional availability for mothers and their prekindergarteners. *Attachment & Human Development, 2*(2), 188–202.

Bosquet, M., & Egeland, B. (2001). Associations among maternal depressive symptomatology, state of mind, and parent and child behaviors: Implications for attachment-based interventions. *Attachment & Human Development, 3*(2), 173–199.

Bouchard, G. (2014). The quality of the parenting alliance during the transition to parenthood. *Canadian Journal of Behavioural Science, 46*(1), 20–28.

Bowlby, J. (1973). *Attachment and loss: Vol. 2. Separation: Anxiety and anger*. New York, NY: Basic Books.

Bowlby, J. (1979). *The making and breaking of affectional bonds*. London: Tavistock.

Bowlby, J. (1980). *Attachment and loss: Vol. 3. Loss: Sadness and depression*. New York, NY: Basic Books.

Bowlby, J. (1982). *Attachment and loss: Vol. 1. Attachment* (2nd ed.). New York, NY: Basic Books. (Original ed. 1969).

Bowlby, J. (1988). *A secure base: Clinical applications of attachment theory*. London: Routledge.

Brennan, K. A., Clark, C. L., & Shaver, P. R. (1998). Self-report measurement of adult romantic attachment: An integrative overview. In J. A. Simpson & W. S. Rholes (Eds.), *Attachment theory and close relationships* (pp. 46–76). New York: Guilford Press.

Busch, A. L., Cowan, P. A., & Cowan, C. P. (2008). Unresolved loss in the adult attachment interview: Implications for marital and parenting relationships. *Development and Psychopathology, 20*(2), 717–735.

Cassidy, J., & Kobak, R. R. (1988). Avoidance and its relationship with other defensive processes. In J. Belsky & T. Nezworski (Eds.), *Clinical implications of attachment* (pp. 300–323). Hillsdale, NJ: Erlbaum.

Cassidy, J., & Shaver, P. R. (Eds.). (2016). *Handbook of attachment: Theory, research, and clinical applications* (3rd ed.). New York, NY: Guilford Press.

Cassidy, J., Stern, J. A., Mikulincer, M., Martin, D. R., & Shaver, P. R. (2018). Influences on care for others: Attachment security, personal suffering, and similarity between helper and care recipient. *Personality and Social Psychology Bulletin, 44*(4), 574–588.

Collins, N. L., Guichard, A. C., Ford, M. B., & Feeney, B. C. (2006). Responding to need in intimate relationships: Normative processes and individual differences. In M. Mikulincer & G. S. Goodman (Eds.), *Dynamics of romantic love: Attachment, caregiving, and sex* (pp. 149–189). New York: Guilford Press.

Collins, N. L., & Read, S. J. (1994). Cognitive representations of attachment: The structure and function of working models. In K. Bartholomew & D. Perlman (Eds.), *Advances in personal relationships: Attachment processes in adulthood* (Vol. 5, pp. 53–92). London: Jessica Kingsley.

Conde, A., Figueiredo, B., & Bifulco, A. (2011). Attachment style and psychological adjustment in couples. *Attachment & Human Development, 13*(3), 271–291.

Crowell, J. A., & Feldman, S. S. (1989). Assessment of mothers' working models of relationships: Some clinical implications. *Infant Mental Health Journal, 10*(3), 173–184.

Crowell, J. A., Warner, D. E., Davis, C. R., Marraccini, M., & Dearing, E. (2010). The influence of childhood adversity on mothers' behavior with preschoolers: Role of maternal attachment coherence, dissociative symptoms, and marital behaviors. *Research in Human Development, 7*(4), 274–291.

DeOliveira, C. A., Moran, G., & Pederson, D. R. (2005). Understanding the link between maternal adult attachment classifications and thoughts and feelings about emotions. *Attachment & Human Development, 7*(2), 153–170.

Edelstein, R. S., Kean, E. L., & Chopik, W. J. (2012). Women with an avoidant attachment style show attenuated estradiol responses to emotionally intimate stimuli. *Hormones and Behavior, 61*(2), 167–175.

Edelstein, R. S., Stanton, S. J., Henderson, M. M., & Sanders, M. R. (2010). Endogenous estradiol levels are associated with attachment avoidance and implicit intimacy motivation. *Hormones and Behavior, 57*(2), 230–236.

Fillo, J., Simpson, J. A., Rholes, W. S., & Kohn, J. L. (2015). Dads doing diapers: Individual and relational outcomes associated with the division of childcare across the transition to parenthood. *Journal of Personality and Social Psychology, 108*(2), 298–316.

Fonseca, A., Nazaré, B., & Canavarro, M. C. (2013). Parental psychological distress and confidence after an infant's birth: The role of attachment representations in parents of infants with congenital anomalies and parents of healthy infants. *Journal of Clinical Psychology in Medical Settings, 20*(2), 143–155.

Fraley, R. C., & Shaver, P. R. (2000). Adult romantic attachment: Theoretical developments, emerging controversies, and unanswered questions. *Review of General Psychology, 4*(2), 132–154.

García-Ruiz, M., Rodrigo, M. J., Hernández-Cabrera, J. A., & Máiquez, M. L. (2013). Contribution of parents' adult attachment and separation attitudes to parent-adolescent conflict resolution. *Scandinavian Journal of Psychology, 54*(6), 459–467.

George, C., Kaplan, N., & Main, M. (1996). *Adult attachment interview* (Unpublished interview), University of California, Berkeley.

Gilbert, P. (2014). The origins and nature of compassion focused therapy. *British Journal of Clinical Psychology, 53*(1), 6–41.
Haft, W. L., & Slade, A. (1989). Affect attunement and maternal attachment: A pilot study. *Infant Mental Health Journal, 10*(3), 157–172.
Hamilton, W. D. (1964). The genetical evolution of social behavior. I and II. *Journal of Theoretical Biology, 7*(1), 1–52.
Howard, K. S. (2010). Paternal attachment, parenting beliefs and children's attachment. *Early Child Development and Care, 180*(1–2), 157–171.
Iles, J., Slade, P., & Spiby, H. (2011). Posttraumatic stress symptoms and postpartum depression in couples after childbirth: The role of partner support and attachment. *Journal of Anxiety Disorders, 25*(4), 520–530.
Jones, J. D., Brett, B. E., Ehrlich, K. B., Lejuez, C. W., & Cassidy, J. (2014). Maternal attachment style and responses to adolescents' negative emotions: The mediating role of maternal emotion regulation. *Parenting: Science and Practice, 14*(3–4), 235–257.
Jones, J. D., & Cassidy, J. (2014). Parental attachment style: Examination of links with parent secure base provision and adolescent secure base use. *Attachment & Human Development, 16*(5), 437–461.
Jones, J. D., Cassidy, J., & Shaver, P. R. (2015). Parents' self-reported attachment styles: A review of links with parenting behaviors, emotions, and cognitions. *Personality and Social Psychology Review, 19*(1), 44–76.
Kohlhoff, J., & Barnett, B. (2013). Parenting self-efficacy: Links with maternal depression, infant behaviour and adult attachment. *Early Human Development, 89*(4), 249–256.
Kohn, J. L., Rholes, W. S., Simpson, J. A., Martin, A. M., III, Tran, S., & Wilson, C. L. (2012). Changes in marital satisfaction across the transition to parenthood: The role of adult attachment orientations. *Personality and Social Psychology Bulletin, 38*(11), 1506–1522.
Kunce, L. J., & Shaver, P. R. (1994). An attachment-theoretical approach to caregiving in romantic relationships. In K. Bartholomew & D. Perlman (Eds.), *Advances in personal relationships* (Vol. 5, pp. 205–237). London, England: Kingsley.
La Valley, A. G., & Guerrero, L. K. (2012). Perceptions of conflict behavior and relational satisfaction in adult parent–child relationships: A dyadic analysis from an attachment perspective. *Communication Research, 39*(1), 48–78.
Lang, S. N., Schoppe-Sullivan, S. J., Kotila, L. E., & Kamp Dush, C. M. (2013). Daily parenting engagement among new mothers and fathers: The role of romantic attachment in dual-earner families. *Journal of Family Psychology, 27*(6), 862–872.
Lionetti, F., Pastore, M., & Barone, L. (2015). Parenting stress: The roles of attachment states of mind and parenting alliance in the context of adoption. *Parenting: Science and Practice, 15*(2), 75–91.
Mikulincer, M., Gillath, O., & Shaver, P. R. (2002). Activation of the attachment system in adulthood: Threat-related primes increase the accessibility of mental representations of attachment figures. *Journal of Personality and Social Psychology, 83*(4), 881–895.
Mikulincer, M., & Shaver, P. R. (2001). Attachment theory and intergroup bias: Evidence that priming the secure base schema attenuates negative reactions to out-groups. *Journal of Personality and Social Psychology, 81*(1), 97–115.
Mikulincer, M., & Shaver, P. R. (2016). *Attachment in adulthood: Structure, dynamics, and change* (2nd ed.). New York: Guilford Press.
Mikulincer, M., & Shaver, P. R. (2018). An attachment perspective on family relations. In B. Fiese (Ed.), *APA handbook of contemporary family psychology*. Washington, DC: American Psychological Association.
Rholes, W. S., Simpson, J. A., & Blakely, B. S. (1995). Adult attachment styles and mothers' relationships with their young children. *Personal Relationships, 2*(1), 35–54.
Rholes, W. S., Simpson, J. A., Blakely, B. S., Lanigan, L., & Allen, E. A. (1997). Adult attachment styles, the desire to have children, and working models of parenthood. *Journal of Personality, 65*(2), 357–385.

Rholes, W. S., Simpson, J. A., Campbell, L., & Grich, J. (2001). Adult attachment and the transition to parenthood. *Journal of Personality and Social Psychology, 81*(3), 421–435.
Rholes, W. S., Simpson, J. A., & Friedman, M. (2006). Avoidant attachment and the experience of parenting. *Personality and Social Psychology Bulletin, 32*(3), 275–285.
Rholes, W. S., Simpson, J. A., Kohn, J. L., Wilson, C. L., Martin, A. M., Tran, S., et al. (2011). Attachment orientations and depression: A longitudinal study of new parents. *Journal of Personality and Social Psychology, 100*(4), 567–586.
Riem, M. M. E., Bakermans-Kranenburg, M. J., van IJzendoorn, M. H., Out, D., & Rombouts, S. A. R. B. (2012). Attachment in the brain: Adult attachment representations predict amygdala and behavioral responses to infant crying. *Attachment & Human Development, 14*(6), 533–551.
Scharf, M., & Mayseless, O. (2011). Buds of parenting in emerging adult males: What we learned from our parents. *Journal of Adolescent Research, 26*(4), 479–505.
Schoenmaker, C., Huffmeijer, R., van IJzendoorn, M. H., Bakermans-Kranenburg, M. J., van den Dries, L., Linting, M. … Juffer, F. (2015). Attachment and physiological reactivity to infant crying in young adulthood: Dissociation between experiential and physiological arousal in insecure adoptees. *Physiology & Behavior, 139*, 549–556.
Shaver, P. R., Mikulincer, M., Gross, J. T., Stern, J. A., & Cassidy, J. (2016). A lifespan perspective on attachment and care for others: Empathy, altruism, and prosocial behavior. In J. Cassidy & P. R. Shaver (Eds.), *Handbook of attachment: Theory, research, and clinical applications* (3rd ed., pp. 878–916). New York: Guilford Press.
Shaver, P. R., Mikulincer, M., & Shemesh-Iron, M. (2010). A behavioral systems perspective on prosocial behavior. In M. Mikulincer & P. R. Shaver (Eds.), *Prosocial motives, emotions, and behavior: The better angels of our nature* (pp. 73–92). Washington, DC: American Psychological Association.
Sheftall, A. H., Schoppe-Sullivan, S. J., & Futris, T. G. (2010). Adolescent mothers' perceptions of the coparenting relationship with their child's father: A function of attachment security and trust. *Journal of Family Issues, 31*(7), 884–905.
Shlafer, R. J., Raby, K. L., Lawler, J. M., Hesemeyer, P. S., & Roisman, G. I. (2014). Longitudinal associations between adult attachment states of mind and parenting quality. *Attachment & human development, 17*(1), 83–95.
Simpson, J. A., Rholes, W. S., Campbell, L., Tran, S., & Wilson, C. L. (2003). Adult attachment, the transition to parenthood, and depressive symptoms. *Journal of Personality and Social Psychology, 84*(6), 1172–1187.
Snell, W. E., Jr., Overbey, G. A., & Brewer, A. L. (2005). Parenting perfectionism and the parenting role. *Personality and Individual Differences, 39*(3), 613–624.
Spangler, G., Maier, U., Geserick, B., & von Wahlert, A. (2010). The influence of attachment representation on parental perception and interpretation of infant emotions: A multilevel approach. *Developmental Psychobiology, 52*(5), 411–423.
Strathearn, L., Fonagy, P., Amico, J., & Montague, P. R. (2009). Adult attachment predicts maternal brain and oxytocin response to infant cues. *Neuropsychopharmacology, 34*(1), 2655–2666.
Talbot, J.A., Baker, J.K., & McHale, J.P. (2009). Sharing the love: Prebirth adult attachment status and coparenting adjustment during early infancy. *Parenting: Science and Practice, 9*(1), 56–77.
Taubman – Ben-Ari, O., Ben Shlomo, S., Sivan, E., & Dolizki, M. (2009). The transition to motherhood: A time for growth. *Journal of Social and Clinical Psychology, 28*(8), 943–970.
Taubman – Ben-Ari, O., & Katz-Ben-Ami, L. (2008). Death awareness, maternal separation anxiety, and attachment style among first-time mothers: A terror management perspective. *Death Studies, 32*(8), 737–756.
Trillingsgaard, T., Elklit, A., Shevlin, M., & Maimburg, R. D. (2011). Adult attachment at the transition to motherhood: Predicting worry, health care utility and relationship functioning. *Journal of Reproductive and Infant Psychology, 29*(4), 354–363.
Vasquez, K., Durik, A. M., & Hyde, J. S. (2002). Family and work: Implications of adult attachment styles. *Personality and Social Psychology Bulletin, 28*(7), 874–886.

Verschueren, K., Dossche, D., Marcoen, A., Mahieu, S., & Bakermans-Kranenburg, M. J. (2006). Attachment representations and discipline in mothers of young school children: An observation study. *Social Development, 15*(4), 659–675.

Whipple, N., Bernier, A., & Mageau, G. A. (2011). A dimensional approach to maternal attachment state of mind: Relations to maternal sensitivity and maternal autonomy support. *Developmental Psychology, 47*(2), 396–403.

Wilson, E. O. (2014). *The meaning of human existence*. New York: Liveright/Norton.

Wilson, C. L., Rholes, W. S., Simpson, J. A., & Tran, S. (2007). Labor, delivery, and early parenthood: An attachment theory perspective. *Personality and Social Psychology Bulletin, 33*(4), 505–518.

Index

O. Taubman – Ben-Ari (ed.), *Pathways and Barriers to Parenthood*,
https://doi.org/10.1007/978-3-030-24864-2

Q

R

S

Printed by Printforce, the Netherlands